THE BUILT ENVIRONMENT AND PUBLIC HEALTH

THE BUILT ENVIRONMENT AND PUBLIC HEALTH

RUSSELL P. LOPEZ

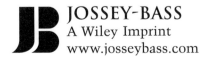

JOSSEY-BASS
A Wiley Imprint
www.josseybass.com

Published by Jossey-Bass
A Wiley Imprint
One Montgomery Street, Suite 1200, San Francisco, CA 94104-4594—www.josseybass.com

Jossey-Bass books and products are available through most bookstores. To contact Jossey-Bass directly call our Customer Care Department within the U.S. at 800-956-7739, outside the U.S. at 317-572-3986, or fax 317-572-4002.

Wiley also publishes its books in a variety of electronic formats and by print-on-demand. Some material included with standard print versions of this book may not be included in e-books or in print-on-demand. If the version of this book that you purchased references media such as CD or DVD that was not included in your purchase, you may download this material at http://booksupport.wiley.com. For more information about Wiley products, visit www.wiley.com.

Library of Congress Cataloging-in-Publication Data

Lopez, Russ.
　The built environment and public health / Russell P. Lopez. – 1st ed.
　　p. cm.
　　Includes bibliographical references and index.
　ISBN 978-0-470-62003-8 (pbk.); 978-1-118-12210-5 (ebk); 978-1-118-12211-2 (ebk); 978-1-118-12212-9 (ebk)
　1. Urban health. I. Title.
　RA566.7.L67 2012
　362.1–dc23

　　　　　　　　　　　　　　　　　　　　　　　　　　　2011032063

Printed in the United States of America
FIRST EDITION
PB Printing　　　10 9 8 7 6 5 4 3 2 1

CONTENTS

Preface   xi

The Author   xv

Part One   Background and History

1   **Introduction to the Built Environment and Health**   3

Dimensions of the Environment   4

Is the Built Environment Really an Environmental Factor?   6

How to Evaluate the Built Environment?   7

Public Perceptions and Assumptions Regarding the Built Environment   8

Cross-Disciplinary Nature of the Study of the Built Environment   9

Placing the Analysis of the Built Environment into a Broader Context   11

Influences on the Built Environment   13

2   **History**   17

The Pre-Industrial Era   18

The Era of Industrialization and Urbanization: 1825–1930   19

Reform Movements, New Technologies, and Changes in Urban Planning and Architecture: 1825–1930   25

Later Reforms and New Initiatives 1930–1980   32

The Current Era: 1980–2010 and Beyond   38

Part Two   Community Design

3   **Planning and Urban Design**   43

Demographic, Economic, and Social Trends   44

Land Use and Planning Controls   48

Metropolitan Structure and Health   54

4 **Transportation Policies**   67

Current Patterns of Transportation in the United States   68

Automobiles and Health   73

Highways and Health   77

Mass Transit and Health   78

Bike Safety and Infrastructure   81

Walking and Health   82

5 **Healthy Housing and Housing Assistance Programs**   91

The Housing Problem   92

The Regulatory Framework   93

6 **Infrastructure and Natural Disasters**   115

Natural Disasters: An Introduction   116

Natural Disaster Response   125

Part Three   Environmental Media

7 **Indoor and Outdoor Air Quality**   137

Overview   137

Land Use, the Built Environment, and Air Quality   139

Air Pollutants   141

Air Pollution–Associated Health Conditions   149

8 **Water**   155

Impact of Water on Health   155

Infrastructure   157

Drinking Water   159

9 **Food, Nutrition, and Food Security**   171

Foodborne Illnesses   172

Food Insecurity   174

Environmental Effects of Farming and Food Production   182

Part Four   Population Health

10 **Vulnerable Populations**   193

The Built Environment and Vulnerability   195

The Definition of Race   195

Poverty   200

Children and Environmental Health   203

The Elderly and the Built Environment   205

Persons with Disabilities   207

11 **Mental Health, Stressors, and Health Care Environments**   209

The Beginnings   210

Biophilia   212

The Role of Stressors and Allostatic Load   219

12 **Social Capital**   227

Theory and Historical Beginnings   228

Measuring Social Capital   231

Improving Social Capital   236

13 **Environmental Justice**   247

The Environmental Justice Movement   248

A History of the Environmental Justice Movement   249

Disproportionate Burden   256

Additional Limitations of Environmental Justice Actions   262

Lessons   265

Part Five   Tools and Applications

14 **Assessment Tools and Data Sources**   269

Tools to Inform Decision Making   270

Information Tools   275

15 **Health Policy and Programs**   287

Public Health Interventions   289

Community Interventions   292

School-Based Interventions   293

Individual Level Interventions   296

Legal Basis for Built Environment Regulation   297

Inserting Health into City General Plans   298

16 **Sustainability**   301

Defining Sustainability   302

Sustainability and Equity   303

Measures of Sustainability   304

The Local Sustainability Movement   307

The Role of Environmental Design in Sustainability   308

Global Climate Change and Greenhouse Gases   316

Glossary   321

References   329

Index   401

To my mother, Jo Lopez

THIS BOOK HAS several target audiences. It is intended to provide information on a variety of topics to students, researchers, and others concerned about the impacts of the built environment on health. In addition, it is meant to be used by public health practitioners, urban planners, and others who may need a quick reference text on issues that often arise regarding health and the environment. It was written under the assumption that most people do not have familiarity with both urban planning and public health and therefore would benefit from the inclusion of detailed information on both. Although every attempt was made to discuss the various debates regarding individual topics and issues, this book tends to adopt the generally accepted consensus regarding the current state of theory and evidence. However, readers are provided sources for further information in each chapter.

The Organization of This Book

This book is based on a model curriculum developed by Nisha Botchwey[1] and colleagues that grew out of the experiences of teaching courses on the built environment and health at a number of colleges and universities. It represents one way of dividing up the study of the built environment into topics and chapters. For more information, readers should see http://www.bephc.com/.

The book begins with a general description of the background of the field of the built environment:

Chapter 1: Introduction

Chapter 2: History

Part Two covers key elements of the built environment:

Chapter 3: Neighborhood and metropolitan design issues

Chapter 4: Transportation

Chapter 5: Housing

Chapter 6: Infrastructure

Part Three discusses specific media and how the built environment is shaped by and influences these factors:

Chapter 7: Air quality

Chapter 8: Water

Chapter 9: Food

Part Four highlights types of outcomes and includes:

Chapter 10: Vulnerable populations

Chapter 11: Mental health

Chapter 12: Social capital

Chapter 13: Environmental justice

Part Five focuses on methodologies and policy outcomes

Chapter 14: Assessment tools

Chapter 15: Health policies and interventions

Chapter 16: Sustainability

Acknowledgments

Many people helped bring this book to publication. They include my colleagues at Boston University, particularly H. Patricia Hynes and Greg Howard, who helped to put together our course on the built environment. Their lectures and research informed much of this book. The many students who took my classes, asked questions, and responded to assignments helped shaped this book as well.

Nisha Botchwey and other professors around the country who shared their syllabi were also essential in the development of this book. Other colleagues, many heavily involved in researching, teaching, and advocating for more healthy built environments, provided encouragement as this project went through research, writing, and revisions. In particular, Andrew Dannenberg of the CDC was most supportive during this process. Friends and family were also very encouraging and I would like to thank all the Lopezes, Shermans, and other members of my extended family for their kind words and support.

Very important: Andy Pasternack and the other people at Jossey-Bass were wonderful to work with. I wish to thank the following individuals for their feedback on the initial plan and approach for this book: Jason Corburn, Gretchen Kroeger, Laxmi Ramasubramanian, Karen Gay Mumford, and Troy Steege. I also wish to thank the following individuals for their many thoughtful and helpful comments on the completed manuscript: Jason Corburn, Bree Kessler, Troy Steege, and Fritz Wagner. Their suggestions, words of wisdom, and edits were most appreciated.

THE AUTHOR

Russ Lopez, DSc, MCRP, a native of California, has an undergraduate environmental degree from Stanford University, a master's of City and Regional Planning from the Harvard University Kennedy School of Government, and a doctorate in Environmental Health from Boston University. He has taught courses in environmental health, urban health, sustainability, and the built environment at Brown, Tufts, Northeastern, and Boston Universities. Dr. Lopez has delivered presentations on the built environment to organizations ranging from the Federal Highway Administration and the American Public Health Association to the American Planning Association. Funding support for his research has included the National Institute of Environmental Health Sciences (NIEHS), the Fannie Mae Foundation, and the Robert Wood Johnson Foundation's Active Living Research. His publications include articles on the health and environmental impacts of income inequality, racial residential segregation, and urban sprawl. His research interests range from the scale of schoolyards' effects on children to the social and health impacts of metropolitan development patterns. Dr. Lopez lives in Boston.

BACKGROUND AND HISTORY

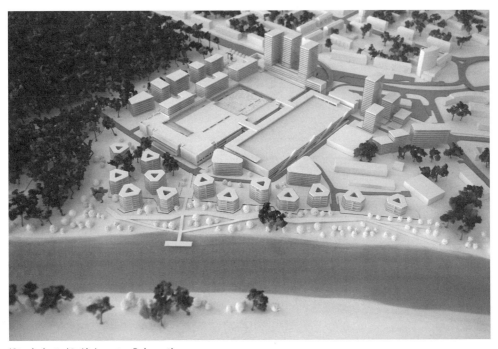

iStockphoto/© Algimantas Balezentis

CHAPTER 1

INTRODUCTION TO THE BUILT ENVIRONMENT AND HEALTH

LEARNING OBJECTIVES

- Compare the three domains that make up the broader concept known as the environment.
- Assess whether the built environment is consistent with the defining characteristics of environmental health.
- Describe the health, equity, and sustainability framework for evaluating the built environment.
- Name some of the professions that are associated with built environment research and practice.
- Describe the processes that shape the built environment.

How does the built environment affect your health? Consider the many different ways. Your apartment, home, dorm, or other place you spend the night protects you from the cold and rain. Curbs separate pedestrians from cars, and schools and commercial buildings have fire alarms, emergency exit signs, and other safety features. For the next twenty-four hours, look around and try to identify the many ways the built environment has been modified for your protection. Were you aware of all of these features? Do you think most people know how much the built environment shapes their daily lives? We will come back to these factors of the built environment in more detail later in this book. For right now, just consider the range and variety of built factors specifically added to the environment for your health and safety.

This book is a survey of the many pathways between the built environment and health, with an emphasis on issues in the United States. The built environment refers to all the many ways humanity builds or manipulates the world around it. The health effects of the built environment occur on multiple scales, including houses, streets, neighborhoods, metropolitan areas, regions, nations, and beyond.

Some impacts operate on very large geographic and temporal ranges, including international or national effects on millions of people over multiple generations. The U.S. interstate highway system, for example, transformed landscapes across the country and contributes to global climate change.[1] Other effects operate at a very local level and may only affect a few individuals for relatively brief moments in time. For example, a temporary sidewalk closing due to building construction may force pedestrians to walk in the street, potentially putting them at risk from passing cars. Including large- and small-scale impacts, those transitory and permanent, the collective impact of the built environment on health may be large.[2]

The built environment provides the framework for how daily lives are conducted, influences health across life spans, and represents important pathways through which individuals come into contact with many health risks. Though the associations between the built environment and health have only been subject to modern epidemiological scrutiny for the past two decades, and efforts to use the power of built environment interventions to address our current health concerns are only in their infancy, there is growing evidence that some environments can promote health while others increase morbidity and mortality.[3] This book provides an overview of the evidence that links the built environment with health, and it describes some of the program, policies, and projects that have been used to modify the environment to promote health.

Dimensions of the Environment

The term *environment* is very broad and can mean many things to different people. Even scientists from different disciplines can utilize varying conceptions of what constitutes the environment. To the geneticist, for example, the environment can be everything outside the genome including features operating on or below the cellular level that influence gene expression or modify genetic material.[4] To the sociologist, however, environment might mean factors beyond what is physically existent in an individual's body and describes the interactions between and among individuals, groups, and societies.[5]

For the purposes of this book, the environment is divided into three broad domains: the physical, social, and built environments. The **physical environment** includes all the various features that are part of mainstream environmental literature: forests, prairies, watersheds, plants, animals, and so on. It also includes the factors that are of concern to classic environmental health: air and water pollutants, radiation hazards, and so forth. These exposures are well known to be associated with certain diseases and to be linked to better or poorer health. Many of these physical environment problems are discussed in this book because the likelihood of exposure to them can be influenced by the built environment. For example, factories, prominent features of the built environment, can influence the degree to which an individual who lives near these facilities may be exposed to air pollutants, and thus impact health.[6] Physical environment attributes may arise from a built environment feature.

The **social environment** represents the many features that result from or are part of how humans interact with each other. These include the distribution of income, the role of race in society, political power, and other similar factors. There is a large body of evidence showing that the social environment can have profound impacts on health, a field that is also known as social determinants of health. For example, even though race is a social rather than a biological construct,[7] how an individual's race is perceived can have important lifelong impacts on health, from the risk of infant mortality to the incidence of prostate cancer in later life.[8] Race interacts with the built environment in many ways. It can influence income and wealth, which can then lead to an individual's ability to live near parks and other environmental amenities.[9] It may limit access to certain neighborhoods, affecting an individual's exposure to hazardous wastes or influencing access to nutritious food.[10] Thus the social environment is also included in this book.

The **built environment** itself consists of all the many features that have been constructed and modified by humanity. These include everything from how rooms are laid out, to the construction of homes, to the various land uses in a neighborhood, to the structure of neighborhoods and metropolitan areas, to the way regional and national geography and infrastructure interact to protect (or not protect) people from natural disasters. All of these levels of the built environment will be discussed here.

These three domains are not totally discrete, that is, there is considerable overlap between them. For example, racial residential segregation, the degree to which racial groups are concentrated in certain neighborhoods in many metropolitan areas, is both a social and a built environment factor.[11] It is a social factor because race itself is a social construct, only defined in the context of the society in which an individual lives. But when individuals can only buy or rent in certain neighborhoods, and thus their access to supermarkets, pharmacies, and hospitals is constrained, then it is also a built environment factor. Furthermore, when the influence of segregation is considered in the study of the distribution of environmental hazards and amenities, it includes the physical environment as well.

Is the Built Environment Really an Environmental Factor?

For those who consider the term *environment* in a more traditional manner, for example, those who think of the word in the context of narrow national pollution laws, there may be concern that the built environment is not a part of the environment at all. Some may believe that the term *environment* should be restricted to those attributes that exclude human-made features completely, or they at least place cities and intensely developed areas at the bottom of a hierarchy that places natural areas yet untouched by human influence at the pinnacle of desirable environments; others, however, have long advocated for the inclusion of humanity when considering the natural environment. But traditionally, the field of environmental health, the branch of public health from which concerns regarding the built environment first reemerged in the 1990s, has defined its agenda by posing a series of questions that set out to include or exclude certain health risks from consideration. By applying these criteria to the health effects of the built environment, we can determine whether or not the built environment is properly considered to be part of environmental health studies. These questions include:

Does the risk occur outside the body? The source of the problem should originate externally for it to be considered environmental. For example, even though environmental health is very concerned about environmental features that promote hypertension, high blood pressure itself is not traditionally considered to be an environmental disease and is rarely discussed in environmental literature. The proximal causes of hypertension, and its health effects, are observed internally; thus, hypertension is not an environmental health risk. In contrast, some distal factors are environmental stressors for hypertension and are within consideration here, including noise exposures, the distribution and availability of healthy food choices, the influence of the built environment on physical activity, and so on.[12] Therefore, sodium consumption, a major risk factor for high blood pressure, is not often discussed in the context of environmental health, but neighborhood food environments that offer few healthy options yet have ubiquitous sources of high-sodium foods are considered here. In general, though the health consequences of the built environment are almost always internally observed, their causes lie outside the body: in a person's home, neighborhood, metropolitan area, or rural community. Thus built environmental factors are not internal to the body—the risks are external.

Is the exposure or health risk voluntary? Generally, environmental health includes involuntary rather than voluntary risks. Smoking is considered to be voluntary (though, as will be discussed in this book, there are features of the built environment that affect the likelihood that someone will smoke), and thus it is not generally considered to be an environmental health problem. In contrast, exposure to secondhand smoke is considered to be an environmental issue, as suggested by secondhand smoke's alternative name, environmental tobacco smoke.[13] Nonsmokers exposed to tobacco smoke do not cause the exposure but rather become exposed because of the actions of others.[14] Considering the built environment, though, there is some individual choice regarding in what sort of environment one lives. For the most part, the broad parameters of the built environment—streets, the need to use a car to get to work, the construction of public works, and so forth—are set by society and an individual has little control over these features.[15] Thus the health risks and benefits of the built environment are not voluntarily accepted or individually produced.

Is the health risk caused by a biological agent? Though very concerned about malaria and other vector-borne diseases as well as diseases spread by contaminated water, for the most part environmental health does not address diseases caused by viruses, bacteria, and other organisms. Thus, as important an issue as it may be, HIV/AIDS is not a major subject in the environmental health literature. However, the built environment's influences on risk behaviors are considered here.[16] In general, the risks outlined in this book act on individual health without the intervention of biological agents.

Taken together, built environment to health pathways tend to originate outside an individual's body and health issues associated with the built environment tend to result from involuntary exposures to nonbiological factors. Based on these criteria, the built environment may be properly considered to be part of environmental health. This does not mean that everyone will agree about this application of these guidelines, only that built environment factors are consistent with the generally accepted parameters of environmental health.

How to Evaluate the Built Environment?

A recurring theme of this book is how do we measure and assess the built environment? How can we objectively describe its features and impacts? As will be seen, there are many ways to evaluate the built environment. For the most part, this book uses epidemiological evidence whenever possible. These include peer-reviewed articles published in academic journals that use standard health research methods. Among the epidemiological tools included here are case-control studies; cohort designs; and qualitative, ecological, and multilevel analysis. The book also uses engineering reports, case studies, architectural assessments, theoretical texts, and other sources as well.

Public Perceptions and Assumptions Regarding the Built Environment

The modern study of the built environment is a fairly new field of research. Although there have been concerns that some environments were healthier than others even back in ancient times[17] and the fields of urban planning and public health had common beginnings that resulted from problems posed by urbanization in the nineteenth century, the majority of research on the built environment that meets current standards of scientific validity dates back to the last two decades.[18] Thus it is likely that the full range of health effects may not yet be identified and it is always possible that a connection between the built environment and health accepted today may prove to be discounted in the future when additional evidence is analyzed. This is a growing and evolving field. The public tends to want certainty, however, particularly when theories of the built environment to health connection could result in expenditures of billions of dollars or more on infrastructure. But it is not always possible to provide guarantees in this field.

Many laypeople may not know about the health risks of the built environment or simply assume that these issues have been long studied and all major controversies resolved. Therefore, a common assumption may be that the suburban environment in which most U.S. residents live is the best possible built environment in terms of health, even if some research suggests this may not be true.[19] Part of this disconnect is the result of the lack of dialogue between researchers and the public. As with most health research, findings are couched in precautionary language, published in scientific journals, and rarely presented in standard English. A related misconception is that many people assume that rural environments, or living away from the rest of humanity on a deserted beach or mountaintop, are among the healthiest place to live—never considering the certain eventual need for medical care, the day-to-day need to purchase food, or the health value of contact with supportive family and friends.[20] Actually, evidence suggests that rural living is less healthy than urban living despite the noise, crowding, and congestion of cities.[21] But these findings are buried in journals unknown to the public.

Another issue is that research findings can contradict the rationale for past decisions. Millions of families moved to the suburbs to provide healthier environments for their children. To suddenly suggest that urban living, or at least living in communities that promote alternatives to cars, might be healthier may challenge these people. In the absence of public education, accessible data, and the time to absorb the implications of new research, it is difficult to expect that new research findings and new theories of health will be broadly accepted. There is much more to be done to educate the public about the health impacts of the built environment.

Cross-Disciplinary Nature of the Study of the Built Environment

From its very beginning in the mid-nineteenth century to its revival at the end of the twentieth century, the study of the built environment has transcended the boundaries between academic disciplines and incorporated theories and research from a wide variety of research approaches.[22] In some respects, this has been a rewarding process and the level of knowledge in participating fields of study has been enhanced. Health research has informed urban planning and economists now study human behavior, for example. But the cross-disciplinary nature of built environment study can also lead to confusion, particularly when two separate disciplines use a term in two very different ways. For example, in ecology research a *community* represents the totality of the animals, plants, and microbes in a given place; the trees, birds, mammals, fungi in the leaf litter, underground microorganisms, and so forth in a forest.[23] Humanity's consideration in this ecosystem schema may be limited to their ability to shape the system by setting fires, building roads, or promoting global climate change. In health and sociology, a *community* represents the collection of individual people in an area, their collective power to effect change as well as their individual characteristics and group interactions, but this may say nothing about the ecosystem they inhabit and the other species that coexist in this environment, differently defined. Still others have placed humanity inside a larger ecological complex that combines these two worlds.[24] The result can be confusion when attempts are made to communicate findings from one discipline to another. But despite these problems, the study of the built environment has been marked by a great deal of cooperation and collaboration across disciplines.

There are also crosscurrents of ideas within the broader disciplines of design and health. Some architects who are best known for their iconic buildings have also informed neighborhood design as well. For example, Frank Lloyd Wright may be better known for his Prairie style residential homes and the Guggenheim Museum in New York, but he also wrote extensively on the layout of suburbs in his Broadacre City work.[25] Lewis Mumford was an influential architecture

FOCUS ON

Disciplines Associated with the Built Environment

Public Health. Closely related to but broader than medicine, public health is concerned with the health of groups as well as individuals; practitioners focus more on prevention of disease and preservation of health than they do on diagnosis and treatment of individual illnesses. Public health professionals conduct studies, design interventions, administer programs, and evaluate services.

Epidemiology. This subfield of public health focuses on the factors that cause, prevent, and may influence disease. Epidemiology is a technical field that uses a number of statistical and other techniques that aim to provide basic scientific evidence that may inform health practice and public policy.

Sanitary Science. Taking their name from the great sanitary surveys of the nineteenth century, sanitarians are those professionals involved in implementing laws and regulations meant to protect public health, including food safety, water quality, and other similar types of inspections and enforcement.

Medicine. Physicians are on the front line of diagnosing and treating disease. Though many doctors also have public health degrees and work extensively in public health, most physicians' preventive health services are performed on the individual rather than the population level.

Nursing. Nurses work with physicians and others to provide direct care to patients. Many nurses also work on the population level to help address health risk behaviors and other types of preventative interventions.

Urban Planning. This field aims to shape and influence the overall nature of neighborhoods, cities, and metropolitan areas. Many urban planners focus on designing and implementing policies and programs that promote economic development, create affordable housing, provide emergency services, administer public programs, manage infrastructure, plan transportation improvements, and so on.

Architecture. Architectural practice can range from the design of open spaces (usually referred to as landscape architecture) to the design of individual buildings, neighborhoods, or cities. As will be seen, architecture is heavily influenced by theories of design and has a long history of trying to improve health. However, it should be noted that architects are not the only designers of buildings. Many are designed by engineers, and the design of buildings in developed societies is heavily shaped by building and other safety codes.

Urban Design. An urban designer often works on the overall physical appearance of, and relationships between, buildings, streets, and open spaces over an area that can range from an individual parcel to an entire community. In contrast to urban planners, who tend to focus on programs and policies, urban designers usually produce plans and design guidelines targeted to a specific location.

Landscape Architecture. Landscape architects tend to design the outdoor spaces for a given project or for a larger community. They may often work closely with architects and urban designers in these efforts.

Sociology. Sociologists, along with their colleagues, anthropologists, study the rich texture of human interactions and how individuals see themselves in relationship to others. They also study human behaviors and the behaviors of groups.

Economics. There are many subfields within economics and though some may seem far removed from the study of the built environment, even the most distant can provide insight on the impacts of the built environment. For example, macro economics, which includes the size and rate of expansion of the money supply, can have an impact on the built environment through interest rates, which can either promote speculative building or severely curtail construction activity.

Ecology. Ecological analysis and environmental science have played an important role in shaping the built environment. Through its tools that include the concept of an ecosystem being a series of energy flows, for example, it assists in the understanding of how the built environment can shape human behavior.

Law. The legal framework of a society profoundly impacts what can be built where. Therefore the study of the law, the identification of how laws are made and how they have been implemented, can assist in our understanding of how the built environment is constructed or how it can be improved.

critic for *The New Yorker* magazine, an author of key urban planning texts, and a cofounder of the Regional Plan Association of New York. Similarly, public health informs medical practice and medicine is central to public health research. In general, this book uses urban planning as a shorthand way to include all the design professions and public health to include all the medical professions. See Focus on: Disciplines Associated with the Built Environment.

Placing the Analysis of the Built Environment into a Broader Context

The environment is more than the sum of an area's trees, cars, people, and wildlife. It represents the totality of life and the broad mixture of interactions among people and between any one small area and the planet as a whole. Furthermore, there will be profound impacts on the environment of future generations that are derived from decisions made in the past and today. Therefore, assessing the impact of the built environment should be greater in scope than simply looking to see if a given single attribute affects the incidence of disease or the prevalence of risk factors at one time. It is important that the assessment of the built environment be placed into a broader context.

In this book, there are three primary areas in which the built environment is assessed: health, sustainability, and equity. All three are highly interconnected. For example, inequality is a risk factor for poor health, and countries, states, and metropolitan areas with higher levels of income inequality tend to have higher infant mortality, higher overall mortality, and lower life expectancy.[26] Thus equity influences health. But health also influences equity, as disability and disease can result in lower incomes and increased exposures to environmental hazards. Therefore it is useful to consider these factors both in isolation and as interconnected constructs.

Health

Over time, there has been a broadening in the concept of what health is. Today, it is considered to be more than just the presence or absence of disease. It includes the overall well-being of an individual, the ability of an individual to fully participate in the social interactions of a community, and a lack of barriers to good health across a life span.[27] Some of the health outcomes of the built environment are easier to characterize than others. Though there are ongoing controversies regarding the definition of obesity and the quality of its measurement, ultimately obesity is fairly easy to identify. But other factors can be more difficult to quantify. The measurement of "connectiveness" of an individual to his or her surroundings, the degree to which individuals feel part of the society around them or even have interactions with others living near or passing by their home, is more difficult to assess. For example, some architects and planners argue against high-rise residential buildings because they believe that living above the fifth floor results in a disconnect from the street.[28] But how to operationalize and measure this type of connectiveness is difficult.

Equity

This factor refers to the distribution of risks and assets between groups as well as the distribution of diseases and good health.[29] This book often highlights inequities in exposures and health that appear to be associated with race, income, or both. The individuals and groups can be located in one place, as in the unequal access to supermarkets between poor and wealthy communities in metropolitan Detroit, or it can reach across countries, as in the case of the transport of hazardous waste from developed countries to less developed nations. An environment can be healthy in many ways that also negatively affect equity.

A gated community, for example, may well provide important recreational opportunities to its residents. But if, as a result, a community votes down a bond issue to support the construction of a public park for its low-income neighborhoods, then the result may widen inequities.

Sustainability

Through sustainability, the concept of equity is broadened to include persons in the future. The impacts of development must not just be analyzed in terms of their effects on current populations, but the very long-term impacts must be considered as well. For example, given the problems associated with greenhouse emissions from coal-powered electricity generation, there have been suggestions that nuclear power plants should once again be built in the United States. But one important consideration must be the long-term impacts of nuclear power generation, including the very large problem of how to secure the safe disposal of radioactive wastes. These may require a site that can be isolated and free from accidental releases for hundreds of thousands or more years. Furthermore, although nuclear power might help reduce carbon emissions today, its wastes might also burden future generations who will not have benefited from our current energy use.[30] In addition, as will be discussed in Chapter Sixteen, the inclusion of equity in sustainability issues has had a controversial history, with some proposing that the very concept of sustainability could be suspect if it meant the perpetuation of existing inequities.[31]

Influences on the Built Environment

The study of the built environment should be broader than the consideration of individual factors themselves; it should also include an understanding of the processes that create these environments. To a certain extent, what we see in an area today is the result of a multitude of short- and long-term processes and decisions that have left a legacy in the design of buildings, neighborhood features, and metropolitan form. Part of the underlying conceptual model used here is derived from Henri Lefebvre's theory that urban space is the result of social processes.[32] In other words, the features of the built environment reflect the interplay of economic, political, and other similar factors. Some of these factors directly influence the shape of the built environment; others are more indirect influences. These include, but are not limited to:

- Laws: development takes place within a legal and constitutional framework
- Geology: soils, coastlines, tectonic factors

- Economics: economic trends, incomes, local economic factors
- Personal and societal values: neighborhood preferences, social factors
- Health assumptions: beliefs regarding causes of morbidity and mortality
- Ideology and political theory: theories of poverty, personal liberty, private property
- Technology: automobiles, Internet, pollution prevention
- Science: research, theories

Summary

The broader concept of the environment can be divided into three domains: the physical, the social, and the built environments. The built environment is consistent with what is traditionally considered to be environmental health because it is concerned with issues that are involuntary, arise outside the body, and are caused by nonbiological agents. The study of the built environment is multidisciplinary and draws on urban planning, architecture, public health, medicine, economics, and other fields.

Key Terms

Built environment	Physical environment
Equity	Social environment
Health	Sustainability

Discussion Questions

1. List five environmental features and classify each as belonging to the built, social, or physical environment. A feature can belong to more than one domain.
2. Describe the place where you would most like to live. What do you think would be the health benefits of this place? What might be the health problems?
3. Discuss why health is more than just the presence or absence of disease.
4. Name three factors that might contribute to the growth of a city or contribute to the form of the built environment.

For More Information

Centers for Disease Control and Prevention. *Healthy Community Design Initiative*. http://www
.cdc.gov/healthyplaces/

Frank, L. D., Engelke, P. O., & Schmid, T. L. (2003). *Health and community design: The impact of
the built environment on physical activity*. Washington, DC: Island Press.

Frumkin, H., Frank, L. D., & Jackson. R. (2004). *Urban sprawl and public health: Designing, planning,
and building for healthy communities*. Washington, DC: Island Press.

CHAPTER 2

HISTORY

LEARNING OBJECTIVES

- Discuss the impact of the Industrial Revolution on the health and environment of nineteenth-century cities.
- Describe how reformers used sanitary surveys to help prompt new health and environmental laws.
- Identify the role of miasma theory in the beginning of efforts to improve health by modifying the built environment.
- Explain the contribution of public health to the development of zoning and building codes.
- Discuss the features that modern architects believed would promote health.
- Identify the social and health impacts of urban renewal programs.

How old is the neighborhood you live in? Have you any idea when the buildings and streets in it were built? Consider some of the clues to the age of a community. These might include the architectural style of the buildings, the density and intensity of land uses, the pattern and layout of the streets, the availability of public transportation, and other features. Keep in mind the clues that help you estimate how old your neighborhood is while we discuss the history of using the built environment to promote health. As we will see, many of the features of community and housing design that have been adopted over the decades have resulted from changing ideas as to what constitutes a healthy neighborhood.

This chapter provides a brief overview of the many ways that the association between the built environment and health has been characterized and addressed over time. This is not intended to be a definitive history; rather it is meant to provide a background on some of the factors of the built environment that exist today but date back to previous decades. In addition, detailed historical background will be provided in other chapters as relevant. As will be seen here, there have been important changes in how the problems associated with the

THE BUILT ENVIRONMENT AND PUBLIC HEALTH

built environment were understood, and the policy and programmatic responses to health issues posed by the built environment have undergone important shifts. This history can be divided into four broad, overlapping, time periods: a pre-industrial era before approximately 1825; the age of large-scale industrialization and urban growth from 1825 to 1930; a reform era that began in 1840 and lasted until 1980; and our current time, roughly from 1980 to 2010, when we have become concerned with the association between the built environment and chronic diseases.

The history of the study of the built environment and health extends back almost two hundred years but even in ancient times there was a consensus that the environment of cities helps shape the health of residents. The famous Roman architect Marcus Vetruvius suggested that cities be founded so that they could maximize their access to helpful sea breezes and minimize the health effects coming from foul-smelling swamps.[1] This concern for fresh air has persisted for millennia. The word malaria, for example, comes from Latin for bad air and is based on the assumption that decaying vegetable matter in marshes is responsible for that disease.

The Pre-Industrial Era

Western urbanism has an almost ten-thousand-year history; readers should consult texts such as Lewis Mumford's *The City in History* for better understanding of ancient and near-modern trends that influence urbanism in the United States today.[2] This historical account, however, begins approximately in 1800 because, despite conscious efforts to plan U.S. cities by colonial powers and entrepreneurs, few cities existed in the United States before 1825, and these were mostly small— many form the central cores of metropolitan areas today. Despite their strategic locations, the geographical extent is limited and their overall influence has been supplanted by over 150 years of other actions. Thus this history will concentrate on the issues after 1825.

Health in Pre-Industrial Revolution Cities

Cities in Western Europe before 1800 and cities in the United States prior to and just after the Revolutionary War had very primitive sanitation and infrastructure.[3] For the most part, human waste was dumped in the streets or nearby open areas; animals, including pigs, cattle, and horses, were ubiquitous and contributed their manure to the streets; and the garbage produced by day-to-day activities piled up as well.[4] The stench was overwhelming. Though epidemics could occasionally provoke cleanup campaigns, most city residents were fairly complacent about what they could do to make their environments cleaner once a crisis passed.[5] The only factor that kept the cities from being even greater health catastrophes was that they were small. In the Western world, for example, only London and Paris had significant populations.[6] There were other problems with the built environment: fires were frequent; congestion caused by carts, carriages, and pedestrians was a major issue; and violence was an everyday occurrence. Cities were seen to be very dangerous and dysfunctional places and the health conditions in this era were very bad, life expectancy low, and infant mortality high. But conditions were about to deteriorate. For more information of the health conditions of this era, as well as how societies sought to respond to these issues, see *A History of Public Health* by George Rosen.

One prominent feature of the American built environment that will be mentioned here, because it developed well in advance of the founding of the United States, is the grid.[7] The health effects of gridded developments will be discussed in Chapter Three. What is important to consider here is that the grid is at least as ancient as Roman times. It was brought to the United States by the development of William Penn's Philadelphia and Charles Oglethorpe's Savannah, among other cities. Another influence was the Spanish Law of the Indies that called for grids to be used in the layout of cities in that country's Western Hemisphere possessions.[8] After the Revolutionary war, the grid fit in well with the U.S. land survey system, which placed a large north-south east-west grid across most of the country to the west of the Appalachian Mountains. New York City established its grid for Manhattan north of the older central core as a way of assisting its growth.[9] L'Enfant used the grid overlaid by diagonals in his plan for the new U. S. capital, Washington, D.C. Thus the grid was very influential during a time of large-scale city building in the United States.[10]

The Era of Industrialization and Urbanization: 1825–1930

The Industrial Revolution had profound impacts on U.S. cities, changing how they were built and vastly increasing their scale. Part of this resulted in cities expanding and overflowing their preexisting infrastructure; eventually, the health and environmental problems of this time would lead to a series of reforms and innovations. Obviously, the growth of manufacturing in the United States continued well beyond 1930, but after that time there was also a dramatic expansion in the role of government in regulating industry and transforming the economy. The 1825–1930 era was also a time of rising prosperity and technological change that contributed to the improvement of health as well.

The Industrial Revolution

Beginning in Great Britain at the end of the eighteenth century and then spreading to Continental Europe and the United States in the nineteenth century, the Industrial Revolution was to have a profound impact on city living and health.[11] Three factors—industrialization, immigration, and urbanization—were to substantially remake cities and to cause them to grow to sizes never before seen by humanity.[12] At first, new industries were dependent upon waterpower and cities began to grow along rivers, where they could take advantage of water-driven mills. With the invention of the steam engine, new industrial enterprises could locate almost anywhere, but they had to be close to where they could find large numbers of workers. Thus the growth of new industries was to propel people into cities.[13]

This was a time when there were no environmental laws to control what a factory discharged into the air, water, or surrounding land.[14] Many of the new industrial processes were fired by coal, which polluted the air, and a developing chemical industry introduced many new chemicals and compounds into the environment. We know now that many of these chemicals were highly carcinogenic and they were toxic to lungs, neurologic systems, and other organs, but at the time, these health effects were not well known or understood. Meanwhile, the industrialization of agriculture and the large numbers of people who could no longer grow their own food led to the development of slaughterhouses and feedlots in urban areas. These were large because their potential markets extended across entire continents and beyond, and they also contributed to the pollution of the era as millions of livestock passed through these facilities.[15]

Much of this development was made possible by the invention of the railroad. For the first time, humanity was no longer dependent upon humans, animals, wind, or water for the power to transport goods, and a factory could ship its goods long distances. But the railroads themselves caused problems. They used coal to fire their steam engines, which produced smoke and cinders. They were noisy and they consumed vast amounts of land for tracks, stations, and service yards.[16] So even as they facilitated the development of cities and contributed to rising incomes, they polluted and caused problems.[17]

The Industrial Revolution depended upon the hard work of unskilled and semiskilled labor, but the low wages paid by the factories were not sufficient for these workers to buy adequate housing and feed themselves. Furthermore, the new consumer goods replaced goods made by skilled artisans and as the Industrial Revolution progressed, the wages of many city dwellers fell.[18] So as these large numbers of impoverished workers and the unemployed congregated in cities, rents rose, and wages fell. Thus, though many people profited from the new economic growth, at the same time cities began to be the home of large numbers of poor workers and their families. It should be remembered that though it would ultimately raise living standards for millions of people, the Industrial Revolution and the processes on which it depended increased the dirt, pollution, and misery in cities.[19]

Immigration

The labor needs of these growing industries were very large and it was impossible to meet the demand for new hires from among the existing pool of poor and semiskilled residents of cities. Thus, as factories clustered in cities, they began to draw in immigrants from rural areas. Many of these new immigrants had been pushed off the land by the beginning of industrial agriculture and the mechanization of farm work. Others were drawn to cities because, as bad as conditions were in the newly growing cities, they were still better than economic opportunities in rural areas and cities at least offered the hope of a better life.[20]

Many countries, particularly the United States, England, and places as diverse as Argentina and Bohemia, quickly found themselves unable to find adequate labor among their indigenous rural populations and had to recruit workers from other countries to staff their machines. Thus London found itself importing workers from Ireland, Barcelona sought workers from France and the south of Spain, and the United States opened its doors to people from around the world. Millions came to the United States, another million went from Ireland to England, and the map of the world's demography quickly changed. Cities became known for their ethnic and cultural diversity.[21] By 1950, Chicago was to be the home of more Poles than Warsaw, and New York City had more Irish residents than Dublin.

Many U.S.-born people did not like these new immigrants. Often, they were perceived to be a different race even if they were of European ancestry, an example of how race is socially rather than biologically determined (see Chapter Ten for a discussion of how race is a socially determined construct). They were devotees of different religions, and they spoke other languages. Thus, even though there was a great economic dependence upon the labor of these immigrants, some upper- and middle-class natives disliked and feared them. Ultimately, the immigration of these groups into the United States was stopped by laws passed after World War I, but the last half of the nineteenth century and the first 15 years of the twentieth saw large-scale immigration and a continuing controversy about whether these groups could ever assimilate.[22]

Urbanization

The result of industrialization and immigration was that cities grew in size. New York City had 60,000 residents in 1800, 515,000 in 1850 (not counting the

96,000 residents of the independent city of Brooklyn), and 3,400,000 in 1900. Chicago, which barely existed in 1850, grew to be the country's second-largest city by 1900. It was just after 1900, when immigration to the United States was at its peak, that the highest ever population concentration in the history of humanity was reached in New York City's Lower East Side. Over 500,000 people lived in one square mile at a time when the neighborhood consisted of three- and four-story walk-ups.

The effects were seen not just in the very largest of cities but also in midsize cities such as Boston, Edinburgh, Buffalo, and Pittsburgh, and included over-crowding, lack of city services, incredible pollution, and the stench of garbage and feces in the streets.[23]

Health Effects

It is difficult to describe the horrendous conditions of cities in the nineteenth century because we lack the vocabulary to express and the ability to imagine what urban conditions might have looked and smelled like.[24] These conditions were not confined to the poor though they were most extreme in the tenement districts. Even the British Parliament was forced to move some of its sessions when the stench from the River Thames became too great for it to bear. In the absence of building codes and zoning laws, houses were cramped and dark, often with rooms that had no windows, and there was no place to dispose of human waste. Houses could abut factories, bone renderers, tanneries, and other noxious land uses. Also important was the tremendous overcrowding caused by the poverty of the time. Entire families lived in a single room, often taking in boarders to help pay for the expense of the rent of the room, and sometimes rooms were occupied in shifts, with one person sleeping in a bed while the other person worked. Almost none of these units had sinks or indoor plumbing and many were in cellars that dripped grime and flooded during wet weather.[25]

It should be no surprise that this was a time of great epidemics. One of the most frightening diseases of the era was cholera, with global epidemics in 1832, 1846, and 1854. Spreading from its source in India, cholera killed large numbers of people and panicked most of the others when it struck. Cholera is a dramatic disease: it kills by dehydrating its victims through intense diarrhea. We know today that it is spread by contaminated water, but at the time of the great cholera epidemics there was still widespread belief that cholera was spread by foul odors (often called miasmas). Not only did these outbreaks sicken and kill thousands, they also severely disrupted commerce because at the first sign of the disease anyone with resources would abandon a city, shutting down commerce and industry.[26] Cholera seemed to strike at the very stability of civilization itself.[27] A single cholera epidemic in St. Louis killed 25% of the population and a cholera epidemic in New York City struck so lethally that there were insufficient coffins to bury the dead.[28]

Another much-feared disease of the era was tuberculosis. Though it was romanticized at one time as a disease of poets and young women in love, it quickly became apparent that it was a disease of the poor in overcrowded tenements. Tuberculosis is caused by a bacillus that is spread by airborne droplets or contaminated food. Most people, if they are healthy, can easily control a tuberculosis infection because the body simply walls off and contains the infection. But if the individual is not healthy, and many workers and their families were underfed and suffered from health conditions caused by malnutrition and constant contact with contaminated food and water, the infection continues to be active and, over time, the disease can progressively destroy lung tissue, the kidneys and other organs, the bones, and the brain. In this era before the advent of drugs to control or kill the infection, only a strong immune system could save tuberculosis victims. Almost everyone was exposed to the disease and millions died.[29]

But it was not just cholera and tuberculosis that had a negative impact on health. There were a multitude of infectious diseases that swept through cities and the tenement districts of this time. Measles and diphtheria killed many, particularly the young, and typhoid fever, another waterborne illness, was a major killer. All of these diseases weakened their survivors so that they were more susceptible to any new illness that might strike or less able to fight off the greatest killer of them all, tuberculosis. There was controversy about the health of this nineteenth-century era that played out in the middle of the twentieth century. Thomas McKeown famously calculated that death rates declined throughout most of the nineteenth century and that most of this decline was the result of rising incomes, not medicine or public health interventions.[30] But a reexamination of the data by others suggested that there was a significant rise in mortality rates in the second quarter of the nineteenth century and the differences in mortality between urban and rural areas did not begin to converge until after 1880. These reassessments suggest that there was a large contribution to increased mortality from the newly industrializing cities and that public health interventions in the later part of the century, along with rising incomes, ultimately led to improving health.[31]

In an era of poor nutrition and long work hours, even for children, the suffering was great. Death rates were high for most segments of the population, but it was the young who were most at risk. In some districts infant mortality, death before the age of one year, was as high as 25% or more. This compares to

FOCUS ON
Contagion Versus Miasma Theory

The nineteenth century was a time of great controversy between two competing proposals on disease causation: contagion versus miasma theory. Miasma theory held that the bad smells caused by decaying organic matter and arising from marshes and rotting feces caused disease. Contagion theory holds that it is germs—bacteria, viruses, and the like—that cause disease. Obviously contagion theory eventually triumphed, but why did miasma theory remain influential for so long?

Miasma theory is older, having first been proposed in ancient times so that when science revived in the Renaissance, it dominated popular and scientific belief. Miasma theory also appeared to be supported by epidemiological evidence: the worst-smelling parts of a city were often the poorest sections where morbidity and mortality were highest. Furthermore, even though van Leeuwenhoek had identified microbes in the seventeenth century, no one linked these microbes to disease until nearly the end of the nineteenth century when Pasteur published his theories on disease causation. So there was no mechanism to support contagion theory.[32]

Slowly the evidence for contagion accumulated. First there was the experience with smallpox vaccination. Then John Snow demonstrated that water spread cholera. By the beginning of the twentieth century, miasma theory had been discredited, but the idea that a healthy built environment should try to maximize access to sunlight and fresh air dominated architecture and planning for most of the next one hundred years.

an infant mortality rate in the United States today of less than .1%. If the crude death rate from tuberculosis in the United States at the end of the nineteenth century was applied to the current population of the United States today, it would suggest that there would be over 400,000 deaths from tuberculosis annually. This compares to the current U.S. mortality of approximately 2,000,000 deaths a year, including deaths from cancer of about 500,000. (See Figure 2.1.)

A major legacy of this era is that cities were seen to be unsafe and unhealthy. Death rates may have been high in rural areas but there wasn't a dramatic clustering of deaths as was seen in cities. Reformers and medical personnel quickly realized that it was in the slum districts, the places where workers were overcrowded in tenements, where death rates were the highest. Suburbs were seen to be healthier and suburban living was thought to be the antidote to the health problems of cities.

FIGURE 2.1 Life Expectancy at Birth

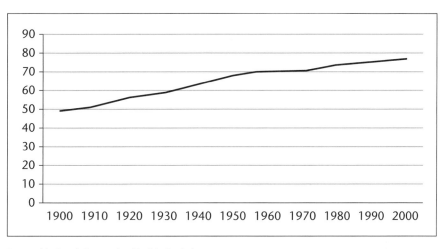

Source: National Center for Health Statistics

Reform Movements, New Technologies, and Changes in Urban Planning and Architecture: 1825–1930

A growing reform movement, often based in the growing middle class and with significant ties to business, began in England about 1848 and quickly spread to the United States. The nineteenth century saw the gradual emergence of the public health profession in a series of design and development theories and practices that would contribute to the growth of city planning. By 1900, modern housing regulation was introduced, quickly followed by zoning and building codes. Again, prosperity and technological change played an important role in the health improvements of this era.

Age of Reform

In response to the horrific conditions of the time, reform movements developed in Great Britain, the United States, and elsewhere. One of the first efforts of these activists was to graphically describe conditions in working-class neighborhoods in order to prompt new laws that would establish the right of government to regulate housing and environmental conditions. Perhaps because England was the site of some of the worst slums and tenement districts, these efforts began there. One of the earliest sanitary surveys, as these reports were called, was conducted by

Sir Edwin Chadwick, who had first come to prominence through his controversial reforms of workhouses. In his report, published in 1843, Chadwick cataloged the filth, overcrowding, and horrendous health conditions.[33] He combined this information with the generally accepted health ideas promulgated by, among others, the noted physician Thomas Southwood Smith, and then argued for a series of reforms that were to revolutionize urban planning and public health. It should be remembered that Southwood Smith and Chadwick believed in the **miasma theory** of disease causation (see page 24). This is the now dismissed belief that it was foul odors that cause disease, not infectious agents such as bacteria and viruses. The way to disperse miasmas and protect health was to ventilate buildings and expose rooms to sunlight.[34] Southwood Smith's theories propelled Chadwick to advocate for new laws regulating living quarters to reduce the health impacts of miasmas; even though these reforms were to eventually result in great public-health advances, they were based on what are now discredited ideas. Despite this, Chadwick's report led to the establishment of a system of local public health professionals who had the legal authority to clean up the worst of the open cesspools and dilapidated housing. It eventually became accepted that protecting public health was a legitimate role of government and that it could even override the rights of property owners. Though it would take almost a hundred years before housing was finally fully upgraded in the United States and England, the effort began with Chadwick.

The use of the sanitary survey spread to the United States. In Massachusetts, Lemuel Shattuck conducted a sanitary survey in 1850 and the result was the first state public health department in the country.[35] New York City's John Griscom helped prompt efforts to clean up that metropolis, and a similar effort led by Frederick Law Olmstead helped address the conditions in the Union army camps during the Civil War. At the end of the nineteenth century, Jacob Riis conducted his own form of a sanitary survey, and the resulting book, *How the Other Half Lives*, helped spark a new wave of housing reform at the beginning of the twentieth century.[36] Because these efforts generally relied on sanitary surveys, their advocates and the professionals who were hired as a result of this advocacy were called sanitarians. This was the beginning of the modern profession of public health.

There were other efforts from this era that were to substantially influence public health and urban planning through to our age. Struck by the extent of substandard housing endured by many working people, an effort began in England in the 1860s that was to be known as the **model tenement movement**. Its early founders included Octavia Hill, the granddaughter of Southwood Smith, and it was to continue to influence how we provide housing for the poor up until our own day; it is essentially the model used by community development corporations and other similar types of organizations to build and finance assisted housing. The model tenement's underlying idea was that landlords were not intrinsically bad nor were tenants fundamentally unable to live in healthy surroundings. The problem was seen to be that developers simply did not know how to build and maintain adequate housing for the working poor; by developing model tenements, their proponents could demonstrate both best building practices and how to successfully provide safe and healthy accommodations for the poor. Ultimately, the movement was not totally successful because developing housing was expensive and it was difficult to guarantee the 5% return on investment that the model tenement movement thought was necessary to attract investors. There were no government subsidies for this housing and, given the high profits that could be secured in other ways, finding investors was a problem. Perhaps the major failing of the movement was that it simply could not provide enough affordable housing to meet the demand; large cities needed millions of units to house their workers and only a relatively modest number were developed.

Confronted by the daunting problem of urban slums, some cities turned to large-scale urban renewal projects to provide public works and eliminate the tenement districts. The most famous of these efforts were those of Baron Haussmann in Paris, where he created beautiful boulevards to connect the various monuments and focal points of that city. In the process, he displaced almost 10% of the city's population. This set a precedent that was to dramatically remake U.S. cities in the twentieth century through urban renewal program: one way to address poor housing was to bulldoze it.[37]

The second half of the nineteenth century also saw the development of the great urban parks that are a major amenity in many U.S. cities today, including New York's Central Park and Boston's Emerald Necklace. Frederick Law Olmsted and his colleagues strongly believed that parks were a vehicle for promoting health and a way of bringing nature into cities. It should be noted that landscape designs of the era were evocative of nature but not necessarily natural in and of themselves. Olmsted prided himself on his ability to create a highly stylized and formal re-creation of the natural world.[38]

Another great public works movement of this era was the provision of clean public water supplies.[39] Cities could not grow unless they could secure safe water for drinking, industry, and fire suppression. Unfortunately, the cesspools, dumping of garbage, and industrial pollution so common in the nineteenth century meant that the aquifers under cities were badly polluted. The solution was to tap distant water supplies and bring them into cities. Often the only treatment of these waters was to simply filter them, but even this was effective in dramatically reducing the risks of cholera, typhoid fever, and other diarrheal diseases—once the public had access to this water.

The effort to bring water into housing was not without problems. At first, only the wealthy could afford to access these water supplies. They brought the water into their homes and used it for cooking and to operate their new indoor toilets. But there was no place to send the wastewater because few cities had sewers and those that did had only sized them for storm runoff and they were not adequate for connections to houses. Homeowners tried draining their wastewater pipes into their backyards but this only resulted in the flooding of sewage-infested waters into backyards, cellars, and streets. They next tried connecting them to the storm sewers but these also could not solve the problem because sewage would back up into the houses. An early fix was to resize the storm sewers so that they were sanitary sewers and then collect the wastes from neighborhoods or entire cities and dump it into convenient waterways such as lakes, rivers, or bays. Eventually, many cities developed dual drainage systems, one for wastes and one for storm runoffs, that were only connected during times of high rainfall when excess effluent in the sanitary system would be released into the higher capacity storm drain system; these connections continued to be a public health problem during periods of high rain in many cities up to our present time. By 1900, clean drinking water was the norm in most cities even if not every unit had its own indoor plumbing, but the dumping of raw sewage into lakes, rivers, and the ocean was still common.[40] This situation remains a problem even though the Clean Water Act was passed in the 1970s.

Ultimately, all these efforts led to the beginnings of the professions of urban planning and public health and great strides were made in reducing morbidity and mortality in growing cities.[41] Conditions and health status may not have been up to present-day standards, but they were substantially improved and the health of the population, even the poor, began to rise. It should be noted that this improvement in health occurred even before the development of modern medicine's ability to diagnose and treat illnesses. Improved nutrition and rising incomes played very important roles in promoting better health, but the modification of the built environment was central to the rise in health standards.[42]

Codes and Zoning

Despite these improvements in health, reform had stalled by the beginning of the twentieth century; however, a new generation arose to renew work to improve the built environment. One of the features of many of the various reform and architecture movements was that they facilitated a substantial learning exchange between Europe and the United States. This exchange began even before 1900 when events such as Chadwick's sanitary report and the model tenement movement sparked similar efforts in the United States; it continued as architects in the United States influenced those in Europe, and European ideas on housing and urban planning spread to the United States.[43]

One of the more interesting and influential movements was the idea of **garden cities**, or model suburbs, first put forward by Ebenezer Howard as a way to address the still tremendous problem of overcrowding in London.[44] Howard was a newspaper reporter who lived for a time in the United States and was influenced by the work of Frank Lloyd Wright, among others. Howard synthesized the ideas for how to plan model neighborhoods into a proposal to build an entire set of satellite communities a few miles from London. These new towns were not disconnected from the surrounding metropolis and Howard's idealized plan included rail connections to the center city and neighboring towns. But inside each new town there were to be spacious and well-ventilated homes for workers and their families, cultural amenities, and factories and other sources of employment within walking distance of housing. It took years to find investors, but eventually Howard acquired wealthy backers for his ideas and the first garden city, Letchworth, was developed in 1903.[45] Raymond Unwin, the architect of Letchworth, would eventually publish an influential text of suburban design.[46] Over the next hundred years, a series of new towns sprang up around London and though they never totally solved the problem of the inner-city tenement districts, Howard's ideas can be seen in places as distant as the United States, Brazil, and Australia. Another innovative theory was the concept of the neighborhood as a unit for organizing and understanding the built environment. As described by Clarence Perry and others, a well-designed neighborhood would have housing, employment, and all the services necessary for day-to-day living without residents having to leave.[47] This did not mean that neighborhoods should not be integrated into the larger city and metropolitan area, only that amenities should be within walking distance of residences.

By 1900, it was becoming clear that there were limitations of the first laws to regulate housing and building form.[48] In general, these laws could dictate how buildings were built but said little about how they were used or lived in. Despite generations of reform efforts, millions of the urban poor continued to live in substandard housing, suffered relatively high rates of disease, were more at risk for what were seen as the moral problems of alcohol use and prostitution, and felt the effects of shoddy construction. Many continued to be particularly vulnerable to fires.[49] The effort to improve housing and cities was not yet complete.

In the United States, a new reform program to upgrade housing was begun by Lawrence Veiller and his allies. Veiller, a follower of Jacob Riis, was a social worker disillusioned by the dreary housing conditions in New York City's tenement districts. Everywhere, he saw a lack of enforcement caused by inadequate laws and a substandard municipal workforce. Influenced by the efforts of

Chadwick and Griscom fifty years before, Veiller and his associates produced a survey of housing conditions; Veiller used this report to introduce legislation that gave New York City the right to regulate housing conditions and ultimately resulted in a complete rebuilding of the city's slums.[50] The law mandated minimum room and window sizes, prohibited the use of one room as egress for another, and required that new construction have indoor bathrooms and that existing buildings be retrofitted so that there was a minimum of one bathroom for every two units. Also important, Veiller placed responsibility for the enforcement of these new laws in public health departments. Because public health professionals had been responsible for visiting tenements to address epidemics for the past fifty years, Veiller thought that with adequate supervision and training, these professionals could also address housing problems.[51] This assignment of responsibility was to have important consequences during the urban renewal era in the United States fifty years later.

Veiller did not limit his efforts to New York City. Along with the support of the Russell Sage Foundation, he published a model housing ordinance and traveled across the United States to lobby legislatures and municipal governments to adopt these laws.[52] In the process he created a national housing movement and contributed to the idea that housing laws should be uniform across the country even if their adoption and enforcement was the responsibility of state and local government.

The congestion and pollution of the early twentieth century led to another innovation, **zoning**. This idea began in Germany, and was adopted to meet the challenges in the United States. Like the model housing ordinance, it sprang from concerns with conditions in New York City. It also had a series of champions, individuals who built coalitions to support reform. Benjamin Marsh, Edward Bennett, and others were very concerned that congestion and traffic was choking the ability of New York City to be a place of commerce and that the increasing number of high-rise buildings was destroying access to sunlight and ventilation. There was also the problem of incompatible land uses. For example, there was nothing to prevent a factory from locating adjacent to housing. In fact, there were incentives for this because being near housing meant having access to workers. But in the absence of antipollution laws this also meant that air emissions, water discharges, smells, and noise could destroy the livability of almost any neighborhood at any time. Property values were potentially unstable.[53]

The solution to these problems was zoning. Cities would identify which areas were appropriate for industry, commerce, and various types of housing, and prohibit incompatible land uses in these districts. Each area would have a carefully defined set of maximum densities and allowed uses. The first zoning ordinance was adopted in New York City in 1916 and, with the help of a model zoning ordinance, was quickly adopted by municipalities across the country.[54] The use of zoning was not always benign. Baltimore, for example, adopted zoning as a way of preserving racial residential segregation by zoning certain areas for blacks and certain areas for whites and not allowing integration. Race-based zoning was declared unconstitutional by the U.S. Supreme Court not because it interfered with the rights of African Americans to live wherever they wanted, but because it was seen as an unnecessary restriction on the rights of property owners to rent or sell to whomever they pleased.[55]

The power to use zoning to regulate land uses was upheld by the U.S. Supreme Court in a landmark decision in the case of *Euclid v. Ambler*. The legal dispute arose in the town of Euclid, Ohio, located on the outskirts of Cleveland, when it sought to protect itself from the encroachment of industry from that city. A property owner, Ambler Realty, sued the city, claiming that the town had no right to regulate what it did with its property. The court ruled for Euclid, in part because it held that the protection of public health was a fundamental responsibility of government and that the rights of property owners could be restricted in the effort to protect health.[56] Thus public health was present at the very beginning of zoning and was a major reason why it was declared legal. This case is also why conventional zoning is often referred to as Euclidean zoning. It is not because of its geometric properties but because it was upheld in Euclid, Ohio. After Euclid, almost every city in the United States eventually adopted zoning as a way to regulate land use and, along with model building codes, the power of zoning helped improve living conditions, at least in certain districts that were newly built for middle-class and wealthy residents. But even as zoning was becoming widespread, there was also an early warning sign of one of the most critical issues that was to affect U.S. cities for most of the twentieth century: the ongoing segregation of African Americans and the resulting social and built environment problems. Even as early as 1899, there was evidence that housing for African Americans was inferior to that for whites.[57] Still, the power of zoning was immediately grasped; empowered by the idea that they could produce ideal cities, planners used these zoning and similar tools to shape development.[58] Along with growing prosperity and growing numbers of middle-class families, these initiatives were to result in a startling increase in the quality of housing in the United States. These codes also become rigid and would contribute to the health and environmental problems of U.S. suburbs at the end of the twentieth century.

Race and the American City

Readers will note that segregation is discussed in several chapters. Segregation's impact on housing quality is described in Chapter Three and race is important in the discussions of environmental justice, vulnerable populations, mental health, and other issues. The topics of segregation and African American health has been extensively covered by authors such as Nancy Denton and Douglas Massey in their landmark book, *American Apartheid*,[59] and readers may also be interested in the works by Anthony Polednak.[60]

The role of race in U.S. cities intensified in the period between 1919 and 1950 just as large-scale immigration into Northern and Western cities was beginning. Racial discrimination and segregation was used to contain growing African American populations and helped establish the physical form of cities during that time. In the South, Jim Crow legislation also contributed to the problems that African Americans would face in housing and neighborhood quality and also to the great migration to the North. Segregation in the United States peaked in 1950, and has only slightly declined since that time.

Later Reforms and New Initiatives 1930–1980

The second half of this reform era, roughly from 1930 to 1980, was a time of large-scale expansion of government, particularly the federal level. First the public housing program was introduced, as part of the expansion of government during the New Deal. Later, the federal government helped fund urban renewal, highway construction, and extensive building of sewers, water supplies, and other infrastructure.

Twentieth-Century Architectural Movements

Accompanying the waves of reform were dramatic changes in architectural styles, materials, and designs. One of the most influential architects of the twentieth century was Frank Lloyd Wright.[61] His designs for houses, including his prairie style and Usonian homes, changed domestic architecture by emphasizing volumes rather than walls, conceptualizing buildings as integrated wholes, and using new materials such as concrete and glass to make houses appear dramatically different from those built before his time.[62] After early successes, personal scandals, and the triumph of a taste for neoclassical designs eclipsed his work in the United States, Wright went on to rethink the design of the American suburb. In a theoretical plan for what he called Broadacre City, Wright articulated the themes of individual houses on large lots set off and away from streets, self-contained communities connected by highways, and the provision of the few items that could not be produced locally being the responsibility of stores along off-ramps of large-scale connecting roads. Wright thought that the city was obsolete and would be eventually replaced by low-density suburban development across the landscape. This was a 1930s vision of United States suburbia that would predominate at the end of the twentieth century.[63] Wright did not conceive of all of these ideas himself, but he brought them together and synthesized them into a coherent whole.

Though Wright fell out of favor in the United States, his ideas were to contribute to development of the most influential architectural movement of the twentieth century, **Modernism**, or the International Style.[64] Wright was not the only source for Modernism; part of it grew out of the tremendous disillusionment with European civilization that resulted from World War I. Because classical architecture was the preferred building form of Europe's prewar elite and because reform-minded architects blamed these elites for the horrendous destruction and suffering of that war, they came to reject neoclassical architecture itself. Modernism also had a substantial public health justification. Still based on the old Southwood Smith idea that miasmas caused disease (though the germ theory was well established by this time), Modernist architects believed that they could improve humanity and help reduce the burden of disease by designing buildings that maximized ventilation and access to sunlight.[65] Modernism had a number of very specific guidelines. For one thing, it rejected ornamentation and believed that austere buildings without cornices or decorative detail were the most pure.[66] Facades were reduced to flat plains, colors were muted, and a building's relationships with the neighborhood around it were minimized. To maximize the health benefits of new construction, buildings were to be sited away from streets and housing clustered in high-rises. This would allow for the maximization of open space.[67] The idiom of the skyscraper in the park, which was to heavily influence urban renewal and the development of suburban office parks in the United States, was idealized. It was in these early decades of the twentieth century that the ideas that were to dominate conventional urban and suburban development for most of the post–World War II era came together: suburbs of single-family homes dominated by cars and separate from employment, along with downtowns of high-rise buildings, connected by highways to these distant suburbs.[68]

One the most influential architects of this era was Le Corbusier, a Swiss national who moved to Paris and helped spark the Modernist movement.[69] In Germany, the famous Bauhaus school of design and architecture developed a new course of study that emphasized craftsmanship, utility, and health. Later, when the Nazis shut down the Bauhaus, many of its architects moved to the United States and helped Modernism triumph in this country.

Modernism was to dramatically change urban form in the United States. Building codes were quickly adapted to require the large setbacks and open space that Modernism thought best for surrounding apartment buildings and offices. In the United States, this often meant acres of parking lots around mid- or high-rise buildings. Downtowns, often being redeveloped under problematic urban renewal programs, also applied Modernist principles to shape new development, resulting in buildings often not much more than plain glass-sheathed boxes set next to empty concrete plazas. For the most part, Modernism did not influence domestic architecture in United States, but there was the very important exception of public housing, which often adopted the model of high-rise buildings set in large open spaces.

By the 1980s, the era of Modernism in United States was beginning to fade. In part this was because of opposition from the public, which had a negative reaction to many famous Modernist buildings such as Boston's City Hall, San Francisco's Embarcadero Center, and the Pan Am building over Grand Central

FOCUS ON

Le Corbusier's Ville Radieuse

One of the most influential Modernist proposals for city building was Le Corbusier's proposal to demolish most of Paris's Right Bank and replace it with a series of large, cross-shaped skyscrapers set in a large expanse of open space. Highways and a central train station were to serve the transportation needs of the city. Rather than a city of narrow streets, broad avenues, and mixed uses, Le Corbusier saw a city maximized for efficiency and order. Retail and commercial uses were to be provided along upper-story hallways. Every unit was to look out on open space and have access to sunlight and ventilation. But the units were small, only about 150 square feet per person. Le Corbusier published several versions of his plan, variously called Ville Radieuse (Radiant City) or Plan Voisin (after its French auto company sponsor). This idea and other parts of theories were accompanied by often quoted phrases such as "a house should be a machine for living" and "the city that is built for speed is built for success."[71]

Le Corbusier purposely meant to create controversy; that was probably his intent rather than to really bulldoze the city. This Modernist-inspired plan may represent a high point in the goal of city planning to rationalize the city and cleanse it of dirt and disorder. Though obviously never implemented in Paris, the plan inspired a countless number of smaller projects from many public housing developments and urban renewal projects to many suburban office parks.[72]

The plan fell out of favor after Jane Jacobs and other urban theorists pointed out that rather than setting up cities for greater efficiency, it actually harmed what cities do best: bring people together in unpredicted ways. Today, there are relatively few proposals to implement plans based on this proposal.

Terminal in New York City. There were also changes in architectural theories that had once favored Modernism but now saw ornamentation and building design itself to be one way in which buildings connected with their surroundings and conveyed meaning to passersby.[70] Though Modernist-inspired projects continued to be built, as a major design influence it has passed.

Public Housing and the New Deal

Public health and urban planning began to drift apart after the triumph of zoning and housing codes in the years after World War I.[73] But in conjunction with Modernism, there were two major programs resulting from the two disciplines' collaboration that were to dramatically change U.S. cities in the decades from 1930 to 1970: public housing and urban renewal.

Public Housing. The movement to fund and build public housing began after the consequences of Veiller's housing laws began to be seen. Though they were becoming very effective in shaping new construction, they had limited ability to improve the conditions in slum districts. One problem was that in the compromises necessary to get legislation passed, existing construction was often exempt from the regulations. In addition, most new construction was for middle-class and wealthy people and little new housing was constructed directly for housing the poor; thus housing in the slums continued to be substandard. In trying to understand why housing was so difficult for the poor, an influential reformer named Edith Elmer Wood demonstrated that it was impossible for a family to afford decent housing on an industrial worker's wages. Their rents were insufficient to pay for mortgages and maintenance. With that idea, housing became a financial problem.[74]

In another example of learning from European experience, Catherine Bauer traveled to understand how Germany, France, and England were solving their post–World War I housing problem. She found that governments were building housing for the working classes and the poor. Bauer brought this idea back to the United States, establishing a new movement that became known as the Housers. A major goal of the Housers was to persuade state and federal governments to allocate funds for construction of new housing for the poor.[75] With the beginning of the Great Depression, the idea gained traction as a way to provide jobs for construction workers as well as to assist the one-third of the country that continued to live in substandard housing.

In the compromises necessary to pass the law providing for public housing, the foundation of the problems of the public housing program was laid. One major issue was that the enabling legislation dictated that public housing should be of inferior quality so that potential tenants would not be tempted to abandon private market housing unless they were truly destitute and desperate. This resulted in poor-quality construction and finishes that would eventually mean that the housing built would be difficult and expensive to maintain. Another problem was that though the program was funded by the federal government, it was administered by authorities established by cities and often appointed by mayors. The planning and siting of these developments became a highly political process; when the program as a whole began to be seen as highly likely to house African American people (because black residents were more likely to be poor, they were often most in need of housing assistance—but in the racial climate of this era, many white communities resisted integration and thus opposed building public housing in their neighborhoods), cities tended to site such developments on marginal land, dooming their residents to be isolated from jobs and services. The final issue was that many of the developments were planned and designed using Modernist principles. Buildings were set on superblocks far away from streets and often used high-rise construction methods to minimize land costs and maximize access to open space. Though this last feature is most often regarded as responsible for the failures of public housing in this country, the contributions of the two earlier problems cannot be dismissed. The consequences were that almost as quickly as the units in the program were built, they deteriorated. The program did not begin in large scale until after World War II, but by 1960 the problems were severe enough to begin to bring it to an end. Relatively little housing was ever provided for the poor by the government in this country and most of it was substandard by design. The result, however, was to discredit both Modernism and government-provided housing.[76]

The public housing movement was only one piece of a set of comprehensive programs that dramatically changed the built environment that began with the New Deal. A response to the large-scale deprivation and unemployment of the Great Depression that began in 1929, President Franklin Roosevelt and his advisers developed a wider range of programs that included the Works Progress Administration, the Federal Housing Administration, the Tennessee Valley Authority, and many other government assistance projects that resulted in new waterworks, the building of schools and hospitals, flood control, rural electrification, and other features that would improve health.[77] Though many of the programs ended by the beginning of World War II, government programs continued in the 1950s with new innovations such as the federal highway program.

Urban Renewal. Though we may now think that American cities were at their peak of vitality in the years right after World War II, observers at the time were very concerned with congestion and deterioration. The rise in the use of automobiles was causing traffic jams and congestion, the streets were too narrow to accommodate them, and the high density of the downtown areas seemed to be attracting even more car users. The continuous exodus to the suburbs by wealthy and middle-class people was alarming city leaders who saw great belts of slums threatening both their quality of life and the quality of city budgets. Most troubling to many city administrations during this era of massive racial discrimination and segregation of African Americans was the great migration of southern blacks into Northeast and Midwest cities. In those racist times when housing discrimination was rampant, city governments thought that the best way to handle the growth in the population of African Americans was to eliminate their neighborhoods. The stage was set for one of the most tragic periods in the history of American cities: urban renewal.[78]

The steps in urban renewal were to set up a redevelopment authority, declare an area blighted, take properties by eminent domain, and either sell these properties to private developers or use them for stadiums, health care facilities, universities, or other institutions or governments. Public health played a key role in these projects because in many cities it was the branch of city government that was responsible for declaring a community blighted. Since the time of Veiller's housing laws, public health departments had been responsible for housing inspections, and so it was logical to turn to them for blight designations. To help facilitate this process, the American Public Health Association published guidelines for a healthy neighborhood and trained local authorities how to use these guidelines to make a designation of blight. In many places, the local health department was also charged to inspect replacement housing so that tenants displaced from urban renewal projects would have decent alternative housing.[79]

As implemented, urban renewal ended up displacing millions of people, the vast majority of them African American, and few of these families received compensation or assistance in finding replacement housing. City administrations quickly began to use the program to target African American neighborhoods and the program earned the nickname of "Negro removal."[80] By design, urban renewal sought to replace low-income housing with housing for the wealthy and the middle class; it was never meant to be a program for the poor. The program began in earnest in 1948 and important parts of cities were bulldozed in the 1950s and 1960s. Many of these parcels are still vacant. Worse, the disruption failed to address the decline of cities and may have even accelerated it.[81] In conjunction with highway building, which may have displaced an additional 15% of urban populations, cities were sent into a spiral of decay from which many never recovered.[82] There were benefits from urban renewal; many cities saw important government, cultural, medical, and educational complexes built. Some wealthy households were attracted to the new housing and new downtown developments.[83] But these positive effects accrue to the community at large and must be balanced against the detriment to the individuals displaced.

The Current Era: 1980–2010 and Beyond

After 1980, the role of the federal government began to change. Although many mandates remained, funding was often constrained by changing fiscal priorities. Prosperity continue to increase, at least at the beginning of this period. But U.S. incomes stagnated after 1990 for the majority of the population. Most of the changes in the built environment in this era are covered later in this book. What is important to consider here is that urban planning and public health were eventually to reconnect after 1990.

Reunification

The details of our current era in the history of the relationship between public health and the built environment are covered in each of the relevant chapters in this book. For the purposes of the review here, it should be noted that for several decades, public health and urban planning were distinct and separate. Urban planning worked on housing and city development; public health sought to address infectious diseases, pollution, and worker safety. But just as urban renewal, including highway construction in urban centers, was reaching its climax, a book was published that was to dramatically change how Americans looked at cities and would ultimately contribute to the reconnection of public health with urban planning. As will be discussed in further detail in the next chapter, Jane Jacobs' *The Death and Life of Great American Cities* would change urban planning and inspire the movement we now call **new urbanism**.[84] By the time the twentieth century ended, mainstream planners no longer believed that the solution to urban problems was to pull down large sections of the city and rebuild them along Modernist or suburban-inspired designs. The new idea was that diversity of land uses was good, density was empowering, and walkable cities were desirable. Beginning in the 1990s, the rise in obesity helped spark a renewed interest of public health professionals in the built environment. Urban planners sought to use new epidemiological findings and new ideas about health into their urban designs. Within a few years, public health professionals adopted the language of new urbanism and urban planning sought to remake neighborhoods in ways that were better for physical activity and social capital.

Once public health adopted these new ideas as ways to meet the health challenges of the twenty-first century, the disciplines of urban planning and public health each began to move to embrace the procedures and principles of the other. Public health professionals now advocate for mixed-use communities and urban planners talk about the health-related virtues of pedestrian circulation and bike transportation. These efforts have been accompanied by cross-disciplinary efforts that include joint courses, joint degree programs, integrated planning, and public health programming.

Summary

The modern history of the built environment and health begins with the industrial revolution when increasing industrialization, immigration, and urbanization vastly increased the scale of cities and exacerbated preexisting problems with sanitation and pollution. Reformers used sanitary surveys to motivate the public and help pass new laws that gradually resulted in cleaner cities and better health. These efforts also led to the development of the professions of public health and urban planning. By the beginning of the twentieth century, new efforts resulted in the adoption of housing laws and zoning codes that dramatically affected urban and suburban development. New ideas about model suburbs and the role of architecture in promoting health influenced architecture, planning, and health. Later, failures of public housing and urban renewal, along with concerns with the problems associated with suburbs, contributed to a reassessment that produced many of the design and health ideas that shape development today.

Key Terms

Garden cities   Modernism

Miasma theory   New urbanism

Model tenement movement   Zoning

Discussion Questions

1. What are the three types of effects that resulted from the Industrial Revolution?
2. How might the problems faced by rapidly growing U.S. cities in the nineteenth century be similar to those faced by rapidly growing cities in developing countries today?
3. Why did the sanitary reformers want to mobilize public opinion to meet the problems in urban tenement districts?

4. What is miasma theory?
5. What are the advantages of using zoning to control land use?
6. Describe the types of land uses you would like to see in your neighborhood. What land uses do you not want in your neighborhood?
7. Can you name buildings near where you live, work, or go to school that seem to be Modernist buildings or influenced by Modernist design principles?

For More Information

Boyer, C. M. (1986). *Dreaming the rational city: The myth of American city planning*. Cambridge, MA: MIT Press.

Duffy, J. (1992). *The sanitarians: A history of American public health*. Urbana: University of Illinois Press.

Hall, P. (1988). *Cities of tomorrow: An intellectual history of urban planning and design in the twentieth century*. Malden, MA: Blackwell.

Jacobs, J. (1961). *The death and life of great American cities*. New York: Vintage Books.

Lubove, R. (1962). *The progressives and the slums: Tenement house reform in New York City, 1890–1917*. Pittsburgh, PA: University of Pittsburgh Press.

Melosi, M. V. (2000.) *The sanitary city: Environmental services in urban America from colonial times to the present*. Baltimore, MD: Johns Hopkins University Press.

Rosen, G. (1993). *A history of public health*. Baltimore, MD: Johns Hopkins University Press.

Rosner, D. (1995). *Hives of sickness: Public health and epidemics in New York City*. New Brunswick, NJ: Rutgers University Press.

Tarr, J. (1996). *The search for the ultimate sink: Urban pollution in historical perspective*. Akron, OH: University of Akron Press.

COMMUNITY DESIGN

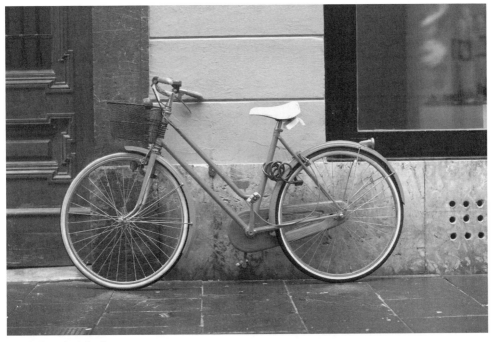

iStockphoto/© Nikada

CHAPTER 3

PLANNING AND URBAN DESIGN

LEARNING OBJECTIVES

- Describe the general features of conventional development.
- Identify the health and environmental issues associated with conventional development.
- Describe the changes in characterizing desirable urban development postulated by Jane Jacobs.
- Compare the features of New Urbanism with that of conventional development.
- Evaluate the degree to which New Urbanism produces healthy communities.
- Analyze the state of evidence linking urban sprawl with obesity.
- Explain the features of a healthy neighborhood.
- Identify solutions for improving the health of neighborhoods.

Look around the neighborhood where you live or think about the community where you grew up. Let's look at some of the features that might promote health or inhibit your ability to adopt or maintain healthy behaviors. Is the street where you live walkable? Do you feel safe walking on it during the day? At night? Is there any place to walk to? Can you access food stores, restaurants, post offices, drug stores, and all the other places you need to go? In this chapter, we will discuss how having these factors is more than a matter of convenience; their presence or absence, along with your ability to access them, help contribute to what is a healthy neighborhood.

How neighborhoods and metropolitan areas are designed and how they impact health are central focuses of this book. To understand the impact of community design on public health, it is necessary to describe the general form of U.S. metropolitan areas and neighborhoods as well as how this form came about. Once the issues posed by conventional development have been identified, solutions to these problems can be developed and implemented.

Demographic, Economic, and Social Trends

Since 1950, there have been profound changes in U.S. society, some of which have been nearly national in impact, whereas others have affected some communities and not others.[1] The second half of the twentieth century saw major changes in the United States' built form that reflected large- and small-scale demographic, social, and economic changes. Nationally, the economy moved from manufacturing to services and factory production first shifted from inner cities to suburbs, then to the West and South, and finally overseas.[2] Millions of African Americans moved into center cities in the great migration from 1914 to 1980, followed by large-scale immigration, predominately from Latin America and Asia, after the reform of the nation's immigration laws in the 1960s.[3] By 2000, immigrants were often directly moving to suburban and rural locations as well.[4] White populations moved from center cities to suburban areas and there has been a much faster rate of overall population growth in the West and South than in the East and Midwest.[5] Another trend that accelerated after 1970 was **gentrification** as affluent, often childless households and single people moved into select neighborhoods and cities.[6] Income inequality increased after the mid-1970s and racial residential segregation of African Americans slowly declined from its 1950 peaks.[7]

Collectively, these trends had profound impacts on the built environment. Many communities suffered from disinvestment and became plagued by vacant buildings and empty lots.[8] The decline put pressure on city services and led to problems with street, sidewalk, and park maintenance in many areas.[9] Some cities saw a high demand for housing, straining low- and moderate-income household budgets and causing displacement, homelessness, and overcrowding.[10] Some fast-growing suburban areas have seen their infrastructure for sewers, schools, parks, and other services overwhelmed. Many areas have seen a growth in populations beyond the reach of transit systems.[11] Overall, the scope of these impacts are yet to be fully identified.

Conventional Development

As noted in Chapter Two, architects, theorists, and others, including Clarence Perry, Raymond Unwin, and Frank Lloyd Wright, proposed suburban development forms intended, in part, to promote health. These ideas had been influenced by the urban problems of the late nineteenth and early twentieth centuries. Along with increasing affluence, new technologies, and a number of other factors, these new suburban ideas helped produce a form of the built environment that dominated most of the United States during the second half of the twentieth century.[12] For the purposes of this book, we will call it **conventional development** and though there were variations in this form, mostly the result of the legacy of development that predated the triumph of this development pattern or changes in suburbanization that occurred as it progressed through a variety of development waves, it characterizes most of the development in rural, suburban, and urban areas in these decades.[13] In general, conventional development consists of single-family homes on lots of at least 6,000 square feet, but often on lots of a quarter acre or larger. These houses are set back from the street with a substantial landscaped front yard and a driveway leading to a garage that can accommodate two or more vehicles. Views of the street from most of the house are not possible. Many residential streets are cul-de-sacs or partly closed off so that through traffic is discouraged. These streets open on to collector streets, which feed into arterials and then highways. Most housing is distant from any commercial, industrial, or other nonresidential uses, though there may be a park or recreational space in the neighborhood.[14] Schools may or may not be present, and similarly, sidewalks and other pedestrian amenities are optional.[15]

Commercial uses tend to be either in strip developments or in malls, but in both cases, stores are separated from streets by large areas of parking.[16] These commercial areas sometimes have sidewalks, but these are far from building entries and often along arterials built to promote the travel of high volumes of traffic at high speeds.[17] Walking to or between commercial developments is difficult and rare. Making them even less pedestrian-friendly, an important percentage of commercial development is oriented toward highway off-ramps rather than residential development. Offices are often in large suburban developments that include a number of discrete buildings, each surrounded by substantial parking lots.[18] These office parks are not accessible by walking or bicycling, either.[19] In center cities, many office and commercial developments are designed on the assumption that suburban users and visitors fear inner-city crime and will only visit and use downtown buildings if they are heavily separated from surrounding neighborhoods. Many mid-twentieth century urban office buildings favor blank facades at street level, entries that are tightly monitored, and surface and structured parking that are subsidized to make driving easier.[20]

Problems with Suburban and Urban Form

For millions of Americans, this conventional development paradigm has many advantages.[21] It maximizes personal freedom while minimizing reliance on government.[22] Privacy is prioritized, the designs have been highly effective in promoting access to sunlight and ventilation, and in conjunction with the great rise in income and living standards in the United States in the fifty years after

World War II, it has helped contribute to improved health. But there are problems with conventional development.[23]

Concerns about the quality and social, economic, and environmental effects of conventional development preceded the identification of its health impacts.[24] By the early 1980s, there was a growing dissatisfaction among many sectors of society with how inner cities and suburbs in the United States were being designed and built. First and foremost, it was clear that many U.S. cities were in serious decline.[25] If conventional architecture and design were not responsible for this decay, they were faulted for not having helped to reverse or slow it.[26]

Conditions were also unsatisfactory in many U.S. suburbs. While they were rapidly growing, attracting population, industry, and new commercial growth, the energy shocks of the late 1970s caused by sudden shutoffs of imported oil demonstrated that suburbs were heavily dependent upon cheap gasoline.[27] Decades of highway construction had shown that simply building more roads would not reduce traffic and residents were now realizing that despite this massive investment in infrastructure, they still had to endure long commutes.[28] Environmentalists were alarmed by the vast consumption of land that had once been used for farming or that had once provided crucial habitats for endangered species.[29] State and municipal finance administrators saw that suburban development relied on large subsidies from federal, state, and municipal governments, subsidies that were hard to provide during the long recessions of the era.[30] Worst of all from the point of view of many architects and urban planners, much of the suburban landscape was ugly, featuring arterials lined by poor signage and vast parking lots, low-slung office parks devoid of character, and mass-produced housing that offered little variation from one part of the country to another.[31]

There were changes in how conventional developments were designed. Over time, the use of the grid as a way of shaping new development was more or less abandoned and after 1975 or so, the percentage of new gridded developments began to rapidly decline.[32] In its place was the dendritic pattern of development where houses were clustered around cul-de-sacs, which led to feeder streets, which led to arterials, which led to highways. This new pattern was thought to be better for small children and pedestrians, and it was thought that it would reduce traffic exposures for most people.[33] As we know now, while children may be safer playing in the street on a cul-de-sac, dendritic street patterns are almost totally unusable for pedestrians and bicyclists and sharply decrease the utility of nonmotorized transport.[34] The only way to reach destinations outside the home in a dendritic subdivision is to use a car.[35]

Thanks to the work of environmentalists such as Ian McHarg, planners after 1964 were emboldened to identify crucial environmentally sensitive habitats and force developers to set aside these areas.[36] It should be noted that in the

FOCUS ON

Rural, Suburban, Urban: Which Is Healthier?

Despite the fact that there has been a great deal of interest over the past few centuries in whether or not certain types of built environments are more healthy than others, there has not been much research in recent years on whether rural, suburban, or urban areas are the healthiest. Many people may assume that rural areas are most healthy, followed by suburban environments, with cities being the least healthy of all. But this may not necessarily be the case.

In the nineteenth century, rural areas tended to be healthier than cities and mortality rates were much greater in urban areas than they were in the countryside. It was not until the end of the nineteenth century that these urban health problems began to subside as cities became cleaner and incomes began to rise. By the 1940s, the **rural health advantage** had disappeared.

Today, there is some evidence that rural areas are less healthy than metropolitan living. This may arise from the lack of access to health care, the overall lower incomes in rural areas, or the changing rural economy that finds more people employed in activities that do not require physical activity rather than farming. In any case, some evidence suggests that rural areas now have higher rates of obesity, drug use, depression, physical activity, and other conditions.

It is not clear that there are substantial differences in the health of residents of urban versus suburban areas. Many urban residents are less healthy, but these may be attributed to poverty, discrimination, and other factors that are not related to place. Based on much of the information in this book, one might assume that suburban residents are less healthy, but to date there has been little research done to determine whether the lower densities and greater amounts of sprawl in suburban areas have combined to make health decline. Again, the differences between areas may be highly dependent on income, race, and other factors that must be controlled in order to determine how living conditions affect health.

For a more detailed discussion of this issue, see Vlahov, Galea, and Freudenberg (2005).[43]

1970s, the production of carbon dioxide and other greenhouse gases were yet to be identified as a major pollution problem and, at the time, many hoped that new innovations such as the catalytic converter would solve the problem of air pollution from cars.

Another trend after 1950 was toward ever lower residential densities in many communities.[37] As incomes rose, consumer preference for suburban living reached a climax, zoning codes became ever more restrictive, and the standard suburban lot increased in size.[38] When the first suburban home guidelines were adopted just before World War II, the standard suburban lot size was set at 6,000 square feet or about seven houses per acre. But in many areas, the minimum allowable lot size grew to a quarter acre, an acre, or even two acres. Thus, even though more land was set aside to preserve open space, the total amount of land consumed by development vastly increased.[39] Another change in development patterns was the increasing size of single-family homes. Even as the baby boom ebbed, the number of single-person households increased, the median household size of the United States decreased, and houses became increasingly larger. The total amount of space per person increased. Because there are fixed energy costs per house, this increase in house size was to result in higher energy costs. The U.S. public may not have been alarmed by these changes, but there was growing concern about these trends among planners and architects. A search for alternatives began to take form.

Residential development in the last half of the twentieth century generally reflects the parameters of conventional development. Though some cities saw growth in high-density housing, many cities, such as Detroit and others, saw their housing markets decline.[40] Other cities, such as Phoenix, saw large population increases, but their new neighborhoods are largely indistinguishable from suburban development.[41] It should be noted that rural development has had greater variability, sometimes including an isolated single or cluster of subdivisions, sometimes having large areas of five-acre lots or larger development, or a mixture of land uses along rural roads and interstate highways, to name just a few types.[42]

Land Use and Planning Controls

Zoning and building codes are the primary way in which local governments control development and urban form.[44] The federal government has a limited role in local development design and most states give their regulatory power to cities, town, or counties to manage and enforce codes, though states often will pass laws or establish guidelines. Most localities have adopted a version of a national zoning code and, though it can be modified to meet local conditions, there is a broad degree of uniformity across the country.[45] These zoning ordinances mandate maximum housing and office densities, require minimum parking capacities, establish setbacks from streets and property lines, and most important, describe what are permissible uses in a given area.[46] Good planning in the post–World War II era thought that nonresidential uses should be sited as far as possible from where people lived.[47] As described in Chapter Two, there was a health basis for granting governments the power to regulate land use, but these regulations were based on nineteenth-century ideas of the need for sunlight and ventilation.

Jane Jacobs

A fundamental paradigm shift for both suburban and inner-city development was assisted by the work of Jane Jacobs.[48] She was an observer and theorist who built on her experiences in the Greenwich Village neighborhood of New York City and her battles with Robert Moses, the powerful head of the Triborough Bridge Authority and many other New York City area development agencies. Moses's design ideas reflected many of the features of conventional development: superblocks, separation of pedestrian circulation from streets, single-use districts, large open spaces, no shared walls between buildings, prioritization of automobiles, and so on.[49] Jacobs promoted housing over stores, aligning buildings so that they were close to and overlooked streets, fine-textured development that took place over decades rather than through large-impact projects, a diversity of land uses, pedestrian circulation, and other features very different from conventional development.[50] Jacobs and Moses fought over several issues, including plans for reconfiguring Washington Square by proposing to extend Fifth Avenue through the park, replacing a portion of Greenwich Village with a development on a large superblock with Modernist-inspired housing, and the construction of a highway across lower Manhattan.[51]

Jacobs and her allies won these battles, and she went on to write a very successful book that was to contribute to a change in mainstream thought regarding what was desirable about cities and urban living.[52] Though it took decades for these ideas to be accepted, they are well represented in planning theory today. When Jacobs published *The Death and Life of Great American Cities* in 1962, many critics at the time reacted to it very negatively, perhaps because she purposely condemned conventional urban planning or because she was largely self-taught and outside the prevailing academic thinking of her age.[53] The great urban planner and theorist, Lewis Mumford, for example, used sexist language to put down Jacobs's ideas and a review in the *Village Voice* focused more on Jacobs's difficult personality than her revolutionary ideas.[54]

Up to the time of Jacobs, urban planners had held to the belief that density was bad for health and cities, and one of the two main goals of zoning was to reduce congestion by reducing density.[55] The other main purpose of urban planning at the time was to eliminate so-called incompatible land uses and cities strove at every opportunity to reduce complexity and minimize mixed uses.[56] Jacobs, based on her observations on life in Greenwich Village, proposed that density and complexity were the very things that made city living desirable.[57]

Early Alternatives

Many planners had come to be dissatisfied with the conventional building and zoning codes even before Jacobs's ideas triumphed. In addition to the problems outlined above, these codes stifled innovation.[58] The conventional building and zoning codes made any deviation difficult.[59] Furthermore, the national codes also made local adaptations rare and they were partly responsible for making one part of the United States look very much like any other.[60] Planners were also beginning to realize that the codes were causing an excessive separation of land uses. The prohibition against mixed uses may have been appropriate for separating housing from slaughterhouses and heavy industry, but they seemed overly strict when it came to keeping residents away from corner stores, locksmiths, and other necessities of life.[61]

Planners and architects sought alternatives, at least so they could implement dendritic street patterns or produce more environmentally sensitive designs. The first new innovation was the **planned unit development** (PUD). This innovation allowed planners to consider an entire development that consisted of multiple dwellings and land uses as a single unified proposal. The older, traditional code would have required each building to be set on a subdivided lot with each building subject to standard setback and density requirements.[62] A PUD enabled developers to cluster their buildings on a portion of their property and allowed for the preservation of wetlands and other sensitive areas, saved the developers money because they could reduce the amount of roads and parking they had to provide, and was also useful for attracting upper-income land uses.[63] Over time the use of PUDs has spread, but although they were initially seen as innovative, their reputation has been tarnished. In part this is because the results of their use have been mixed. In some localities the PUD has become abused and developers propose them as a way to get around the difficulty of applying for a variance. In other communities, PUDs have simply been used to allow for conventional type developments.[64] Few advantages over pre-PUD building were seen and, overall, PUD-permitted developments have accomplished little to improve the health and environment around them.

New Urbanism

The early 1980s, the effort to find alternatives to conventional development produced a range of new types of development, some of which crystallized into what is known as new urbanism.[65] New urbanism began by embracing Jacobs's ideas about the value of density and complexity and by capitalizing on the dissatisfaction with what was seen as the sterility of conventional development.[66] New urbanists looked to Europe for inspiration as well and they expressed admiration for the density and complexity of European urbanism. The new urbanists also consciously looked back, with a certain sense of nostalgia, at small-town America and traditional older urban neighborhoods, and they sought to re-create these types of neighborhoods as a way of building community.[67] One of the first important new urbanist developments was Seaside in the Florida Panhandle. The developer, Robert Davis, had inherited the property and proposed a number of alternative developments before turning to the already famous Miami-based architects of Andres Duany and Elizabeth Plater-Zybeck to design a new resort community.

Seaside combines traditional Southern architecture with a New England influence to place small, carefully designed cottages on small lots set back from the beach and close to commercial uses. Blocks are small, as are streets, so that there are multiple ways of moving around the development and the use of cars is minimized. There are strict architectural guidelines that establish the architectural theme of the development and ensure that everything built contributes to a harmonized whole.

Several of these features would become standards for what Duany and his associates were to call new urbanism. Though there is a wide range of styles, in a new urbanist development, densities can be higher, open space is minimized for individual properties and maximized for the development as a whole, street lengths are kept short and blocks small, buildings are moved closer to the street, and pedestrian circulation is maximized while the use of cars become secondary. Also important, mixed uses are allowed and small stores and offices, along with restaurants and other types of similar destinations, are encouraged.[68]

The new urbanists went on to found the Congress for New Urbanism (CNU) to promote this new form of development. CNU was consciously modeled on CIAM (Congrès International d'Architecture Moderne), the influential association of Modernists of the mid-twentieth century.[69] CNU also adopted a charter of principles putting forth their underlying values and how they envisioned proper development.[70] Since its founding in 1993, CNU has grown to over 3,000 members and by 2010 there were over 1,000 new urbanist kinds of developments across the United States and elsewhere. New urbanism, though it may not have influenced as many units as conventional development, is now an important planning ideology in this country.

New Urbanism and Public Health

It should be noted that the rise of new urbanism predates the return of interest of public health in the built environment. It was not until the beginnings of the obesity epidemic, and the realization that the built environment was potentially

FIGURE 3.1   Age-Adjusted Obesity Rates—United States

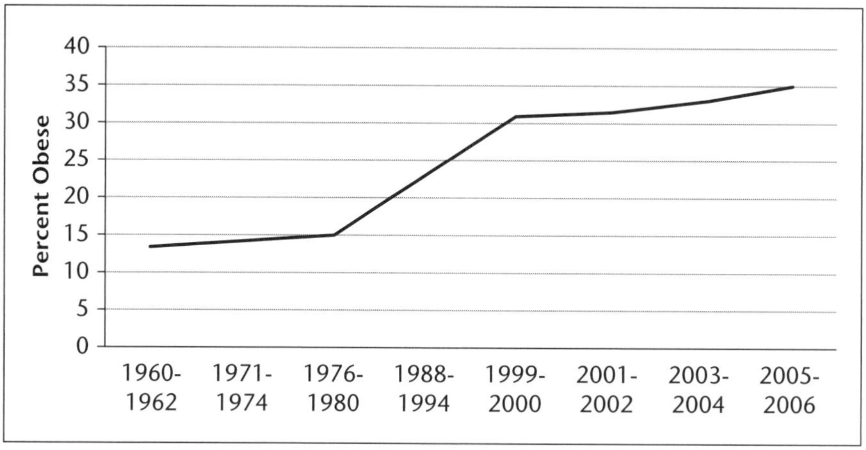

Source: CDC-NHANES

playing a key role in promoting obesity (see Figure 3.1), that public health returned to the study of the built environment. Rather than influencing new urbanism, public health adopted new urbanist principles as its own, even before the availability of any epidemiological evidence to support their utility. The Charter for the New Urbanism does not mention health except in the very most broad terms and a close reading of other new urbanist texts, such as the early book by the new urbanist architect Peter Katz and Andres Duany's model new urbanist code, finds that the concept of health is promoted in a narrow manner that would be recognizable and approved by Southwood Smith in the early nineteenth century—that is, the goal is to promote access to sunlight and ventilation.[71]

But in practice, it appears that new urbanist developments do indeed promote health. In particular, their emphasis on pedestrian circulation and bicycling rather than automobile transportation fosters physical activity. Their incorporation of mixed uses and their embedding of retail and food providers into what in traditional development would be exclusive residential districts create an environment that also appears to reduce obesity risk. Their allowance for higher densities is also important, because density is seen as a key factor for promoting more physical activity. More controversial, but perhaps just as effective, is new urbanists' promotion of interaction among residents so as to improve social capital. Evidence suggests that individuals with greater social capital have a higher health status and are more able to withstand negative events.[72]

There has been criticism of new urbanism. Some critics have maintained that new urbanist developments are too expensive because new urbanist codes are difficult to comply with. Others have maintained that the U.S. public does not want to live in a highly dense and highly interactive environment, and that these kinds of neighborhoods have been rejected by most of the public for many decades.[73] Some find the codes too restrictive, particularly when they have been accompanied by very stringent design guidelines that even may control the choice of paint for exteriors.[74] Some architectural critics have maintained that new urbanism's architectural idioms are fake, too suburban, and promote nostalgia for a time and place that was never as workable as we now believe.[75]

New urbanists have countered that their high prices reflect high consumer demand for these types of developments which indicates that a substantial portion of the U.S. public does indeed want to live in these types of development. They point out that the design guidelines that frame how many new urbanist developments have been built are no more restrictive than the design guidelines for many contemporary conventional developments which also limit exterior options. New urbanists believe that their choices of architectural idiom are valid and reflect long-standing ways of building this country. The debate continues.

From a health perspective, a larger concern centers on the external connectivity of new urbanist developments. They may well have great internal connectivity and accessibility with their short blocks and mixed uses, but they are often not well connected to the surrounding neighborhoods, communities, and metropolitan areas. Many new urbanist developments have been built at relatively low densities and may lack parks, retail uses, and other amenities. This criticism surfaced even as early as the 1990s when architecture critic Vincent Scully suggested that the movement be called "new suburbanism" because that was where the majority of projects had been built and how many looked.[76] Many of the developments, like the original Seaside, are built in rural areas and are only accessible after long drives from metropolitan centers. Others are built in suburban or peripheral metropolitan locations and are a distance from other populations and only accessible by car. Even some of the urban developments are almost walled off from the surrounding streets and inaccessible to neighbors. To the extent that these developments lack external conductivity or mimic conventional development, this limits their health-promotion ability.

Form-Based Codes

The new urbanist codes and similar development guidelines are known as **form-based codes**. The conventional zoning code has grown into a document of more than 1,000 pages, with standards for almost every imaginable land use. In contrast, a form-based code focuses on general outcomes rather than on detailed allowances and prohibitions for how each land use is accommodated. Form-based codes encourage architects and land owners to think creatively on how to meet the goals and guidelines.[77] A form-based code will describe the outcome for an area and allow each new development to meet these goals however it can. Rather than detailed lists of what is permitted, setbacks, and so on, the process is much more open.[78] The result is a much shorter code and one that focuses on outcomes rather than process.

Metropolitan Structure and Health

By the end of the twentieth century, the U.S. population was experiencing an alarming rise in obesity.[79] This increase happened too rapidly to be attributed to genetic causes, so researchers began to study the built environment to see what might be contributing to increased obesity risk. There are most likely many different factors including, but not limited to, stress, diet and access to healthy food, exposure to chemicals, and so on. Some of these factors are related to the built environment and are discussed elsewhere in this book, such as access to supermarkets, fast food policies in schools, walkability, and the like. Others, such as television watching, may be very important obesity risk factors but are less related to the environment, and are not included in our discussion.

In terms of metropolitan form, the most studied factor is the potential association of obesity with urban sprawl. Heavily influenced by the urban planning literature, researchers looked at the overall level of urban sprawl in metropolitan areas and began to research whether sprawl was associated with increased obesity. *Sprawl* is an old term, first coined in the 1920s, and could have imprecise meanings; the first thing researchers had to do was to come up with measures of sprawl that were objective, adequately described existing conditions, and structured in such a way that they could be used in epidemiological research. One of the first sprawl measures was developed by an organization called Smart Growth America, which combined 24 measures into one overall measure. Though this measure was complex and difficult to calculate, it was available for over 75 large metropolitan areas using 2000 data.[80] Other measures followed, some of which were simpler, but available for all metropolitan areas and for other years besides the year 2000.[81]

Public health researchers were aided by new data sources and new technologies that allowed them to analyze risk factors on both the individual and metropolitan level. Individual factors that might influence obesity risk included age, sex, race/ethnicity, smoking, and other similar factors. But now multilevel modeling allowed for simultaneous inclusion of individual metropolitan areas' sprawl factor into regression equations.[82] The first data source for these studies was the Centers for Disease Control and Prevention's (CDC) Behavioral Risk Factor Surveillance System (BRFSS), an annual telephone survey overseen by the CDC but conducted by the states, which is available at a minimum in both English and Spanish.[83]

The BRFSS, like many other surveys, uses self-report to calculate body mass index or BMI.[84] The use of BMI to determine obesity status is controversial. For one thing, there is evidence that self-reported height and weight may not be reliable. There are also concerns that the cutoffs used by the CDC to determine who is overweight or obese are not appropriate. In general, an adult is considered to be overweight with a BMI over 25 and obese with a BMI over 30. Critics have suggested that this can cause those individuals who are overly muscular or athletic to be considered obese or overweight when they are merely very physically fit.[85]

In general, studies have found a link between the level of sprawl in a metropolitan area and the risk of obesity: as sprawl rises, so does obesity risk. The sprawl-to-health pathway hypothesis suggests that sprawl increases the need for driving, reduces physical activity, increases distances to sources of healthy food, and ultimately results in increased obesity. The individual components of this pathway have been tested against sprawl and the preliminary evidence appears to support this hypothesis.[86]

But it should be stressed that the sprawl–obesity link is yet to be definitively established. Critics have pointed out that cross-sectional studies cannot test causality. In the case of sprawl versus obesity, it is not known whether obese people seek out sprawled metropolitan areas or whether the increased obesity risk is really the result of living in these sprawled communities.[87] There have been attempts to use longitudinal databases, studies that track individuals over time, but these tend to have relatively small numbers of subjects and may not be sensitive enough to identify increased risks from sprawl.[88]

Features of a Healthy Community

More than a decade into the twenty-first century and fifteen years after planners and public health professionals began to restudy the built environment, a growing body of evidence is suggesting, but is not yet providing definitive proof, that certain types of features are associated with increased physical activity and a decreased risk of obesity, two of the most important factors influencing health in our time. In general, almost everything that promotes walking and reduces the need for using a car has health benefits. There are also additional benefits for the environment, including improvements in the overall health status of individuals and communities, and the strengthening of community ties (social capital). Many of these factors are also discussed in the chapters on transportation and housing.

In the general order from the largest to the smallest scale, these features include:

Compact Metropolitan Area. Though the evidence is not yet conclusive, more compact, less sprawled metropolitan areas appear to have residents with greater physical activity levels and lower rates of obesity. This may suggest that persons in these metropolitan areas have lower rates of diabetes, cardiovascular disease, and other conditions associated with those risk factors. Most likely, sprawl harms health because residents drive more and are less likely to walk or bicycle to work.[89] Sprawl may result in longer ambulance response times as well.[90]

Higher Densities. The public often opposes density because they fear it will create traffic congestion, foster crime, or lower property values. The conventional health argument was that higher densities make access to sunlight and ventilation more difficult and therefore density is harmful to health. Though higher densities may be associated with increased traffic, it also appears to be associated with lower obesity risk, lower risks of traffic-related accidents, and increased social capital.[91]

Public Transportation Systems. In general, communities that rely solely on cars have lower health status than those where people have a variety of transportation options (See Chapter Four). People who use mass transit to commute to work are more likely to report walking as well. This may be because riders often walk to and from transit stops as opposed to traveling by car, which is more likely to be door to door.[92]

Access to Employment, Goods, and Services. Most walking is purposeful; people walk to a destination rather than just for the sake of walking. Therefore, having destinations within walking distance, having something to walk to, is associated with increased physical activity. This concept is often operationalized as mixed use. Different land uses within close proximity to residential areas encourages walking in those neighborhoods. The conventional alternative is the strict separation of land uses that many late-twentieth century communities mandated through their zoning codes. This may reduce the utility of nonautomobile transport.[93] Evidence also suggests that having walkable destinations also increases social capital.[94]

Parks and Playgrounds. Large-scale regional parks may be visited by people from long distances, but most neighborhood parks are primarily used by neighbors. Similarly, surveys of residents suggest that most will not use a park or playground unless it is within a quarter mile of their house. These facilities are important because they help promote physical activity.[95]

Connected Street Networks. Conventional developments, particularly those built after 1975, are more likely to use what are known as dendritic street networks, a pattern of cul-de-sacs, collector streets, and large arterials that make it almost impossible for pedestrians and bicyclists to access destinations. The more traditional gridded street pattern, which predominated until well after World War II, facilitates walking and biking because it simultaneously slows down traffic and creates many pathways between homes and potential destinations. Therefore, connected street networks facilitate physical activity.[96]

Lower Traffic Speeds. Pedestrians and bicyclists tend to fear high-speed traffic because it makes them feel unsafe. When cars speed, they may dramatically increase the risk of injury and death. Thus anything that can lower traffic speeds can encourage people to feel safer and make them more likely to walk or bicycle.[97]

Sidewalks. Many suburban and most rural areas lack sidewalks. Some sidewalks found in many urban areas may be in extreme disrepair. Where there were no sidewalks or sidewalks are poorly maintained, pedestrians may be forced to walk in the street, placing them at risk of passing cars. This also discourages walking.[98]

Pedestrian-Friendly Street Crossings. Some of the greatest sites of pedestrian-automobile accidents are street corners where pedestrians are crossing busy intersections. Many intersections have been highly engineered to promote easy turning by cars, but these can be problematic for pedestrians. Solutions range from the simple to the complex and can include everything from stop signs to pedestrian countdown signals that alert both drivers and pedestrians of how much time is left for individuals to get across the street.

On-Street Parking. Given the profound fear of traffic, any kind of barrier between sidewalks and streets make pedestrians feel safer and thus encourage physical activity. Simply allowing on-street parking can often make the sidewalks appear safer from traffic on the streets. On the one hand, this is another easy way to encourage physical activity or at least make it appear safer to pedestrians. On the other hand, making on-street parking difficult also encourages walking.[99]

Street Trees. Trees can encourage walking and physical activity in several ways. Their shade can help promote physical activity during hot summer days, their bulk helps protect pedestrians from cars, and their very presence can help promote better mental health. All of these factors may help explain why the presence of street trees encourages pedestrian activity.[100]

Streetlights. Streetlights help make streets feel safer for pedestrians at night. They may reduce the amount of crime and thus may promote walking by mitigating fear of crime.[101]

Houses Oriented Toward Streets. As incomes have risen and tastes in domestic architecture have changed, building lots have become larger and the setback from house to street has increased in size. In many communities, the need for larger garages to house more cars has led to garages and driveways taking over more and more of the space in front of the house. Pulling buildings away from the streets tends to make pedestrians feel isolated and more unsafe. Therefore, anything that can be done to make the fronts of houses close to the street along with appropriate façades that emphasize windows from living quarters rather than garage doors, can help facilitate walking and physical activity.[102]

Crime. The fear for personal safety is one of the main reasons why people say they will not walk to work or let their children walk to school. Addressing crime may be critical to encourage people in certain communities to be physically active.[103]

Solutions

There are, perhaps, two main ways of action to create healthier metropolitan and neighborhood environments: retrofit existing communities and change the way new areas are designed. But rebuilding existing communities and shaping the development of new areas so that they promote physical activity and increase interactions between neighbors is not easy. There is a great deal of inertia because many neighborhoods are totally built out using problematic designs and many communities are not familiar with more healthy alternatives. Changing how we build our neighborhoods is going to take actions on many levels. Part of this may involve educating individuals and families on the health consequences of the residential choices. This may result in promoting increased demand for healthier environments. It may include working with state and local government to encourage the adoption of laws, codes, and policies that prioritize and promote healthier designs.[104] Developers need to be educated on the changing taste for communities that promote physical activity. These types of efforts may increase the supply of healthy neighborhoods. Finally, there is a need to rebuild or reengineer existing communities so that they are healthier for their residents. None of these actions will be easy and most will be expensive. However, if we are to improve the built environment they are all vitally necessary. Some of the programs and policies that have been developed in the past several decades are described below. This is not an exhaustive list; it just demonstrates some of the ways people in communities have worked to implement alternatives to conventional development.

Smart Growth. If sprawl is associated with increased obesity and decreased physical activity, then efforts to reduce the levels of sprawl may have positive health effects. Over the past several decades one of the most comprehensive set of policies to change how communities are designed and built has been smart growth. The policies that are part of the smart growth agenda include increasing densities, promoting mixed-use developments, emphasizing the need for pedestrian amenities, prioritizing walking and biking over automobile use, providing incentives for reusing older, potentially contaminated parcels known as Brownfields, pushing for increased development near mass transportation facilities, restricting low-density and peripheral development, encouraging inner-city revitalization, and other similar development strategies. A particular challenge for smart growth has been the lack of regional government in this country. Sometimes, smart growth policies are adopted by a single municipality even though other cities and towns in its metropolitan area have their own conventional development strategies. Other times, smart growth policies have been adopted by county or state governments but not all the local governments that actually control development have signed on. One of the few comprehensive programs to promote smart growth was the effort that began in the late 1990s in the state of Maryland. Under the leadership of Governor Parris Glendenning, state development monies were focused on promoting smart growth at the local level. Though these strategies may be adopted on the local level, they may be more effective if adopted on the metropolitan or state level.[105]

Urban Growth Boundaries. Another way to manage growth and to reign in sprawl is to establish urban growth boundaries which force new development inside the boundary, leaving areas outside the boundary for nonurban purposes. More compact metro areas may ultimately increase physical activity and reduce obesity risk. One of the first urban growth boundaries was in Lexington, Kentucky, but the most famous is around Portland, Oregon. In Portland, a boundary was drawn beyond which government services were not extended and further development not allowed. The adoption of growth boundaries has been controversial and some have claimed that they are an infringement on the rights of property owners to use their land as they wish. Others claim that it has led to an increase in housing costs and reduced affordability in the Portland area. The evidence for both of these claims is mixed. It does appear that the Portland growth boundary has been successful, though there has been a problem because some development seems be pushed across the state border into neighboring Washington state. One lesson may be that a growth boundary must be comprehensive and that any gaps in the boundary will lead to a burst of growth in that area.[106]

Greenbelts. A greenbelt strategy to rein in urban sprawl differs from the growth boundary method in that government or nonprofits purchase land at urban peripheries to keep it from being developed.[107] Again, the goal is to promote physical activity and reduce obesity risk. This has the advantage of guaranteeing that the land will be protected from development in perpetuity but it suffers from the drawback of being very expensive. Perhaps the most comprehensive greenbelt is the one around San Jose, California, which was funded by parcel taxes and other dedicated revenue sources that has resulted in the purchase of several hundred thousand acres of land around that city and its suburbs. The strategy is successful and the metropolitan area has grown substantially in terms of population without consuming significantly more land. Similar to the controversy in Portland, Oregon, this greenbelt strategy has been criticized because it leads to higher housing costs and most of the preserved open space is only accessible to higher-income households on the edge of the metropolitan area. One study, however, has found that the greenbelt strategy in San Jose resulted in only a modest reduction in the size of the housing stock (most preserved land was in areas with steep slopes) and by implication, has contributed very little to that city's high housing costs.[108] Another study has found an association between urban containment programs and physical activity.[109]

Zoning Code Reform. If the conventional building and zoning codes are promoting unsafe and unhealthy development that is highly dependent upon automobile use, then one strategy may be to simply change the code. The goal is to change codes so that they permit and encourage development that is more consistent with new ideas about promoting physical activity or access to amenities. In response to concerns about the quality of conventional development, the conventional codes have been modified so that communities can now adopt standard code language that permits mixed-use development, higher densities, and more pedestrian-friendly street layouts. But there are challenges in reforming building and zoning codes. One challenge is to get them adopted. Some neighborhoods and cities may not want new urbanists or more pedestrian-friendly designs and

FOCUS ON

Eminent Domain

One of the more controversial government powers is what is known as eminent domain. This is the right of the government to take private property, with compensation, to use for a public purpose.[111] Understandably, when someone's home, business, or other property is taken by the government, the experience can be quite emotional.

One major issue is what constitutes proper compensation. The U.S. Constitution establishes the right of government to use eminent domain, but only when property owners are paid for the taking. But establishing value can be difficult. Oftentimes, independent appraisers are used, but property owners may feel that these appraisals do not adequately reflect either the economic value of the land or their long-term emotional ties to the property. Sometimes landowners will challenge the compensation in court.

Another major issue is what constitutes a proper public use. Many communities were devastated by eminent domain that was used for urban renewal and highway construction in the second half of the twentieth century. At least in the case of highway construction, the land and the use were clearly in the public realm even if the people losing their homes for the construction of a new highway neither drove nor had any need to use the new highway. Similarly, taking land for school construction or other similar public use may be difficult for those who lose their properties but is generally more supported by the public as a whole.

More difficult is the case when land taken by eminent domain is to be used for economic development so that it would be ultimately turned over to a private developer or nonpublic enterprise. Is the goal of economic development and providing more jobs in the community a justifiable public use? In a controversial decision in 2005, the U.S. Supreme Court ruled that the City of New London, Connecticut, could take the property owned by Susette Kelo et al., so that it could be used by a pharmaceutical company to build a new facility.[112] In the years since that decision, many states have passed legislation or constitutional amendments to curb the use of eminent domain in their jurisdictions. The controversy continues.

may not want the kinds of pedestrian amenities that are known to foster physical activity. There may be opposition from the government agencies responsible for implementing these codes because they are not familiar with them or do not like these new provisions. Finally, even if the codes are actually adopted they may be difficult to implement. It is often hard to retrofit existing communities, developers may be reluctant to try new untested designs, and communities may oppose any actual changes in the zoning designations on a given parcel. Again, one of the answers to these issues is education for everyone involved.

Density Bonuses. The more houses or square feet of commercial office space that can be built on a given piece of land, the more potential there is for profit for developers because the per-unit land cost is reduced. Therefore, some communities have provided density bonuses as an incentive to encourage developers to produce the designs that they feel will be more healthful.[110] In addition, higher densities themselves will promote walkability. The problem in granting density bonuses is that neighbors are often concerned about the density of the original proposal or may be very against any increased density at all.

Rezoning and Upzoning. If one problem is simply that too much land is zoned at too low a level of intensity of use, then one solution may be to change the zoning restrictions so that more intense use or mixed uses are allowed.[113] The idea is that over time, as parcels are redeveloped, densities will slowly increase. The underlying health concept is that increased density will lead to higher levels of physical activity. This often becomes a political issue because many committees are opposed to any higher-intensity uses, usually because they fear that these higher intensities will bring in increased crime and traffic. Though this technique has been used in certain limited areas in many cities, there has not been a comprehensive upzoning of a major portion of any large city in the United States.

Transit-Oriented Development. As noted above, transit use is associated with physical activity, but users have a limited distance they will walk to a station or bus stop. Increasing density and the scale of buildings near transit centers may lead to an increase in the number of people who use transit. As pointed out in the description of smart growth, one strategy is to encourage development around existing transit nodes such as light rail stops, rail stations, and major bus lines. The idea is that if people have access to good-quality public transportation they will not need to drive as much. Critics have suggested that this has not resulted in increased public transportation use and that car usage in these communities is as high as it is elsewhere.[114] Some studies suggest, however, that although transit-oriented development does not result in eliminating all car usage in a household, it may reduce the number of households that have more than one car and may reduce the number of noncommuting automobile trips.[115]

Rebuilding Commercial Districts. The large-scale parking, lack of access, and other disincentives for pedestrians posed by conventional commercial development may be a barrier to physical activity or access to food. In the country as a whole and in many local communities, there is too much commercial space, resulting in much of it being underutilized or vacant. In particular, older strip developments and abandoned big-box retail stores are problems in many areas and represent underutilized land. This also offers an opportunity. Strategies have been created to redevelop older underutilized parcels and include demolishing existing buildings, rebuilding and refocusing commercial uses at particular nodes, providing wider sidewalks and pedestrian amenities, reducing parking or placing parking in structures rather than on open lots, and increasing the overall intensity of use of these parcels.[116] One of the more ambitious of these types of projects is one covering several hundred acres in the White Flint area of Montgomery County, Maryland. If completed as envisioned, the development would be much more pedestrian friendly, would feed into an existing Washington Metro stop, and would provide more tax revenues for the county.[117]

Building Pedestrian and Other Amenities. As discussed above, pedestrians are very sensitive to street designs and traffic. Thus, if the goal is to increase pedestrian activity as a way to encourage physical activity, the design of streets and neighborhoods must be carefully considered. Retrofitting residential areas can be more difficult than changing how commercial areas are built. There tend to be more property owners, making it challenging to reach a consensus for change. If there is a need to purchase land to create new streets or facilities, this becomes a potentially difficult political process and can be prohibitively expensive. Targeted homeowners may not want to sell or move and, once built, street layouts are difficult to change. Thus there have been few attempts to open up a traditional dendritic neighborhood to create better connectivity and pedestrian circulation. However, some residential areas can still be improved to make them more pedestrian friendly or more amenable to physical activity. Many developments contain small pieces of land that did not end up built on and these can be used for parks, playgrounds, or sitting areas. Residential development that did not initially include sidewalks or street trees can have these amenities added. Streetlights can be installed to make streets safer at night, and traffic patterns can be studied so that car speeds are reduced, and crosswalks and other safety measures are installed. There can be some opposition to installing sidewalks because some communities feel that this would result in an unwelcome change to the rural feeling for that neighborhood. But a bigger problem is cost. It is difficult to find the dollars for capital improvements that these changes often need. Some communities have tried what are known as local improvement districts in which property owners are assessed a tax to pay for the improvements. These have been controversial. It also is difficult for low-income communities to afford increased property taxes even if there is a desire for these new amenities. Some cities have turned to federal and state grants and other funding sources to pay for these improvements.[118]

Summary

For most of the twentieth century, conventional development promoted car use, dendritic street designs, separation of land use, and other norms that are now thought to be associated with increased environmental burdens and increased obesity. A number of alternatives have been proposed that include New Urbanism, growth management efforts, transit-oriented development, and actions that promote pedestrian and bicycle uses.

The issues and solutions outlined in this chapter are closely related to transportation and housing. Indeed, the connections between transportation, land use, and housing are strong; programs to significantly change or improve a neighborhood may have to address all three. As will be seen in the next two chapters, the factors that can lead to healthier populations are very similar across these areas of concern.

Key Terms

Conventional development	Planned unit development
Form-based codes	Rural health advantage
Gentrification	Smart growth
Greenbelts	

Discussion Questions

1. Name the key features of what we call conventional development.
2. Describe the potential benefits and problems associated with conventional development.
3. What is New Urbanism? Why might it promote healthier living?
4. What is urban sprawl? Discuss the evidence linking it to obesity.
5. Describe the features of a healthy built environment.
6. Name five programs or policies that might help promote a healthier build environment.
7. Discuss barriers to these programs and policies. Why might it be difficult to get communities to adopt them?

For More Information

American Planning Association. *Planning and Community Health Research Center*. http://www .planning.org/nationalcenters/health/index.htm.

Congress for the New Urbanism. www.Cnu.org.

Duany, A., & Plater-Zyberk, E. (2001). *Suburban nation: The rise of sprawl and the decline of the American dream*. New York: North Point Press.

Dunham-Jones, E., & Williamson, J. (2009). *Retrofitting suburbia: Urban design solutions for redesigning suburbs*. Hoboken, NJ: Wiley.

Katz, P. (1994). *The new urbanism: Toward an architecture of community*. New York: McGraw Hill.

Smart Growth America. www.smartgrowthamerica.org.

Squires, G. (2002). *Urban sprawl: Causes, consequences, and policy responses*. Washington, DC: The Urban Institute Press.

The Prevention Institute. *The built environment and health: 11 profiles of neighborhood transformation*. http://www.preventioninstitute.org/index.php?option=com_jlibrary&view=article&id= 114&Itemid=127.

CHAPTER 4

TRANSPORTATION POLICIES

LEARNING OBJECTIVES

- Describe the overall pattern of transportation mode choice in the United States.
- Name the groups most at risk for transportation-related deaths and injuries.
- Explain the relationship between land use and transportation.
- Explain why dendritic street patterns may inhibit physical activity.
- Compare the meanings of mobility and accessibility.
- Describe the differences between highway and mass transit funding.
- Differentiate between the strategies of preventing accidents versus reducing injuries caused by accidents.
- List some of the ways that pedestrian activity can be promoted.

How do you travel from your house, dorm, or apartment to school or work? Did you walk, ride a bike, take public transit, or travel by car? Why did you travel the way you did? Do you have options? Now think about how your choice of transit mode might affect your health. Was your trip to work or school stressful? Dangerous? Were you physically active or did you sit the whole time? How did you feel once you arrived at your destination? As these questions suggest, how you travel to and from destinations is highly influenced by the built environment and your choice of travel mode, and your experience while moving to and from a place can have profound impacts.

Transportation has a major influence on health. There are its direct impacts on accidents and injuries and a variety of indirect effects that include transportation's influence on physical activity, air pollution, the production of greenhouse gasses, and the destruction of natural habitats. This chapter begins with an overview of travel behavior and touches briefly on transportation theory. It then covers issues related to individual modes: automobiles, transit, bicycles, and walking. It ends with a summary of design initiatives aimed at promoting pedestrian activity and reducing the risk posed by automobiles.

Current Patterns of Transportation in the United States

Some of the main sources of information on U.S. transportation patterns are the U.S. Census and the periodic National Household Transportation Survey (NHTS) conducted by the U.S. Department of Transportation. These data indicate that the main way people in the United States move around is by automobile. Sometimes there are multiple people in one vehicle, but most people drive alone to their destinations, at least when it comes to traveling to work. The past several decades have seen increases in the share of people who drive and an increase in the number of miles driven per capita. These trends appear to be true for both adults commuting to work and children going to school. It was only when the price of gasoline spiked to over four dollars a gallon followed by a deep recession in 2008 that this trend was blunted. In general, U.S. residents drive even for short trips of less than one mile. Collectively, the U.S. population drove 2.4 billion miles in 2008 and the transportation sector accounts for about 25% of the total amount of greenhouse gases emitted in the United States.[1] In 2007, 75.8% of people traveled to work by car by themselves, 10.4% carpooled, 4.5% took public transportation, 2.8% walked, and .5% rode a bike (see Figure 4.1).[2] Part of the cost of this travel is congestion, which can consume large amounts of

FIGURE 4.1 Workers 16 and Over—Commuting Mode Choice

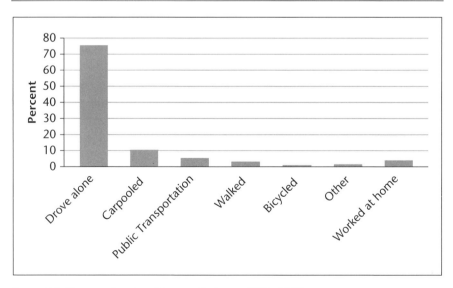

Source: U.S. Census—American Community Survey 2005–2009

time. The Texas Transportation Institute estimates that nationally commuters spent 4.2 billion hours stuck in traffic at a cost of $83.2 billion or $750 per person in 2007.[3]

Mobility Versus Accessibility

Transportation planning has traditionally been concerned with **mobility**,[4] how to get people from point A to point B. This can be thought of as the engineering of pipes that connect people to destinations. In this conventional planning paradigm, there is no questioning of where people want to go or where these destinations should be; the role of the transportation planner is simply to connect various points in a metropolitan area and beyond with the assumption that almost all trips will be made by car. There is also no questioning of why people are driving or how the connection of distant points relates to the needs of individuals and households. One outcome from this type of policy is an emphasis on building roads and improving the ease of automobile-based transportation.

In recent decades, there has been greater attention paid to **demand management**.[5] In a sense this is looking at where and how people join or leave the pipe. Solutions under this type of transportation planning have included limiting access or egress to highways, metering of highway access (putting in lights that slow down the number of cars that enter the highway in a given amount of time), or changing how feeder streets connect to arterials. There have also been movements toward implementing **congestion charges** and tolls, and increasing fees during high demand times.[6] Again, this says nothing about where people live, where they want to go, or why they may want to go there.

Since the 1990s, there has been a movement to change transportation planning away from its focus on mobility toward a concern for **accessibility**.[7] This movement posits that people have no innate desire to travel long distances to get to jobs, shopping, or other destinations. They travel, instead, simply to access these destinations.[8] The goal of people is not to drive, but to access goods, services, and jobs. Therefore, rather than accepting the distribution of housing, jobs, and amenities as a given, resulting in narrowing the focus of transportation planning simply to connecting trip beginning and end points regardless of distance, an additional goal of transportation planning should include reducing the distance between points and thus reducing the need for travel itself.[9] The results for consumers would be more accessibility and a reduced focus on mobility. But the public would not notice this because they are still accessing all the goods, services, and amenities that they need and demand. By focusing on accessibility, the total amount of driving decreases, the time spent on driving diminishes, and ultimately the cost of driving falls. These reductions include direct costs such as gasoline and wear and tear on cars as well as indirect costs, including the amount spent on road construction and the total amount of greenhouse gases produced.[10] The policy responses that arise from this shift in emphasis to accessibility include linking transportation and land use, broadening the work of transportation planning to include how people will live and work in communities, consideration of other transit modes, and incorporation of concerns about the built environment.

Intersection of Transportation with Land Use

The way people use transportation is intimately associated with the type of land use in their community.[11] Most people seldom walk for the sake of walking or even rarely walk to meet physical activity goals; most walk to get to a destination, either for work or for other purposes. But these other types of walking trips are only feasible if there are destinations within walking distance and if walking to and from these destinations is safe.

Studies suggest that people who live in denser communities and those who have nonresidential land uses within walking distance of their homes are more likely to walk. Similarly, most users of neighborhood parks are people who live within walking distance of these amenities and people will not walk if there is no place to walk to. This highlights the importance of coordinating land use and transportation.[12] But transportation planning too often takes place in a vacuum with little consideration of its ties to the walking needs of residents; sometimes routes are selected based on the cheapest available land, rather than on the public health needs, and transit can be dislocated from surrounding residents. For example, many transit authorities seek to maximize their catchment areas for commuters and surround stations with large parking lots and garages. Though these may assist people who drive to a station and then take public transit, they may also discourage walking for those near these facilities.

The answer to these kinds of issues has been **transit-oriented development**, a subset of planning that seeks to integrate land use and transportation, developing higher density housing, retail, and other uses within walking distance of a station, and taking care that the station area is safe and accessible for pedestrians.[13] These types of developments do not necessarily result in residents giving up cars altogether, but they can reduce the number of car trips in the area and reduce the number of households who have more than one car.

The relationship between land use and transportation mode choice is strong. This means that if policymakers desire to reduce the amount of automobile travel, there may be a need to change the underlying land-use patterns in a community. This may not be easy and may be very expensive but ultimately could prove necessary. However, given that so many trips by car are under one mile in length, it may be possible to promote alternatives to cars without massive changes in the built environment, but through small-scale changes such as making streets more connected and safer for walking.[14]

Epidemiology of Transportation-Related Injuries

Given that people in the United States drive so much, it should not be surprising that injuries and deaths from automobile-related accidents are a major public health issue. Though they have declined in recent years, there are over 43,000 deaths annually from automobile accidents and 5 million visits to emergency rooms.[15] Automobile-related fatalities are the leading cause of death for young people in this country and one of the leading causes of death overall.

Among subpopulations, accidents and fatalities are more likely among the younger and older driving populations.[16] This may be related to the greater propensity for risky behavior overall and a lack of experience for younger people and the increased risk of impairment and slower reaction times for the elderly.[17] Driver education, license restrictions, raising minimum drinking age laws, increasing alcohol taxes, and other public health campaigns have been used to address youth driving risks.[18] Some states have called for increased vision and driving testing of elderly drivers and others have advocated for public health campaigns to publicize the special needs of elderly drivers.[19] In addition, people in rural areas are more at risk than those in urban areas, perhaps because urban travel speeds are lower, there is less driving in cities, and more urban streets have appropriate protective infrastructure.[20]

Children, the elderly, and Hispanic people are at increased risk for pedestrian injuries. The greater rate of cognitive problems, lower reaction times, slower walking speeds, and other problems may explain some of the elevated risk for elderly pedestrians.[21] Children's increased risks may be best addressed by parental, driver, and child education programs and modifications of the built environment to promote safety.[22] The reasons for greater Hispanic risk is yet to be well characterized, but their elevated risk suggests a need for more research and programs targeted to this population.[23]

Commuting

Commuting refers to the daily movement of people from homes to jobs and back. Data from the latest transportation surveys indicates that most people drive to work alone or, to a much smaller extent, drive with others. Recent years have seen discussion on what are known as extreme commutes, commutes that take 45 minutes, an hour, or longer. Data from 2000 suggest that almost as many as 10 million Americans have extreme commutes and, given the changes in development patterns in the past decade, where much of the growth has occurred adjacent to or outside metropolitan areas, these numbers may have grown.

Commuting, regardless of transit mode, is not a health-neutral act. On the contrary, there may be a number of health risks that are associated with commuting that may potentially include decreased physical activity, increased risk of obesity, increased stress, greater exposure to pollutants, and increased risk of accidents. It is not just the time spent on commuting that harms health but also the unpredictability of the commute (accidents and traffic jams) and the general level of impedance, all the things that happen along the commute that may slow the trip. Preliminary studies suggest that those individuals with longer, more unpredictable commutes are more likely to suffer from psychological and physiological problems associated with commuting. The type of job may also affect commutes. Some workers have less flexibility at work and may face consequences if they are late. Though some workers can modify their start times to ease their commutes, others do not have this ability.

The effects of commuting may also result in a decreased amount of time available for nonwork and noncommuting activities. Commuting takes away from the amount of time available for families, physical activity, and other actions that might reduce stress. Potentially, these negative impacts could be much greater for those with extreme commutes. Research on these topics is limited, but suggests that those who make trade-offs that result in living far from jobs in order to access more affordable housing may be negatively affecting their health.[24]

Safety Benefits/Problems with Dendritic Street Designs

There is a growing concern that the conventional dendritic street pattern of cul-de-sacs to collector streets to arterials poses safety and health problems. One reason that these street pattern became popular was that they reduce the amount of traffic on cul-de-sacs and they make the residents feel safer because they can identify people who do not belong there.[25] In addition to the problems posed by the lack of street conductivity outlined above, there may be other problems with dendritic street designs.[26] By reducing traffic on the cul-de-sacs they are increasing traffic on arterials and collector streets, making those streets less safe.[27] But cul-de-sacs have also been opposed by firefighters and other emergency responders because it makes it difficult for fire engines and ambulances to access houses along cul-de-sacs during an emergency. In a gridded street design system, if there is a blocked street, responders can quickly find alternative routes to the emergency. But in a dendritic street pattern, a street blockage, such as that caused by an accident or a stalled vehicle, can result in an entire neighborhood being closed off. Thus local fire marshals and other emergency agencies can become allies in efforts to reform how suburban neighborhoods are laid out.[28]

Transportation for People with Disabilities

There are a growing number of people who, because of age or illness, have disabilities. Unfortunately, conventional street designs often do not accommodate the needs of people who have visual issues, difficulty walking, or other types of disabilities that make it difficult for them to maneuver in conventional built environments. To accommodate this growing population, advocates have begun to assess outdoor spaces with the goal of eliminating barriers to people with disabilities. In addition to the many types of pedestrian-friendly designs mentioned above, these can also include carefully monitoring curb heights, increasing the legibility of signage, raising crosswalks at intersections, and other improvements that enable people to use the environment. The result can be areas that are more usable for people with limitations, reduced risk of accidents, and an increase in physical activity for people with disabilities. Note that in the process of designing streets to assist people with disabilities, the walkability of the neighborhood is increased for everyone.

Who Can Drive?

It must be stressed that a substantial percentage of the U.S. population cannot drive. This includes everybody under the age of 16, a significant percentage of the elderly, and an important percentage of those of working age. Many households cannot afford a car, some people can't drive because of medical conditions, and others may have lost their licenses.[29] For these people, living in an environment that is only accessible by car is severely constraining. It makes them dependent on other people and makes it difficult for them to access medical care, food, jobs, and all the other things that we require outside our homes.[30] Therefore, from a public health perspective and from an egalitarian view of urban planning, it may be necessary to address the accessibility needs of such people and households.[31]

Automobiles and Health

Data from the American Community Survey from 2005 to 2009 indicate that over 95% of households had a least one car and 32.5% had three or more cars.[32] As noted above, cars and automobiles dominate the U.S. transportation system

FIGURE 4.2   Total Annual Miles Driven in the United States

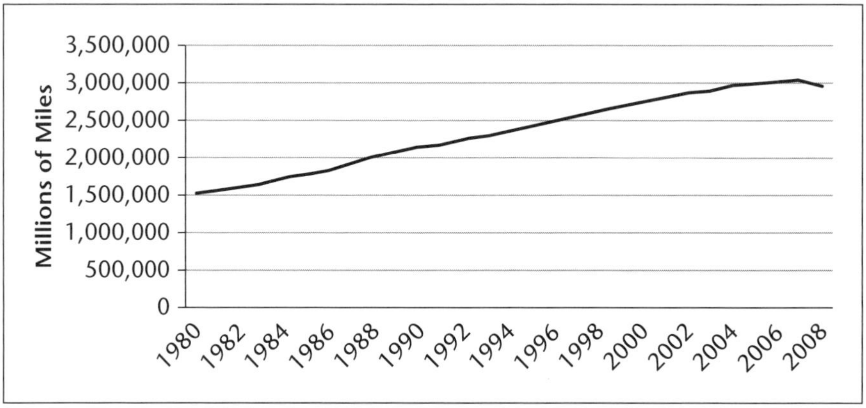

Source: U.S. Department of Transportation

and though there was a small decline in miles traveled by car in 2007 when gasoline prices exceeded $3 per gallon, there is no sign that this dependence on cars is changing (see Figure 4.2). Thus automobiles are of major importance when considering transportation's impact on health.

Driving Safety

Even in the context of the overall growth in vehicle miles traveled in the United States, there has been a long-term, slow decline in mortality associated with automobile use, and driving has become safer since the 1960s. There are three broad categories of actions behind this improvement in safety: roads have been engineered to reduce the likelihood and severity of accidents; cars have been modified to make them safer for passengers in the event an accident occurs; and laws, programs, and policies have been put in place to reduce some of the causes of accidents.

Roads have become safer.[33] For example, better engineering results in smoother mergers on and off highways. This helps reduce the likelihood that there would be a crash at this key conflict point. There has also been a systematic change in the areas along highways so that there are fewer hard barriers that cars can crash into. For surface streets, better design of intersections (for cars), improvements in roadway management, and other types of innovations have also contributed to increased safety.[34] Another reason that traffic fatalities have declined is that cars have become safer. Seatbelts, airbags, better braking systems, and other improvements mean that occupants in cars are safer when crashes occur. The growing use of seatbelts is also an essential component to this effort to make streets and highways safer. Finally, laws to reduce impaired driving, publicize the problem of risk behaviors, and other similar actions have been major public health priorities.[35]

FOCUS ON
Cell Phones

The increase in the use of cell phones over the past two decades has prompted concerns about their health impacts. The potential connection between cell phone use and brain cancer is beyond the scope of this book, but there are other serious problems associated with cell phone use that are more closely related to the built environment. The most important problem is the growing evidence that cell phone use is associated with increased risk of accidents.[36] The problem stems from the way talking on a cell phone distracts drivers. Unlike talking with passengers, which appears to have minimal effects on concentration or accident risk, recent studies suggest that talking on a cell phone is as risky as driving while intoxicated. Drivers on phones can sometimes ignore driving conditions around them, they may not notice pedestrians, other cars, and sometimes even stop signs and stoplights. It is not only distracted drivers who are a potential health risk; some evidence suggests that even pedestrians on cell phones are more likely to stumble or walk into fixed objects because of the distractive potential of cell phones.[37]

Some states have passed laws requiring hands-free headsets or prohibiting drivers from dialing their phones. Unfortunately, talking on a phone may be as risky as dialing and therefore these laws may have limited effects. No state has moved forward to ban all cell phone use while driving, though the federal government has prohibited drivers of public transportation vehicles from doing so. This may be a case where there needs to be more education focused on the general public so that they begin to understand the health risk of this seemingly innocent activity.

The Cost of Driving

One reason why people in the United States drive so much more than residents of other countries is that automobile use in the United States is highly subsidized.[38] The actual cost of constructing and maintaining roads is greater than what is raised by gasoline taxes. Estimates vary on the amount of this subsidy, but some studies suggest that federal and state gasoline taxes pay as little as 20% of the total cost of driving cars in United States.[39] These subsidies come from various sources and include gasoline taxes that support road and highway construction. But there are other, additional subsidies that are more or less hidden so that drivers are not even aware of their benefits; such subsidies are embedded in the free parking provided by both employers and businesses.[40] These include parking in an office park or at a mall, which may seem to be free, but actually includes (1) land costs borne by property owners who must set aside land for parking even though it does not generate revenues, and (2) the foregone property taxes that cities and localities lose because they cannot tax the land under roads—and streets are much wider now than they would need to be if people drove less. There are also the health costs caused by pollution and traffic accidents. Some have suggested that to the extent that foreign and military policy is used to protect petroleum sources, those costs should be added to the total amount of subsidies as well.[41]

The amount of these subsidies matters because of a well-known economic principle that when a good or service is subsidized, people will consume more than if they are paying the full cost. This means people drive more, the negative effects on the environment are greater, and the consumption of land use is greater than if drivers bear the full cost of driving.[42] These subsidies ultimately have helped increase the amount of driving in the United States as well as contributed to urban sprawl.[43] Furthermore, since the extent of the subsidies is not really known to the public, they may be particularly difficult to reduce. For example, if people in the United States believe that gasoline taxes are more than adequate to pay for all the costs of driving, they may be resistant to the idea that taxes should be raised.[44] The reality—that gasoline taxes do not pay for the full cost of road and highway construction, much less their maintenance and other costs—is not well known by the public.

Despite these subsidies, the cost of driving is a major burden on many households in the United States, particularly the poor.[45] It has been estimated that the average household spends approximately $9,000 per year on transportation, almost all of that on driving. This makes driving the second largest budget expense in many households, second only to the cost of owning or renting a house. Though many low-income households and many nonpoor households in inner cities get by with only one car or without a car altogether, most households in the United States have at least one car for each person of driving age. Some have more than one car per person. Not only does this result in costs borne by households; it has major land use implications.

Impact of Highway Construction on Urban Communities

The era of large-scale highway construction in inner cities, which began in earnest in the 1950s, had a profound impact on urban communities.[46] The very siting of these highways was often problematic as they were often purposely used to wall off or destroy African American or low-income neighborhoods. The results of this scale of destruction on long-standing African American business districts were severe and the effects on residents were great.[47] From Miami's Overton district to East Los Angeles, there have been concerns that as highways have been constructed and/or expanded, established communities have been destroyed, businesses lost, and housing left to deteriorate.[48] The fact that these highways have been disproportionately constructed in low-income and minority communities also raises an environmental justice issue.[49]

The effects on cities as a whole were also significant. One of the goals of building highways was to connect downtown business districts to distant suburbs and thus strengthen their economic position within metropolitan areas. However, the effects may have been quite the opposite. Building highways to the suburbs made it easier for upper- and middle-income families to leave the cities, weakening the tax base. The chaos and destruction caused by highway construction further debilitated inner-city neighborhoods and pushed even more people to leave cities. One study suggests that each highway segment into a downtown commercial district from a distant suburb resulted in a population loss of 15% in that city.[50] Thus the overall effects of highway construction were profound.

Partly because of federal, state, and local transportation funding priorities, the building of highways expanded rapidly in the period 1954–1980 while transit systems stagnated.[51] Perhaps this is one reason why transit use is low in the United States.[52] Highways are also barriers in neighborhoods.[53] They often result in only a limited number of crossings, so communities on one side of a highway are isolated from those on the other. This can decrease connectivity, which may further reduce the utility of walking and biking. It may also further exacerbate the decline of neighborhood commercial districts.[54]

Highways and Health

The past decade has seen growing evidence that highways have major environmental impacts on the neighborhoods near them. They are major sources of air pollution; residents who live near highways are more likely to be exposed to higher levels of particulates, oxides of nitrogen, carbon monoxide, and other pollutants. These exposures have been linked to a number of illnesses including asthma, cardiovascular disease, and certain cancers. Reducing these exposures may be problematic.[55] A related issue is that these roads are often alongside or in the middle of low-income and minority communities.[56] Traffic engineers try to increase speeds to reduce idling along stretches of urban expressways but as traffic volume and congestion increase, these efforts become more and more difficult. Another solution is to address the pollution of cars themselves; as cars become more fuel efficient or less polluting, the pollution impact of any single individual car will be reduced. The problem is that as cars become more fuel efficient, the cost of driving decreases and the amount of driving increases, potentially negating some of the gains from lower polluting cars.

Another problem is the noise that highways produce. People who live near highways are more exposed to higher levels of ambient noise and these increased exposures have been associated with stress and illnesses and may be a factor in cardiovascular disease and other health problems.[57] The solution, in many places, has been to construct sound barriers and it is not uncommon to see mile after mile of cinder block or concrete walls lining highways in urban areas.[58] Another way to reduce noise exposures is to bury highways below grade, but this can be very expensive. Perhaps the most problematic roadways in urban areas are elevated highways because (1) it may be difficult to introduce some mitigation measures on these roads, and (2) they have a greater potential for visual blight. Perhaps houses near highways could be retrofitted to reduce exposures to air pollutants and noise, but this would be expensive and wouldn't address outdoor problems.[59]

Mass Transit and Health

Some evidence suggests that public transit has the potential to promote health by encouraging pedestrian activity. A few studies have found that transit riders often walk to and from transit points during their trips. This walking has the potential to provide an important percentage of overall physical activity needs.[60] Transit also has environmental benefits, producing lower amounts of greenhouse gases per passenger mile traveled,[61] and if the transit mode uses electricity, natural gas, or cleaner diesel technology, fewer particulates and other air pollutants.[62]

There are some health concerns regarding transit, however. Though accident rates are low, injuries can still be a concern and there have been periodic calls to require seatbelts on school buses.[63] Air quality can be problematic in subway stations and trains.[64] However, the health benefits of transit may outweigh these issues.

Intermodal Surface Transportation Efficiency Act (ISTEA)

For many decades, the federal government only provided grants for highway construction and localities had limited access to federal funds for mass transit or nonautomobile projects.[65] They either had to agree to the construction of more highways, or else forgo the funds and the jobs they created. This changed in 1991. In that year's highway bill, funds were set aside for the first time to fund other modes of transportation including pedestrian and bike improvements.[66] The law's name, **Intermodal Surface Transportation Efficiency Act (ISTEA)**, reflects its new perspective on transportation policy: it was to be intermodal, not just focused on automobiles, and it connected its broader options to the goal of making the transportation system more efficient. In comparison to funding for automobiles, the funding for alternative transportation is still relatively small. However, ISTEA has survived into later funding cycles and it remains part of the United States' transportation strategy.[67]

Federal Funding of Mass Transit

Federal funding for transit is handled differently from how the government funds highways. Money for highway construction is distributed using a formula that includes population, land area, and other factors. States and localities more or less get the money from the government through a formula that includes population, land area, and other related factors. The only question is how many total dollars have been set aside in the latest highway bill.[68] In contrast, mass transit is funded by a much more cumbersome process. For example, local transportation authorities have to apply to the federal government in a competitive process. Extensive documentation for the application is required and the application process includes an assessment regarding whether revenues are sufficient to maintain and operate the new transportation infrastructure. Funding for mass transit in recent years has been set at no more than 20% of the total federal transportation construction budget, an increase from earlier decades when funding for mass transit from the federal government was essentially zero. Thus transit funds are much more scarce than highway funds and much more difficult to secure.[69] Therefore, local governments have to find alternatives to fund capital and maintenance costs of transit.[70]

Some critics hold that because car use represents well over 90% of all trips, the overconcentration of funds on highways is legitimate and represents proper public policy.[71] These arguments contend that because consumers have decided they want to use cars rather than transit, the federal government should simply support this choice, and that if anything, there is too much money spent on mass transit.[72] These arguments, however, ignore the great amount of subsidies for automobile transportation. And they also ignore the fact that policy should be proactive and focused on planning for future needs, rather than reinforcing past trends.[73]

State and Local Financing of Transit

The majority of dollars for construction, maintenance, and operation of mass transit in the United States comes from state and local governments.[74] The funding mechanisms for transit include fare box revenues, sales taxes, property tax levies, and other sources. One problem with this is that state and local governments have less ability to raise large sums of money than the federal government. Another issue is that these revenues tend to steeply decline during times of recession, forcing local transportation agencies to cut back service during times when people may be more dependent on transit for mobility and accessibility.

The constraints on the fiscal capacity of local transportation agencies mean that they may have limited capacity to expand service to areas that are underserved or may be unable to make the changes that public health and neighborhood activists may have determined are best for their communities.[75] There have also been concerns that the priorities of some local transportation authorities have favored wealthier suburban communities over poor inner-city neighborhoods. The Los Angeles Bus Riders Union, for example, successfully sued the Los Angeles County Metropolitan Transportation Authority because that agency was extending rail service into distant whiter suburbs while systematically draining resources from the bus system that serves predominantly Latino and African American riders.[76] This issue, known as transportation justice, has been raised by communities across the United States.

Role of Active Transport in Health

Current Centers for Disease Control and Prevention (CDC) guidelines for physical activity suggest that adults have 5 hours of moderate activity or 2.5 hours of vigorous physical activity each week. Children should have one hour of physical activity each day.[77] In the context of busy lives for both adults and children, it can be very difficult to meet these minimum standards if physical activity involves a special trip to the gym or a park. It is much easier to meet these guidelines if physical activity is incorporated into other daily activities. Therefore, many public health advocates have been trying to promote more active modes of transportation to meet these activity needs.[78] The fact that many short trips are made by car represents an opportunity for increasing physical activity, if the built environment can promote noncar transportation and if the public can be educated about the value of incorporating physical activity into the routines of daily living.[79] In addition, people who use public transportation walk more than those who use cars.[80]

Bike Safety and Infrastructure

An ongoing concern in the United States is how to best accommodate alternatives to cars in cities and suburbs. Most U.S. cities have fragmented and minimal infrastructure for bikes compared to the extensive systems in many European countries.[81] Amsterdam and Copenhagen, for example, have large numbers of interconnected bike lanes that are heavily used. Some cities, including New York and Portland, Oregon, are also working to develop bike systems. The lack of infrastructure may be one reason that fewer people use bicycles in the United States and why biking is much less safe in this country.[82] A priority public health program in the United States has been to encourage bicyclists to use helmets. This is consistent with the U.S. emphasis given to individual responsibility for maintaining health and is a much lower-cost alternative than the community-level approach of making streets safe for bicyclists. In contrast, few European bicyclists use helmets, but their head injury rate is a fraction of that in the United States.[83] This highlights the relative effectiveness of bike infrastructure versus bike helmet strategies, though given the traffic and infrastructure patterns in the United States, educating the public to wear helmets is essential. These types of interventions parallel the effort to make automobiles safer. Part of the effort involves infrastructure improvements (bike lanes, and so on) to reduce the probability and severity of an accident, and part includes increasing the survivability of an accident (bike helmets).

A comprehensive bike infrastructure program would include separate lanes for bicycles that protect them from both moving and parked cars. It would include special signaling to accommodate bikes at intersections, attention to roads so that streets are smooth for bikes, and places to safely store bikes while they are not in use.[84] Though some communities have a few locations with bike lockers or require business to provide showers and other accommodations for bicyclists, for the most part these types of infrastructure are rare.[85]

Modifying streets for bike lanes, widespread in Europe, is also fairly uncommon in the United States. There are several reasons for this. In addition to the fact that there is rarely political pressure to accommodate bikes in transportation plans, there is a reluctance to implement any program that reduces a street's capacity to accommodate cars. Taking away parking or a lane of traffic for bikes would be very controversial in most communities. Conventional transportation planners and engineers are often against it and as a result, there are few well-connected, extensive, and well-maintained bike networks in the United States.

There has also been a philosophical dispute regarding bike lanes among bike riders. Some bicyclists are very strong advocates of their right to ride in the street in traffic, and they fear building bike lanes will force them out of the street. Others believe that bike lanes are actually less safe than street riding, though the epidemiological and accident evidence contradicts this. In any case, efforts to build bike lanes often face opposition from both car advocates and members of the bicycling community. There is a need to better understand which types of bike infrastructure lead to the greatest increases in safety and use. Though these have not been studied in enough detail to make definitive conclusions, it could be that the greater the separation of bikes from cars, the safer and more used is the infrastructure.[86]

Bike-Sharing Programs

One factor that may discourage bicycling in cities is the lack of places to store them and the high cost of buying and maintaining a bike. In order to address these issues, some cities have started large-scale public bike-sharing programs. These have mostly been implemented in Europe in cities including Paris and Barcelona. They have also been started in Washington, D.C., and Denver. In general these programs work by having would-be riders sign up in advance, paying a small annual fee. Then riders can swipe a card at selected locations, pick up a bike, and travel to a site near their destination where they can return the bike, swipe their cards, and go on with their day. There were fears that these programs would not be very successful because of (1) theft and vandalism of bikes, (2) the prices necessary for the economic stability of the system would be too high to attract riders, and (3) there was little demand for bicycle riding in general. Even though there have been problems with theft and vandalism, these programs appear to be successful and popular.[87] When there are enough destinations around the city so that would-be riders can easily pick up or drop off a bike, these programs tend to be highly used.[88] Though their usage may not be large enough to have a major impact on mode choice, such services may still be valuable for communities wishing to increase physical activity, decrease the amount of automobile traffic, and make an environmental statement.

Walking and Health

The U.S. population has a high rate of sedentary behavior and the number of people who do not meet CDC guidelines for physical activity is high.[89] Walking can provide an important percentage of overall physical activity and has been associated with lower risk or lower severity of cardiovascular disease, obesity, cognitive decline, diabetes, and other health problems.[90] The benefits of walking can accrue to all segments of the population. One study has even suggested that walking may assist children with attention deficit hyperactivity disorder (ADHD).[91] But as stressed many times in this book, walking behavior is highly dependent on the built environment and therefore one way in which public health workers may address physical inactivity is by making changes to walking environments.[92]

Many communities may not be safe for walking. They may lack sidewalks, place pedestrians too close to high-speed traffic, or present other barriers.[93] Intersections are a particularly dangerous place for pedestrians where accidents caused by cars making turns or proceeding through the intersection may be serious.[94] The elderly and people with disabilities may be at particularly greater risk. Given the need to encourage walking, these may be priority issues in some communities.[95]

Encouraging Children to Walk to School

The shifting of travel behaviors in the United States away from walking and biking to automobile-only transportation has not been confined to adults commuting to and from work. Children are much less likely to walk to school than they once were. A generation ago (1969), approximately 42% of children walked or biked to school each day; the percentage was down to about 16% in 2001.[96] The big change has been the increase in the numbers of parents driving their children to school. There are several negative impacts in this mode shift. For one thing, the area around schools has become greatly congested with traffic as hundreds of cars converge on a school each morning and afternoon. This also increases pollution problems and is a potential safety hazard. In addition, walking to and from school is a major source of physical activity and given that childhood obesity rates in the United States have significantly increased in the last two decades, increasing the percentage of children walking to school would be a major policy to address childhood obesity.[97]

The decline in children walking to school has several causes. Very important is safety. Parents feel that their children are at risk for abduction or other safety problems if they walk to school. Increasing traffic is also an issue. As the number of cars increases and the numbers of children walking to school decreases, so does the sense that walking to school is unsafe.[98] The increased number of cars around the school itself may discourage others from walking. Another problem has been changes in where schools are located. Older schools tend to be located closer to housing, but changes in state laws have mandated larger school sites, often forcing the opening of new schools to peripheries that are quite distant from where children live. In addition, land costs are often lower at these more distant locations and this provides another incentive for schools to be located at peripheral locations.

It response to this decline in the number of children walking to school, several policy initiatives have been suggested. One is a change in law so that schools are not forced to move to the edge of towns. This can be accomplished by allowing school districts to petition for waivers to land requirements or through subsidies for school construction in high land cost areas. Another program has been to encourage children to walk to school. Sometimes this takes the form of "walk to school days," schoolwide efforts to have parents accompany their children to school on foot rather than drive them. The idea is that by demonstrating the feasibility of walking to school more parents will feel comfortable letting the children walk. Another idea has been "walking school buses." Under this program, parents are put in contact with each other so that children can walk together and fewer numbers of parents are necessary to walk with a given number of children. Still another initiative involves close scrutiny of the streets around a school with careful consideration given to places where children are potentially at risk from traffic. Then schools and parents work with their local government to make changes at these points in order to reduce traffic risks. The end result is safer walking enhancements for children.[99]

FOCUS ON

Portland, Oregon's Transportation System

Though the oldest, largest cities in the United States have well-developed public transit, most newer and smaller metropolitan areas tend to have limited transit options. Many have built light rail systems in the past fifteen years, but in most parts of urban America, the vast majority of people travel by car. One important exception is Portland, Oregon, which for an American city of its size has a well-used network of transit and bicycle infrastructure.

How did this happen? For one thing, Portland has a strong tradition of land use controls that dates back to the 1970s. Its urban growth boundary is discussed in Chapter Three. Portland has invested in a light rail system, street cars, and a commuter rail system. It has been a leader in promoting transit-oriented development and pushing for increasing densities around transit centers.[100]

Most important, Portland has decided to build an extensive system of bike routes including bike lanes and bike boulevards, streets that permit car use but are designed to prioritize bicycle riding.[101] As a result, in Portland the share of bike commuting to work is the largest in the United States.

Changing Transportation Choices

In general, studies suggest that people in the southern United States, those without access to public transportation, households with higher incomes, and those living in lower-density areas drive more. A major goal of public policy is to find ways to reduce the amount of driving. Given the range and magnitude of transportation impacts on health and the environment, planners and health advocates have developed a number of programs that aim to reduce the use of cars, promote walking and bicycling, and reduce the dangers to pedestrians and others. These options are in addition to promoting compact development, changing land use patterns, building transit, pedestrian, and bike infrastructure, and so forth. Recall that the effort to make cars safer had two options: reduce the risk of accidents and reduce the severity of accidents. Many of the pedestrian-oriented programs and policies discussed here have the goal of reducing the risk of accidents to pedestrians as a way of making them feel safer. It is almost impossible to reduce the severity of accidents themselves, so this is the only set of policy options available for pedestrian travel.

These programs and policies include:

Complete Streets. Begun as a reaction to what appeared to be an overemphasis on facilitating automobile use rather than all other alternatives in conventional transportation planning, some advocates have begun to press for what are called **complete streets**.[102] This is a concept in which streets are designed to accommodate all potential transportation modes including transit, pedestrians, bicyclists, and cars. There is no single way in which this goal can be accomplished but in general these kinds of street designs include broad sidewalks, generous pedestrian amenities, medians, corner bulb-outs, extensive signaling, aids for crossing streets, dedicated lanes for bikes and transit, and other similar improvements.[103] Overall, designing streets to accommodate all users results in safer streets and more pedestrians and bicyclists, and makes the streets more usable for people with disabilities.[104]

Traffic Calming. At one time, street design and neighborhood layouts were almost exclusively focused on promoting the travel of cars on streets. A negative side effect of these efforts was that streets were made so efficient that motorists felt comfortable driving faster. Although this may have been good for car travel, it had a bad effect on pedestrians and bicyclists because people on foot or on bikes feel less safe when there are speeding cars on the streets. In response, a movement has begun to deliberately slow down cars and to make driving less efficient. These efforts have been collectively called **traffic calming**.[105] Among the physical improvements that can be made to slow down traffic and to make drivers more aware of pedestrians or bicyclists are corner bulb-outs, making the sidewalk wider at intersections so that the distance to cross the street is reduced and the sight lines for pedestrians are improved; speed bumps, raised pavement that results in drivers instinctively reducing their speeds; restoring parking to streets because studies suggest that drivers slow down when there are parked cars along a residential street; introducing curves on streets, another physical change that slows down traffic; narrowing travel lanes or the right-of-way, which can also pressure motorists to slow down; and other similar transportation improvements that slow down cars, favor pedestrians, or increase the visibility of pedestrians and bicyclists.[106]

Congestion Charges. Discouraging automobile traffic inside urban cores has been a priority since the 1920s, but few metropolitan areas have been successful at reducing traffic volumes. In 2003, London, England, implemented a congestion charge, targeting vehicles entering Central London with a substantial fee. Using scanning technology that could read license plates as cars pass into the fee zone, drivers are given a certain amount of time to pay the congestion fee. Revenues from the fee are to be used to increase transit service into and within the congestion zone. Despite substantial initial opposition, the fee has appeared to have met its goals: traffic in central London has been reduced and travel times across the core have increased without any substantial negative effects on business inside the congestion zone.[107]

The success in London has prompted other cities to consider congestion pricing. New York City proposed a zone to cover lower and midtown Manhattan. The San Francisco Bay Area is considering allowing single-passenger cars to use commuter lanes based on their paying a fee that rises and falls based on the level of traffic in these lanes. The New York City proposal was rejected in the state legislature because opposition from suburban commuters and urban residents who resided on the edges of the zone proved too strong. The problems with implementing congestion pricing are as much political as they are technical.

Pedestrian Zones. In an effort to re-create the benefits of suburban malls in inner cities, a number of municipalities experimented with banning cars from certain sections of their urban cores. The idea was to encourage shoppers to stroll along downtown retail districts. The effects of these efforts were disappointing: for the most part downtown retail sales continued to decline and merchants complained about the falloff in foot traffic and the loss of revenue. Today, many critics believe that these types of zones are at best ineffective and at worst detrimental to downtown retail districts. A substantial portion of pedestrians drive into central districts and the lack of clear sight lines might discourage shoppers. These types of streets may also heavily disrupt surrounding traffic patterns. Though these features remain popular in Europe, they have fallen out of fashion in the United States.

Eliminating One-Way Streets. Traffic engineers, in their effort to speed traffic in and out of older areas of cities, converted many streets from being two-way to one-way travel. The goal was to increase mobility in and out of the core. The effects of these traffic changes are now thought to be detrimental for the very same reason they were once thought to be successful: they speed up automobile traffic and allow people to quickly enter and exit an urban center. This may be good for the drivers, but it is bad for pedestrians and retail activity. Pedestrians feel threatened by the higher speeds and retail activity declines. Some cities, including San Jose, California, are now reestablishing two-way streets in their downtown areas.

Eliminating All Traffic Signs and Controls. Based on the success of traffic calming, some communities have decided to eliminate all traffic signs and controls altogether. This might seem to potentially create hazards for cars, bikes, and pedestrians, but the impact may be the opposite, because when drivers feel less safe and less sure of how to proceed, they drive more slowly and are more likely to yield to bikes and pedestrians. The evidence for these types of street designs is still being evaluated, however.

Roundabouts. Communities once used roundabouts to accommodate rapidly rising levels of car traffic. Without resorting to signals, roundabouts allow for a smooth movement of traffic around and through an intersection and they reduce the speed of cars as well. In the effort to make streets safer for bikes and pedestrians, some communities have revisited the idea of roundabouts and have built them in residential neighborhoods.[108] Based on preliminary evidence, these improvements do seem to reduce speeds and may reduce accidents. But there have been concerns that the design is unfriendly to pedestrians and bicyclists.[109]

Signal Changes. Crossing busy intersections can be difficult and dangerous and many pedestrians avoid them. Large streets can be major barriers to walking. To make the problem worse, many signals are timed to accommodate cars rather than pedestrians; it can be impossible to cross a street in the time allowed by the pedestrian time signal, pedestrians may still not be able to cross because cars will not yield to them, or the signals can be so poorly timed that pedestrians give up waiting for a light. To encourage walking and make intersections safer for pedestrians, some cities have reevaluated their pedestrian signals. At a relatively low cost, signals can be reprogrammed to provide longer times to cross streets, for example. Another simple but highly effective idea has been to let pedestrians begin to walk before cars can proceed through an intersection. Cars are more likely to yield to pedestrians already in a crosswalk rather than yield to pedestrians about to leave the curb. Other cities have experimented with allowing simultaneous four-way crossing of intersections. Some have made crossing lights automatic and not dependent on someone pushing a button. Retiming lights involves careful analysis of existing traffic and pedestrian patterns. Another helpful innovation is to include countdown signals that let pedestrians know how much time they have left to cross the street.

Eliminating Right-Hand Turn Lanes. One common potential source of conflict between pedestrians and automobiles is at intersections, and intersections with right turn lanes pose a particular problem for pedestrians because cars often feel that these lanes give them the right to turn without stopping and it makes drivers less likely to watch for pedestrians (a hazard for bicyclists as well). As a response, some pedestrian advocates have proposed eliminating these types of lanes altogether. The opposition often comes from motorists and some transportation engineers who fear that eliminating these lanes will result in decreased traffic speeds and more congestion. Of course this is one of the very reasons why pedestrian advocates want these types of lanes in the first place. Eliminating such lanes or at least requiring cars to make a complete stop (difficult to enforce and often just as controversial) may reduce some of the risk but would not eliminate it altogether.

Intersection Safety. Given the dangers posed to pedestrians, improving intersections might be a priority in many communities. Among the strategies that have been implemented are timed pedestrian signals, allowing pedestrians to cross before cars can proceed, curb cuts, bulb-outs, and other similar improvements.[110] The goal is to make pedestrians more visible, reduce accidents, and improve overall safety.

Summary

Transportation is highly related to land use patterns. There has been a shift from an emphasis on promoting mobility to a concern with access. Most U.S. residents travel by car, which has led to increased accident rates, air pollution, and contributions to global climate change. A particular concern is commuting, which can create health and social issues for those with what are known as extreme commutes. Bicycling can be a healthy alternative, but it is important to consider ways to improve the infrastructure that supports bicycling. Promoting pedestrian uses can include a variety of measures that aim to increase safety and help pedestrians feel safe.

Key Terms

Accessibility

Complete streets

Congestion charges

Demand management

Intermodal Surface Transportation Efficiency Act (ISTEA)

Mobility

Traffic calming

Transit-oriented development

Discussion Questions

1. How do people in the United States travel to and from work?
2. What are some of the factors that govern travel behavior?
3. Who is most at risk for traffic accidents?
4. What is the difference between mobility and accessibility?
5. Why do public health advocates place such great emphasis on promoting walking?
6. What are some of the problems associated with long commutes?
7. Name ways we can make pedestrians safer.
8. What are the advantages of "complete streets"?

For More Information

American Public Health Association. *At the intersection of public health and transportation: Promoting healthy transportation policy.* http://www.apha.org/NR/rdonlyres/43F10382-FB68−4112−8C75−49DCB10F8ECF/0/TransportationBrief.pdf.

Centers for Disease Control and Prevention. *How land use and transportation systems impact public health.* www.cdc.gov/nccdphp/dnpa/pdf/aces-workingpaper1.pdf.

Convergence Partnership. http://www.convergencepartnership.org/site/c.fhLOK6PELmF/b.4950415/k.4FF7/Transportation_and_Health_Toolkit.htm.

Kay, J. H. (1998). *Asphalt nation.* Berkeley: University of California Press.

National Center for Safe Routes to School. www.Walktoschool.org.

Shoup, D. C. (2005). *The high cost of free parking.* Chicago: American Planning Association.

Victoria Transport Institute. www.vtpi.org.

CHAPTER 5

HEALTHY HOUSING AND HOUSING ASSISTANCE PROGRAMS

LEARNING OBJECTIVES

- Describe how the "housing problem" has been redefined over time.
- Differentiate the federal role in housing from that of state and local governments.
- Discuss the problems associated with mid-twentieth-century public housing.
- Name the major problems associated with housing today.
- List the seven key features of healthy housing.
- Describe Integrated Pest Management.
- Discuss the contribution of homelessness to poor health.
- Explain how displacement and gentrification may affect the health of individuals and communities.

Let's talk about where you live. Fortunately, most of us live in places that are generally safe. And most dwelling units, if they are up to code, have a bathroom with running water and a functioning toilet, a refrigerator and a place to cook, and each full room has a window. As we have discussed, all of these standard features of homes, dorms, and apartments are now required because public health reformers advocated for their being required in housing. Think of what it would be like to live in a place without these features. Consider how having them makes the place where you live healthy.

This chapter begins with an overview of housing policies including both historical and current practices. It then discusses overall housing quality and concludes with highlights of some of the special issues that affect certain subpopulations.

The Housing Problem

People spend the majority of their time indoors, much of that at home, so the features and quality of their housing can have an important influence on health. At one time in the United States, the quality of housing for many households was quite poor, particularly for those with low incomes.[1] But in the past two centuries we have seen a progressive improvement in housing quality brought on by the general rise in living standards, improved technologies and building practices, and ever-tightening government regulation. There has also been a change in how housing problems are characterized. In the early nineteenth century, housing was seen to be a problem of tenant responsibility—landlords were not held liable for housing problems even after such extreme events such as when a staircase collapsed.[2] Slowly, legal responsibility for housing quality shifted to landlords and property owners and the period from the mid-nineteenth century to the first decades of the twentieth was a time of new laws, codes, and means of enforcement. After the 1920s, housing quality was reenvisioned to be an economic problem: poor people could not afford safe and healthy housing.[3] This prompted a number of new initiatives including the public housing programs of the 1930s to 1970s in addition to the more lasting and much larger-scale program of mortgage subsidies and assistance to home buyers.

As late as 1950, one-third of housing units in United States lacked indoor plumbing, full kitchen facilities, or both.[4] The quality of the U.S. housing stock dramatically improved, as evidenced by the American Household Survey, a biannual portrait of the country's housing stock funded by U.S. Department of Housing and Urban Development (HUD) and conducted by the U.S. Census that provides important information on the state of the country's housing (Table 5.1). In 2007, there were approximately 110,000,000 housing units, of which 32% were rental, 65% were single-family detached homes, and 64% were built before 1980. Approximately 18% of total units had exterior physical problems including 10% with exterior water leakage, about 8% had interior water leakage, and 9% had blown fuses or circuit breakers. About 8% had no working smoke alarm and 67% had no carbon monoxide alarm.[5] Because by 1970 most housing had indoor plumbing and full kitchen facilities, the U.S. Census stopped asking about these features in the decennial census.[6] Housing problems are more likely to exist in units occupied by low-income households, African Americans, and Hispanics. There continue to be issues with the enforcement of standards, an ongoing problem of affordability, and a need to address the health problems associated with conventional suburban development.

Table 5.1   Occupied Housing Units—Reported Housing Problems

External Building Conditions	
Sagging roof	1,888
Missing roofing material	4,640
Hole in roof	1,458
Missing bricks, siding, or other outside wall material	2,323
Sloping outside walls	1,167
Boarded up windows	821
Broken windows	2,984
Bars on windows	3,318
Foundation crumbling or has open crack or hole	2,227
Internal Building Deficiencies	
Holes in floors	1,141
Open cracks or holes (interior)	5,517
Broken plaster or peeling paint (interior)	2,378
No electrical wiring	84
Exposed wiring	355
Rooms without electric outlets	1,274
Total occupied units	111,806

Numbers in thousands

Source: American Housing Survey, 2009

There have been changes in housing features over the past several decades. In general, more housing has been built in the suburbs than in center-cities or in more heavily built-up areas, potentially indicating increased sprawl. Interestingly, the average size of a house has substantially increased over the past several decades even as household size has decreased—or, in other words, smaller households are occupying larger houses.[7] This may have important energy use implications and contribute to problems of long-term sustainability.[8]

The Regulatory Framework

The responsibility for housing reflects the complicated multilevel structure of government in the United States. In general, the federal government has a very strong role in housing finance programs but a very limited one in the regulation and enforcement of housing quality standards at the local level. The overall pattern, on the one hand, is for local governments to be responsible for housing enforcement because they have been given this authority by state enabling legislation. On the other hand, local governments tend to have limited resources to provide financial incentives to promote housing construction, though they may have some powers and abilities to do so in some places. They can help promote construction through their zoning authority by increasing the supply of buildable land or by providing incentives for the development of affordable housing. Though there may be exceptions, states tend to not be directly involved in the enforcement of housing quality because they have delegated this authority to local governments. Many states, however, provide some support for assisted housing.[9]

Federal Housing Programs

Federal programs to promote housing and homeownership date back to the 1930s when the desperate state of the construction industry, along with long-standing concerns regarding tenement conditions, prompted a number of initiatives to promote homeownership. Most famously, the Federal Housing Administration (FHA) and other related federal programs did much to improve the housing stock in the United States since their beginnings during the Great Depression.[10] To qualify for an FHA-approved loan, construction had to meet certain minimum standards and as this was one of the few sources of mortgage money, developers built to this standard. Partly as a result of FHA and other similar programs, almost all the housing built after these programs began is safe and healthy if it has been properly maintained and the building envelope is secure from leaks. There may be a problem with lead paint, asbestos, or other legacies of older building materials used, but buyers and renters of housing can for the most part safely assume that the broader aspects of this housing are healthy. The mortgage-support programs also increased the affordability of housing. Collectively they lowered the monthly cost of owning homes so that many more families could afford to do so and it was only in the past two decades, in select metropolitan areas, that housing prices have been consistently higher than most middle-income households can afford.

But there were also substantial problems with these programs, particularly in the first several decades of their existence. Most serious was the discriminatory nature of the initial programs. FHA guidelines were strongly prejudiced against African American people and the neighborhoods that housed them. For the most part, FHA-backed mortgages were denied to people of color, to anybody who wanted to buy a house in a mixed race or African American neighborhood, or even to people looking to buy houses in neighborhoods that were at risk of becoming mixed-race or predominantly African American. The result was an extremely negative impact on people of color and on inner-city neighborhoods.[11] African Americans were unable to become homeowners, or if they did have the resources to buy a house, they often had to turn to unregulated and often unscrupulous non-FHA financing mechanisms. This led them to be vulnerable to lenders offering very high interest rates, or even worse, forced many to use what was known as contract buying, a system of financing that combined high interest rates with punishing terms that limited the ability of black homeowners to build up equity or often left them at risk of losing their homes altogether. The effects on neighborhoods in inner cities were also very negative. Because certain neighborhoods were off limits to FHA-backed mortgages, their decline was almost guaranteed. These so-called redlined neighborhoods, denied access to capital, saw their housing stock decline because homeowners and investors could not get the loans they needed to buy, maintain, and upgrade homes and apartments. By the mid-1960s, when federal legislation finally guaranteed that all persons had to be allowed to access FHA and other federal housing programs, many inner-city communities had declined to the extent that they were the sites of large-scale abandonment and deteriorated housing.[12] Even after the regulatory barriers were eliminated, there have continued to be problems of access to mortgages and housing.

A related problem resided in the FHA guidelines for what constituted eligible housing. These guidelines resulted from the assumption that single-family homes in suburban-like settings were the only appropriate housing type for families. The guidelines mandated minimum lot sizes, parking, and single-family uses that even in the absence of race-based mortgage guidelines made it very difficult for inner-city properties to qualify for FHA mortgages. Until the guidelines were broadened several decades later to allow for the financing of multifamily properties, condominiums, and cooperatives, FHA mortgages were very strongly tilted towards the financing of suburban homes and away from inner-city housing.[13]

Public and Publicly Assisted Housing

Given the expense of constructing housing and the difficulty that many low-income families have in renting housing, there have been almost seventy years of government efforts in this country to create housing opportunities for low-income households. In general this takes two forms. Some housing is actually owned by a branch of government, usually a Local Housing Authority (LHA), established by state enabling legislation, but often operated by local government. But the United States also has a long tradition of private ownership of housing specifically for low-income people. Some of this may be simply market housing that for one reason or another can be affordable for persons who have low incomes without any type of government assistance. In addition, there is what is known as publicly assisted housing. Private developers, both for profit and nonprofit organizations, use a variety of government programs that all have the aim of reducing housing costs for low-income renters. Typically, developing this type of housing involves an intricate process of putting together the various programs to reduce housing costs so that the offered rent can be affordable. These programs include direct development subsidies, loan subsidies, special tax incentives, and rental subsidies. To a certain extent, this multitude of programs reflects a history of the reluctance to have government intervene in housing markets and a piecemeal approach to addressing the problems of housing affordability.[14]

Public housing, units owned by local housing authorities, also dates back to the Great Depression. There had been opposition to public financing of low-income housing. Real estate and building interests opposed the program because they saw public housing as a rival and a threat to market housing. Others were philosophically opposed to this expansion of government responsibilities, believing that the private sector should be the sole provider of housing. Despite this opposition, in 1937 the United States passed a law that provided for federal support of local area housing for low-income families. But there was limited funding for the construction of public housing in the 1930s, so it was not until the housing act of 1948 that large-scale public housing was funded.[15]

Today, there are still well over one million units of public housing and the quality of these developments varies greatly. Some have been recently rebuilt or have benefited from appropriate long-term maintenance. Others have been deteriorating for several decades and may be abandoned or at the brink of abandonment. Congress typically provides an annual appropriation for the renovation and redevelopment of public housing units, but these funds are only a small fraction of what is necessary for the full-scale upgrade of the total public housing stock. Thus local housing authorities and tenants continue to struggle with the legacies of this underfunded program.

Other Current Housing Programs

Housing affordability remains a major issue because many families do not have sufficient income to pay the prevailing rents in their communities and, though the magnitude of housing assistance programs in the United States is smaller than it once was, there continue to be a range of programs to assist low-income people. There remains, for example, a substantial program for building housing for low-income senior citizens. This housing is popular among communities because it enables many seniors to remain living in their long-term neighborhoods. This program has encountered little public opposition because seniors are seen as nonburdens on government services, senior citizen housing tends to be inclusive of all races, and the quality of the housing itself has been generally well maintained. There also continue to be mortgage subsidies and other programs for private-sector (usually nonprofit) developers of low-income family housing that allow for lower financing and development costs and, when combined with other subsidies, can result in quality housing; however, the demand is much larger than the total number of units available from these programs. A major program for the redevelopment of existing public housing family developments is the HOPE VI program that often results in complete reconstruction or very substantial renovation of developments.[16] This program often results in mixed-income developments, a reduction in the number of units for low-income families, and the incorporation of what are now seen as health-promoting designs including orienting buildings and building entrances toward streets, minimizing the number of units that share entries, reducing densities, and other features.

The other major program for housing assistance for low-income households is called the Section 8 rental assistance program.[17] It currently provides subsidies for 2,000,000 households through what are known as vouchers or certificates.[18] There are two types of Section 8 rental certificates. One type is dedicated to specific units. In return for guaranteed rent payments from the LHA over a certain time period—twenty or thirty years—the owners of these units promise to only rent to qualified low-income families. If a low-income family moves out, they are replaced with another qualified household throughout the lifetime of the Section 8 contract. In the other type of Section 8, the certificate goes to a family in need. That family then uses the certificate as a voucher that promises a landlord a certain rent level. The tenants pay a percentage of their income, usually 30%, toward the rent and the LHA or other administrative agency of the Section 8 program pays the rest. In general, these programs have been a success. But one of the greatest problems for both types of Section 8 certificates has been their limited availability; there are not enough rental certificates to meet demand. Thus the amount of housing that can be built with Section 8 guarantees is limited. Similarly, there tend to be long waiting lists for Section 8 housing vouchers. Sometimes there can be problems with the rent levels set by the U.S. Department of Housing and Urban Development on a metropolitan by metropolitan basis. If the rent level is set too low, landlords will not rent to tenants with certificates because they can receive more money from private market tenants. If the rent levels are set too high, other families may be priced out of the market, exacerbating affordability problems, as well as resulting in too few families receiving assistance. Given that these rates are set by the federal

FOCUS ON

Community Development Corporations

One of the major nonpublic providers of housing for low-income households in the United States are Community Development Corporations. CDCs grew out of community activism in the 1960s and a dissatisfaction with urban renewal and top-down planning.[21]

There are different ways in which CDCs are organized. Many are nonprofit organizations organized under section 501(c)(3) of the federal tax code. This allows them to accept grants and charitable donations to support their work and frees them from many tax liabilities. Some CDCs have for-profit subsidiaries to operate housing and business projects. Some are chartered by states with specially mandated boards, others have been created by local boards of trade or groups of community activists.

Many CDCs have broad goals, including community advocacy, business development, open space creation, social service programs, as well as housing. Most of the housing they develop and manage is for low- or moderate-income families or the elderly. Given the cost of providing housing, these projects take a considerable amount of public resources and the development process often consists of a painstaking bringing together and applying for funds from a number of programs. Funding sources can include federal rental and mortgage subsidies, similar state programs, funds derived from fees on local development, and charitable contributions.[22]

government and that market conditions can fluctuate rapidly, it can be difficult to guarantee that rents are at the right level.

The Section 8 program helps boost health in several ways. Directly, it ensures that families have safe and healthy housing because there is a requirement that units be inspected before a Section 8 rental contract is signed and the tenant is allowed to move in. Therefore, all tenants of the Section 8 housing in the private market should be in safe and healthy housing—though many of the unit-based Section 8 developments have had maintenance and quality issues similar to those that have affected LHA-owned housing.[19] Indirectly, Section 8 housing helps low-income tenants because it reduces the burden of housing costs; tenants with lower housing costs have more resources available to purchase food, clothing, and all the other essentials of modern life.

It should be noted that for the most part a far greater amount of resources are dedicated toward providing assistance to middle- and upper-income homeowners than there is available for low-income renting families. Federal and state mortgage interest deductions on income taxes represent an annual subsidy for homeownership in the hundreds of billions of dollars.[20] In contrast, the total amount of housing assistance available for low-income families is less than $2 billion per year.

Housing and Health Issues

Though housing in the United States is generally safe and the effort to ensure that all households have access to kitchen facilities and indoor plumbing has been long won, there remain a number of problems that can affect housing and health of residents. These include the following:

Mold. Mold in housing has been associated with asthma and a complex of symptoms that range from minor respiratory distress to severe systemic reactions. In general, mold needs a food source such as paper or other organic substance as well as water to grow; its presence reflects too much moisture in a house.[23] There are several ways moisture can accumulate in sufficient amounts to facilitate the growth of mold. One major cause is that there can be leaks in the building envelope, particularly from roofs and around windows. There may be leaking plumbing, including both supply and waste lines; moisture penetration from the exterior; or there may be a buildup of moisture from cooking, cleaning, bathing, and inhabitants that is not adequately ventilated.[24] Sometimes mold is difficult to detect, particularly if it is growing inside walls, behind furniture, or under carpets. However, mold does not have to be visible to cause health problems.

Removing mold can be expensive and difficult. In addition, the moisture source that is driving the growth of mold must be addressed or the problem may recur. This may include sealing leaks in exterior walls where moisture can enter the building; ventilating interiors; fixing interior plumbing problems; or addressing other related housing problems. There is little government regulation of mold, though most building codes say that mold is a violation of standards, but the federal government does not set mold exposure standards.[25] Consumers, particularly homeowners, are often left on their own to deal with mold as many homeowner policies specifically exclude payment for mold damages. Tenants may have rights under local housing codes and laws to require landlords to clean up mold, but these may not be available to help in all individual circumstances.

Lead. Even though lead was recognized as a toxin as early as Roman times, the use of lead in household paint was not banned in the United States until 1978. As a result, much of the United State's older housing stock is contaminated with lead and with the phaseout of leaded gasoline, lead paint remains one of the main sources of lead poisoning. There is a stark geographic pattern to the distribution of child lead poisoning cases: they are heavily concentrated in poor and minority communities with old housing. Newer suburban areas have less pre-1978 housing and more affluent areas tend to have well-maintained homes that reduce the risk of lead paint exposure (or have been deleaded over the years). But inner-city communities with large belts of older housing and many units in various states of disrepair tend to have the most cases of lead-poisoned children.[26]

Lead has been associated with a number of health problems, but its most serious effects are on mental cognition and development in children. The most problematic lead exposures in housing often occur during a critical time in the mental development of children from one to three years of age. This is also the time when children are beginning to explore their environment and often are crawling and beginning to walk as well as touching everything and putting their hands in their mouths. Thus the potential for exposure is at a peak at the same time the potential for cognitive effects is at a maximum. Untreated, exposures during this age can result in a lifetime of cognitive difficulties.[27]

The response has been to develop coordinated programs of education, enforcement, testing, and subsidies.[28] The U.S. Environmental Protection Agency has set standards for lead removal in housing.[29] Enforcement includes the adoption of strict laws that establish landlord liability for ensuring that children are protected and the careful establishment of procedures that guarantee safe removal of lead paint.[30] Testing is one of the main ways that children who have been poisoned by lead can be identified and many states mandate periodic testing of infants, toddlers, and preschoolers so that any children who are found to have elevated blood lead levels are quickly treated and the lead in their environment identified and remediated. Enforcement includes follow-up by local health departments and building departments so that housing is brought up to code and lead laws complied with.[31] Subsidies are necessary because of the high cost of deleading units; many landlords cannot afford to delead, and the presence of programs can be used as an incentive to help bring more units into compliance. Education is necessary so that parents are aware of the need to have their children tested and landlords understand their responsibilities under the law. Though there has been a large decline in the number of children with elevated lead levels (Table 5.2), these rates should be as near to undetectable in as much of the population as possible and there is still much work to be done.[32] One major effort to address childhood lead poisoning on the local level has been childhood lead coalitions, groups that bring together housing code enforcers, health providers, tenant advocates, and others to oversee assistance programs, public education, and other strategies to reduce exposures to lead.[33]

A related problem is lead in soils around housing. This can be a risk to children because they play in yards and outdoor soil can be tracked into homes,

Table 5.2   Percentage of U.S. Children with Confirmed Elevated Blood Lead Levels

Year	Confirmed EBLLs as % of Children Tested
1997	7.61%
1998	6.50%
1999	5.03%
2000	3.96%
2001	3.03%
2002	2.56%
2003	2.27%
2004	1.76%
2005	1.53%
2006	1.31%
2007	1.00%

Source: CDC

contributing to the burden of indoor lead. It can also be a problem if certain foods grown in these soils are consumed. The lead can be the result of exterior paint flaking off buildings or it could be a legacy of lead in gasoline. Solutions can include removing lead-contaminated soils, covering these soils with clean dirt, rock, or other barriers, or using phytoremediation or other protective actions.[34]

Indoor Air Quality. This issue is covered more extensively in Chapter Seven. Typically the sources of indoor air pollutants are mold, chemical releases from building materials or interior furnishes, personal consumer products, tobacco use, or sources outside the home. The health effects of indoor air quality depend on the particular toxicants involved and the sensitivity of the residents inside the home. In general, there is little outside regulation of housing air quality and residents have few resources they can use to identify and remedy these problems. The solution tends to include avoiding problematic materials, guarding against leaks, and ensuring proper ventilation inside units.

Fires. The CDC reports that fires are a leading cause of injury and deaths. In the United States in 2008, there were over 400,000 residential fires resulting in more than 13,500 injuries and 2,700 deaths (not including firefighters).[35] Smoking was the leading cause of fire-related fatalities, and cooking was the leading cause of fires overall. Children and the elderly are at greater risk of fire injuries and deaths, and African American, Native Americans, rural residents, persons in substandard units, and low-income households have a greater risk of fires.[36]

Education and code enforcement are the major ways to address fires and the risk of fire-related injuries and deaths. Education centers on informing the public about the causes and prevention of fires, the importance of a plan to evacuate in case of a fire, and the proper use and maintenance of smoke detectors. Code-enforcement measures can include ensuring that smoke detectors are properly installed and operational and inspecting wiring and heating systems.[37] The well-known national program of using the resetting of clocks for daylight savings in spring and fall as a reminder to check the functioning of smoke detectors is an example of an effective public health campaign.[38]

There has been a movement to mandate the use of sprinklers in residential construction.[39] These have already been required in most high rises, offices, and in many multi-unit residential buildings where their strong contribution to reducing deaths, injuries, and damages caused by fires has been well documented. Residential sprinklering has been opposed by builders who fear it may raise costs and by some property owners who fear it may be a maintenance problem. However, sprinklering can also reduce insurance premiums.

Household Injuries.   Homes are a major location of injuries, with the young and the elderly are most at risk.[40] Injuries include falls, drownings, poisonings, and burns. Falls are a major life threat to the elderly, who can end up hospitalized or at increased risk of medical complications from falls.[41] Children are at risk from drownings and poisonings. The key to injuries is prevention, which may include ensuring that railings and other protective items are well maintained, close supervision of children and persons with impairments that may place them at increased risk of injuries, and the proper storage of toxic household chemicals.[42] Proper lighting may help prevent injuries. Another important action is the identification and remediation of potential safety problems.[43]

Attributes of Healthy Housing

In general, there is a developing consensus as to what constitutes healthy housing that includes factors inside homes and in features of the surrounding community. Healthy and safe housing should mean that units are without substantive housing quality issues and that the housing itself should be in neighborhoods with nonautomobile access to amenities such as parks, schools, grocery stores, medical care, and other features that promote health.[44] Housing should be close to employment so as to reduce the need for long commutes, yet distant from factories, highways, or other sources of pollution. Communities should have good pedestrian, bicycle, and mass transit infrastructure, access to clean water, and well-functioning waste disposal systems. In addition, there should be a variety of housing types that are appropriate for households of different incomes and persons of all ages.[45] The overall ability of housing to meet these goals varies widely from place to place.

Codes and Housing Regulation

In general, the responsibility for the enforcement of housing laws and regulations is given to local government, usually the municipal or county building or code enforcement department. The codes themselves are typically not the product of state or local government, but have been developed by large-scale, independent, nonprofit organizations such as the International Code Council, the International Building Code, Underwriters Laboratory, and the National Fire Protection Association.[46] These organizations have extensive engineering and research departments and have the ability to investigate accidents, fires, emerging health and environmental issues, and other problems that might be affecting housing quality, health, and safety. They can use this information to produce modifications of their codes as necessary.[47] Note that these organizations tend to use engineering evidence, not epidemiological studies, to test and modify their codes. States typically adopt these codes as a whole, though they may include some modifications, because they lack the engineering and other expertise necessary to produce these codes and keep them up to date. The individual codes can be thousands of pages long and may include everything from definitions of what is safe egress to electrical safety to what are acceptable plumbing fixtures. Local governments and builders tend to like these codes because by complying with the code they can reduce their liability in the case that something goes wrong; in addition, the use of the code allows for uniformity of building practices across the United States, easing training, compliance, and enforcement.[48]

This uniformity of codes, along with the standardization of building materials, may have contributed to a decrease in building costs. Individual building materials such as door frames, plumbing fixtures, and other items are standardized and thus can be manufactured in large volumes, making building materials more affordable. This standardization and the resultant lowering of costs had been a dream of architects and urban visionaries since the 1920s.

Housing Code Enforcement

Despite the general improvement in housing quality, there are still many units that are not in compliance with current standards, particularly in lower-income areas. Thus there is an ongoing need to enforce housing regulations. Creating the right enforcement program is not always easy, however. Overly zealous enforcement of housing codes can result in backlash from property owners, which cities often want to avoid. In addition, rigorous enforcement that results in tenants being evicted or displaced is also undesirable. There have also been concerns that enforcement has not always been carried out in ways that really get to the root problems in housing, perhaps focusing so much on details that it may miss overall problems with housing quality. In response, organizations such as the National Center for Healthy Housing (NCHH) have developed new criteria for enforcing housing quality. NCHH has proposed enforcement and inspection methodology that focuses on the seven features that together help ensure that housing is healthy.[49] These are:

Dry. As described earlier, moisture can result in deterioration of finishes and structures and it is a prime factor in the development of mold. Hence careful attention to roofs and windows, repairing outside surfaces, painting, and other potential sources of outdoor moisture penetration should be a major priority. Vapor barriers to prevent outdoor moisture in the air from entering buildings and the careful engineering of building systems can help keep housing safe. Indoors, plumbing should be free of leaks and there should not be overly high moisture content in indoor air.

Clean. Not only is the overall level of cleanliness a potential indicator of housing quality, dirt and left-out food can promote pest contamination or be a factor in injuries.

Ventilated. The proper rate of exchange between indoor and outdoor air can be extremely important. Too much air exchange can lead to high energy costs and may be an indication that the building envelope is unsecured and at risk for moisture penetration. Too little air exchange can result in the buildup of moisture or the concentration of toxics in indoor air.

Pest-Free. Insects and rodents are a major problem in many homes. In addition to posing serious quality-of-life issues, they can exacerbate asthma and other respiratory problems.

Safe. Given the problems posed by injuries and fires, the safety of housing must be a major priority. Thus special attention should be focused on potential safety problems including the presence and proper operation of safety features, the identification of factors that may pose fire, electrical, or other types of injuries, and the quick remedy of any identified problems.

Contaminant-Free. Many household use and store a variety of chemicals that can have important health effects. Cleaning products, pesticides, building materials, and other products can pose poisoning or indoor air problems. Off-gassing from building materials may be a problem. Safer alternatives are often available and can assist in reducing the amount of chlorinated hydrocarbons (CFC), polycyclic aromatic hydrocarbons (PAHs), and other potentially problematic chemicals. The key may be to educate the public about the potential health problems of these products; their proper use, storage, and disposal, and the use and availability of alternatives.

Maintained. Keeping housing safe is highly dependent on the proper maintenance of building envelopes, systems, and interiors. Improper maintenance can result in the deterioration of housing quality and contribute to many of the problems highlighted throughout this chapter. Maintenance needs to be a priority of both property owners and tenants.

By focusing on these factors, inspectors can help ensure that housing is healthy and also avoid some of the problems associated with overzealous enforcement of the highly detailed housing code. Another proposed solution to improve the quality of housing code enforcement is to have professional certification of housing inspectors. Currently, there is no national adopted set of qualifications for being a housing inspector and the quality and expertise of these inspectors may vary greatly from place to place. As a remedy, housing advocates have proposed a national certification program whereby would-be inspectors would receive certification after completing a training course and successfully passing an exam. This has been a slow process to implement due to resistance on the local level but ultimately it may well help improve housing quality across the country.

Community Legal Advocacy

There is an important connection between housing quality and health, and many of these issues first come to the attention of health personnel when children or other residents visit emergency rooms because of asthma exacerbations, injuries, or other housing-related health problems. The traditional response has been to address the individual health conditions by treating the medical problem that is presented. But several inner-city hospitals have developed an advocacy program that works to solve the underlying housing problem that has led to the medical emergency. This can include working with code enforcement departments, filing injunctions and other legal actions, or working to secure adequate housing services for low-income families.[50] The overall goal of these programs is to provide primary prevention and keep the family safe so that further medical emergencies do not happen. These programs can be expensive and may require employing advocates in emergency rooms and clinics. Funding may be difficult, but the positive results may be great.

Integrated Pest Management

The potential health and quality-of-life impacts brought on by cockroaches, rats, and other pests have resulted in a wide range of efforts to address pest infestations. The problem is that some of these efforts may cause health problems themselves. The very chemicals used to kill roaches, for example, may pose neurological, respiratory, and other health risks. In other words, households may be at risk if they have a pest infestation and may be at risk if they take certain actions to address these infestations.[51] Given past uses and current practices regarding chemicals to address pest infestations, it is not surprising that many housing units are contaminated with pesticides of varying potencies and with a range of potential health effects. For example, surveys of public housing in Boston demonstrated that there are a large number of pesticide residues in units, including pesticides that have been banned for a number of years because of health and environmental concerns. It is not known if these residues are the result of current use or are a legacy of past use, but given the number of children who live in such housing, the results were of concern to tenants and the housing authority.[52]

A response to these kinds of problems has been the growing use of what is known as **Integrated Pest Management** (IPM). In general, the features of an effective IPM program include extra-careful cleaning, the control of food sources, the elimination of access points, and the selective use of pesticides. Cleaning routines should include the use of vacuum cleaners that have high-efficiency particulate arresting (HEPA) filters, which have the ability to pick up both particles and other pest residues, the use of special soaps that can eliminate some of the chemical aspects of pest contamination, and routine follow-up to keeping units clean. There must be absolute control of potential food sources because even the remains of a single meal can reinforce a pest infestation. Thus all food must be kept in secure containers and every surface wiped down after every meal. Limiting access points for pests includes identifying leaks that might serve as water sources for pests and plugging holes under doors, around plumbing, and between floors and apartments. Pesticides can be used, but only specially approved pesticides should be applied, sprays and aerosols should be avoided, and whenever possible, pesticides should be applied as gels or other types of products that do not get released into the general household environment.

In all of these practices, is critical that the occupants and managers of housing be involved and engaged. For a single-family home this means every member of the family must understand the goals and principles of IPM and participate in the day-to-day practices that help keep housing pest free. In multifamily housing, there must be extensive education of tenants and maintenance staff, which can take time and money.[53] In both cases, there is a need to ensure that best practices continue to be followed indefinitely. If proper long-term practices are not maintained, an infestation may recur.

Abandoned Properties

A growing issue in many communities is that the housing downturn that began in 2006 has resulted in large numbers of abandoned houses. This is not a new problem in some areas. As populations declined in many center-city neighborhoods from the 1950s onwards, the absolute number of households also declined and properties were abandoned.[54] Making the problem worse, many of these properties had fallen behind in paying property taxes and the owners were difficult to locate, making enforcement actions difficult to accomplish. Abandoned houses can be a major blight in a neighborhood because they attract crime, depress property values of occupied homes around them, deteriorate and become structurally unsafe, and become prime targets for arson.

In response, many cities move to demolish these homes as quickly as possible, but this also poses a number of problems. First of all, the procedures governing local governments' taking ownership of abandoned properties is a legal process that can take years to complete. The process for condemning and demolishing houses can also be lengthy and throughout these processes, the buildings pose hazards to their surroundings. In addition, demolition can release asbestos and lead into the environment; some cities have developed special programs to reduce the environmental impacts of demolition.[55] Further complicating the management of abandoned properties, the problems with do not end with demolition. The resulting vacant land may become overgrown, attract criminal activity, may make neighbors feel reluctant to walk on these streets, become sites for illegal dumping, or otherwise be a detriment to the community at large.

In some cities that have suffered from extensive population loss, abandoned properties, and now vacant land, there have been proposals to consolidate this cleared land, which collectively can be substantial. This situation has led to what is known as the **shrinking city movement**, which in places such as Detroit and Youngstown, Ohio, has proposed returning land to agricultural or natural uses. But abandonment usually happens property by property with residents continuing to live around these eyesores rather than resulting in entire blocks emptying out. This may mean that other, existing residents would have to be bought out and relocated, a difficult and expensive process. There are also concerns about the social justice implications of such programs because these may end up causing forced evictions and may disproportionately affect low-income and minority households.[56] So there is controversy as to what to do with the residents of those neighborhoods that had been selected to be cleared. Fortunately most cities do not have to make these tragic choices.

Abandonment has begun to occur in distant suburbs as a result of the housing crisis that began in 2007. Unlike center-city governments, which often have professional and experienced housing departments that know how to manage these properties, many of these abandoned homes are in peripheral locations that have weak or inexperienced local government. These abandoned homes may experience many of the health and safety issues associated with inner-city abandoned properties but may also have problems with abandoned swimming pools and other potential sources of disease and health problems. Again, there may be the issue that many of these properties will never have the potential to be reoccupied and thus local governments may be confronted with the problem of how to manage and dispose of these properties. This is an issue that may dominate exurban housing policies for the next ten years.

FOCUS ON

Housing for Special Needs Populations

Though in general, housing in the United States is healthy, there are many people who because of disabilities, development issues, substance abuse problems, family status, and so on cannot live in the general housing stock but require special types of housing.

The type of housing depends on the needs of the individuals.[57] Some can live on their own, but they may require special adaptations to meet the needs posed by sensory or mobility impairments. Others may best be housed in group quarters where they can live in a situation that gives them structure as well as personal privacy. Still others may need highly supervised situations. Decades ago, many people with special needs were simply institutionalized, but since the 1970s there is a recognition that these institutions were often dehumanizing, expensive, and subject to abuses.

Two of the major problems that people with special needs face is discrimination and barriers in the built environment.[58] Some landlords may not rent to them; other housing may simply not be appropriate. The goals of housing for people with special needs is to allow individuals to live as independently as possible and to recognize that everyone should be treated with respect and dignity.

Homelessness

The United States has a significant homeless problem. The estimates of the number of homeless people in this country vary but could be over 600,000.[59] A 1994 study found that 14% of the U.S. population had experienced homelessness at some point in life.[60] One issue is that it is very difficult to count the homeless because the population is larger than the number of people who are in shelters; it includes people who are living in temporary and transitory conditions such as moving in with family members or friends when their own housing was lost, those who are living on the streets and are beyond contact with service providers, and others.[61] There are groups who are at more risk for homelessness, including low-income households, people who have just been released from institutions or have aged out of programs for children, people who are unemployed, the elderly, and those with mental illnesses.[62]

There are many causes of homelessness. Very important is affordability and the lack of enough housing assistance programs to reach all the people who might be in need. Given the high cost of housing in many parts of this country, it may be difficult for even some employed people to afford prevailing market rents in certain areas. In other situations, households may be able to afford the rent but they may not have sufficient resources to pay realtor fees, security deposits, and other costs associated with renting an apartment.[63] Some people may not qualify for housing assistance and others may have special needs beyond the ability of service providers to meet.

Homelessness can have serious consequences for health and well-being. Among children it may contribute to problems with asthma, behavioral and development issues, and may have a negative impact on school performance. Being homeless can make it very difficult for individuals to cope with chronic diseases such as HIV, high blood pressure, diabetes, and other problems that need detailed and frequent treatment.[64] Homelessness has been associated with tuberculosis and an increased risk of mortality,[65] and can exacerbate mental health problems because of the stresses associated with it. The stress could also make it difficult to keep other diseases under control.

Addressing homelessness requires a comprehensive set of programs that ideally should work on prevention and on providing safe and effective interventions should homelessness occur. For many reasons, shelters might not be the best way to address homelessness. Shelters can be dangerous for some homeless people, may create new stresses, or may have inflexible rules that make it difficult for some people to acquire the economic resources to find housing. Traditionally, service providers worked to address underlying mental health or substance abuse problems prior to addressing the issue of homelessness. An alternative approach has been to work first on the housing problem and then provide the services necessary to address underlying problems.[66]

Displacement and Gentrification

In a sense, the amount of housing and other activities in a given urban area is fixed. New development can occur but it is often time-consuming, expensive, at the periphery, or otherwise not available or accessible to much of the urban population, particularly those who are poor or lack the resources to compete with others for this limited space. This situation has led to the idea that cities are contested space where different groups compete for communities and neighborhoods; others have proposed that in an ethical city, there is a "right to the city" and that all groups must be accounted for and housing should accommodate households of all incomes.[67]

A consequence of the scarce resource of housing and neighborhoods is that many cities have seen large-scale displacement of people over time. Between 1950 and 1970 this was often the result of intentional government programs that aimed to demolish housing for low-income people and eliminate African American neighborhoods. Since the 1970s, and perhaps earlier in some places, there has been a phenomenon that is called *gentrification*. This is a process by which higher-income individuals and households supplant lower-income households in a given community. Often, there was a race component to gentrification where an influx of more affluent white residents leads to lower-income nonwhite residents having to move out because they can no longer afford to live in the neighborhood.[68] Gentrification is a global phenomenon and has been extensively studied in places such as London and has been identified as a process affecting many U.S. cities, including Boston, San Francisco, and New York City. Gentrification can happen slowly and be a process that takes decades to complete or can be fairly rapid, with a neighborhood changing substantially after only one or two years.[69]

The causes of gentrification may be related to issues such as globalization, other economic changes such as the movement from manufacturing to services, increasing income inequality, or might reflect changes in attitudes toward urban living or the rights of the urban poor.[70] There may be corporate support for neighborhood change and in many cases, government policy and subsidies are directed to encourage gentrification.[71]

As early as the 1960s, there was a growing recognition of the health consequences of clearing entire neighborhoods and dislocating entire populations. Sociologists and psychologists compared the process to grief and documented the physical and mental anguish of those who have been displaced.[72] Furthermore, community psychologist Mindy Fullilove has noted that large-scale displacement caused by urban renewal resulted in entire communities collectively suffering from dislocation in a term that Fullilove called "rootshock."[73] Deborah and Roderick Wallace have observed how displacement in the South Bronx, a process that was in part the consequence of government policy that deliberately withheld services to this low-income community, helped foster the spread of HIV infections from the early center in the Bronx to African American communities throughout Brooklyn and Queens.[74] Gentrification may also have a negative impact on social capital.[75] The full health effects of gentrification are not yet identified, in part because there is much study yet to be done.

Preventing dislocation and gentrification may not be easy. Although large-scale government programs, such as urban renewal, that removed millions of people from their homes are no longer in existence, the total demolition of public housing developments that have hundreds or more units continues.[76] The large-scale movement of people caused by gentrification is a problem in many areas. Preventing gentrification might be more effective than trying to address the problems caused by it; some of the programs that have sought to stabilize communities have included the building of affordable housing, organizing community institutions to own land and buildings, homeowner or renter assistance programs, and other community-based projects.[77] Unfortunately, these necessary programs are expensive and there may not be sufficient funds to pay for some of them.

Segregation and Housing

As noted in many parts of this book, residential racial segregation, particularly of African Americans, is a large problem in the United States.[78] Some of the issues associated with the built environment and segregation are covered in other chapters. For example, the contribution of segregation to unequal exposures to the factory pollution and hazardous waste is covered in Chapter Thirteen, Environmental Justice, and the contributions of segregation to health problems such as infant mortality are discussed in Chapter Ten, Vulnerable Populations. The role of segregation in influencing housing quality is discussed here.

The great migration of African Americans from the rural South to urban areas from California to the Northeast began during World War I and ended around 1970.[79] This was also a time of very high levels of discrimination in housing markets.[80] Thus, at a time when the population was growing rapidly in many communities, African Americans were specifically excluded from many, if not most, parts of many recipient metropolitan areas.[81] Part of the results of segregation has been that African Americans have tended to live in the worst housing in a community, often pay a disproportionate amount of their incomes on rent, overpay to buy housing, and do not benefit from the wealth-producing effects of homeownership that many other segments of the U.S. population receive.[82] The legacy of this nearly hundred years of housing segregation may be one reason why in 2010 African Americans were more likely to live in substandard housing.[83]

As sociologist Bunyan Bryant and others have pointed out, in a sense African Americans have been forced to live in an ecosystem that includes housing that is often contaminated with lead.[84] Their housing often has mold and other problems that exacerbate asthma, they are at increased risk for injuries associated with housing, and they are more likely exposed to the mental health issues associated with poor housing.[85] As discussed elsewhere in this book, African American communities are more likely to lack parks, supermarkets, hospitals, and other features of the built environment that are protective of health. They are likely to be communities that are affected by pollution, unwanted land uses, or other factors that may harm health.[86]

Addressing segregation is not easy. Enforcement of fair housing laws is essential and addressing both overt and covert discrimination is very important.[87] Programs that target housing quality and neighborhood environmental issues are essential if the problems associated with segregation are to be mitigated.

Affordability

As early as 1919, Edith Elmer Wood pointed out that central to the housing problem in United States was affordability and the lack of economic resources to purchase adequate housing.[88] As noted elsewhere, particularly in Chapter Nine on food accessibility, housing affordability can be a major problem for many households, and households that are paying too high a percentage of their incomes for rent or other housing costs are more likely to have problems with food insecurity, and may be at risk for other difficulties as well.[89] Addressing affordability may be important if these issues are to be mitigated.

As noted above, there are approximately 3,000,000 housing units subsidized by federal and state government to be more affordable by the poor. There are approximately 9,000,000 families who were below the official federal poverty line in 2009.[90] Thus many of the poor do not receive any housing assistance. Addressing affordability, which will enable focusing on homelessness, food insecurity, and other associated problems, may require additional resources.

Mental Health and Housing

There are a number of ways that housing may affect mental health.[91] These may include the stresses that are associated with overcrowding and poor-quality housing, the need for housing to accommodate persons with special needs, the effects that living in poor-quality neighborhoods with limited access to services may have on mental health, and the contribution of good-quality housing to overall well-being that manifests itself in better mental health.[92] These issues may indicate that one way to improve the mental health of individuals and communities would be to address housing issues. These issues are further discussed in Chapter Eleven, which discusses mental health.

Summary

Over time, housing has been redefined from being a problem of enforcement to one of affordability. There are a variety of public programs and government responsibilities for housing that include production, subsidies, and code enforcement. In general, maintaining healthy housing includes keeping it dry, pest free, and safe, along with other basic health promoting attributes. In addition, there are problems with past legacies of asbestos and lead paint. Many current housing problems that affect specific vulnerable groups include the effects of homelessness on low-income and handicapped individuals, displacement of longtime residents through gentrification, and the special vulnerabilities of people with mental health issues.

Key Terms

Integrated Pest Management (IPM)

Shrinking city movement

Discussion Questions

1. Describe the various ways the "housing problem" has been defined.
2. In general, what is the difference between federal and state/local government involvement with housing?
3. How might Section 8 and other housing voucher programs help make housing safer?
4. Name the main problems associated with housing quality in the United States.
5. Why is lead in housing a problem?
6. What are some of the policies to reduce lead exposures?
7. What are the advantages of national housing codes?

8. What is Integrated Pest Management?
9. How might abandoned housing affect health?

For More Information

Alliance for Healthy Homes. www.afhh.org.

Healthy House Institute. www.healthyhouseinstitute.com.

Healthy Housing Coalition (formally the National Center for Lead Safe Housing). www
.leadsafehousing.org.

National Center for Environmental Health—Centers for Disease Control and Prevention. *Healthy housing reference manual*. www.cdc.gov/nceh/publications/books/housing/
housing.htm.

National Center for Healthy Housing. www.nchh.org.

INFRASTRUCTURE AND NATURAL DISASTERS

LEARNING OBJECTIVES

- Describe the role of advance planning in addressing public health needs during a natural disaster.
- List the ways a hurricane can harm lives and property.
- Identify the potential health effects associated with flooding.
- Explain the role of building codes in preventing injuries and deaths from earthquakes.
- Describe the role of social isolation in vulnerability to extreme temperature events.
- Name some of the barriers to Brownfields redevelopment.
- Describe the role of maintenance in securing the protective features of infrastructure.
- Identify ways in which parks and playgrounds might promote health.

The news media often has stories about natural disasters: floods, hurricanes, earthquakes, heat waves, and so on. If a crisis were to strike in your community, how might your home or neighborhood be affected? Who in your community might be most at risk? Let's think about the large- and small-scale features of the built environment that keep you safe. In some areas, there are dams and levees. Less obvious, but more ubiquitous, are safety plans, first responders, and other ways that society is organized to meet the challenges of natural disasters. Consider how these contribute to your health and safety.

Though many people would like to think that those of us living in this most modern and wealthy society are immune to the effects of natural disasters, events in the past several decades have continued to highlight the vulnerability of people to natural disasters even in those countries that consider themselves to be the most advanced. In the United States, there have been the repeated disasters caused by hurricanes, most notably Hurricane Andrew in 1992 and Hurricane Katrina in 2005. In addition, portions of the United States are highly vulnerable to earthquakes, with the 1989 Loma Prieta earthquake responsible for 63 deaths

FIGURE 6.1   Annual Number of Declared Disasters

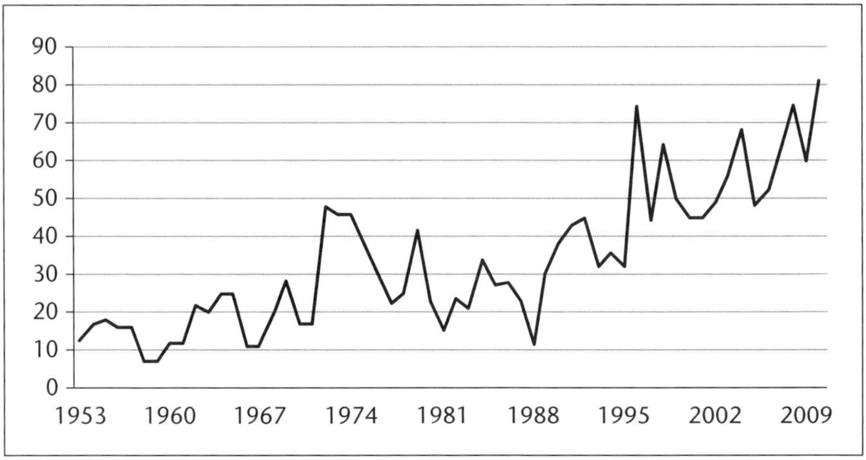

Source: FEMA

and billions of dollars in damages, including the failure of a freeway in Oakland, California. More subtle, but perhaps just as deadly, are extreme weather events, which have killed thousands in the United States and Europe in the past fifteen years. (See Figure 6.1.) While these deaths are perhaps not as dramatic as those caused by earthquakes and hurricanes, collectively they are responsible for many more deaths.

But infrastructure is not just a factor in preventing mortality; well-built and well-maintained infrastructure can be central in the promotion of health. Much of this health-affirming infrastructure is discussed elsewhere in this book, for example, the role of sidewalks in promoting health is presented in Chapter Four and the ability of well-designed communities to promote physical activity is addressed in the Chapter Three. But there are other issues associated with infrastructure and this chapter will begin with a discussion of hurricanes and other types of natural disasters, then move on to a presentation on infrastructure, and conclude with an outline of how parks and playgrounds affect health.

Natural Disasters: An Introduction

A major theme in a discussion of natural disasters and health is that even though the exact timing of many of these events cannot be predicted, their effects can be anticipated, protective measures adopted, responses planned, and deaths and injuries prevented. There is no inevitability about the deadliness of natural disasters.

Hurricanes

Even before Katrina, the destructive power of hurricanes was well known and the history of the United States contains examples of very destructive hurricanes, including the one that struck Galveston, Texas, in 1900 and the New England hurricane of 1938. The former killed over 6,000 people; the latter, over 700. Hurricanes kill and destroy property in several ways. There is the wind, which can tear off roofs, cause buildings to disintegrate, or propel objects into people or buildings. There is the flooding that results from the heavy rains that often accompany hurricanes, and these floods can cause rivers to overflow their banks or flood streets. In addition, these rains and floods can overwhelm storm sewers. But the most dangerous aspect of a hurricane and the feature that is most deadly is the **storm surge**, the rise in coastal waters that can exceed 10–15 feet in height, drive vast amounts of water far inland, and result in high-powered waves smashing into buildings and submerged coastal properties.[1] It was the storm surge that was responsible for the destruction of Galveston and it was a storm surge pushing through the canal system in New Orleans that caused the flooding in that city.

The failure of local, state, and federal government before, during, and after Hurricane Katrina highlights the role of infrastructure and advanced planning in the protection of lives and property. Hurricane Katrina also demonstrated who is most vulnerable during a natural disaster and how these vulnerabilities are not randomly distributed across the population; Katrina starkly showed how disasters reinforce existing vulnerabilities in a society. It was the very poor, the elderly, the nonwhite, and those with other preexisting social and health vulnerabilities who were most at risk of losing their lives and their homes. Katrina also exposed how these vulnerabilities must be anticipated and addressed in advance of the disaster itself.[2]

Although many aspects of Hurricane Katrina remain controversial, several lessons from the destruction in New Orleans have become clear. First of all, the very vulnerability of certain geographic areas can be highly anticipated. It was known for decades, if not longer, that the special geographic location of New Orleans placed it at risk to hurricanes. Much of the city is below sea level and the whole area is sinking even as sea levels are rising. Thus, with each passing year, the danger to the city was increasing. Much of its protective infrastructure of levees, pumps, and drainage canals was poorly engineered and badly maintained. Worse, some of the local infrastructure served to increase the vulnerability of the city rather than decrease it. For example, the Mississippi River Gulf Outlet

(MRGO) has been credited with funneling in the storm surge that caused multiple failures along its length.[3] All these failures had been anticipated or predicted, but over the years little had been done to prepare for the inevitable hurricane. Instead of working to protect the city, there was inertia at all levels.

It was the inability of government to function during the crisis that captured much of the media attention immediately after the hurricane. Evacuations were delayed, hospitals and temporary shelters overwhelmed, and rescue efforts idled while flood waters rose. But again, it was during the planning period before the hurricane struck where many of the failures began. Which layer of government was ultimately responsible for these failures is controversial and beyond the scope of this book. However, some of the broader lessons of these failures include the following:

Inadequate Evacuation Plans. The standard response to an imminent hurricane is to order the evacuation of people from coastal and at-risk areas. In New Orleans, these plans did not anticipate the problems of evacuating very poor, isolated people situated in the most low-lying areas in the city. Many of these people did not have access to cars and could not respond to an evacuation order that did not include assistance to get them out. Many of those who could have left chose to stay because they feared that leaving would place their properties at risk from looting and vandalism, or they feared leaving because they had no place to go and no money to provide for necessities during the evacuation.[4] Then there were those who were in such frail health that they could not move themselves, so any evacuation of these people would have had to be carefully planned. For all these groups, the proper response of government should have been to identify in advance who would be most at risk during an evacuation, develop a plan to get these people out safely, preassign responsibilities to specific individuals to carry out evacuations, monitor the evacuation while it was going on, anticipate the needs of vulnerable peoples while they are evacuated, and finally, plan for an evaluation so that the response to the next disaster will be improved.[5]

Inadequate Protective Infrastructure. The failure of New Orleans's protective levee system was obvious, but less well known and just as problematic was the failure to protect the surrounding wetlands that could have served to blunt some of the impacts of the storm. Development and erosion have caused thousands of square miles of marsh and low-lying land in the Mississippi Delta to disappear. If these lands had been maintained they would have provided space for the storm surge to dissipate or at least lose some of its force. But in their absence the full force of the storm could move closer to the city. An important lesson in this failure is that the preservation of natural areas, particularly critical environments

FOCUS ON

The San Francisco Bay Delta

The region where the Sacramento and San Joaquin Rivers enter San Francisco Bay is illustrative of many of the problems with infrastructure in the United States. At one time, the delta was subject to large-scale seasonal flooding by winter rains and by spring snow melt from most of interior central California. This was probably a very productive ecosystem that supported migrating flocks of birds and provided breeding grounds for aquatic life.[8]

But over the past 150 years, substantial changes both in the delta itself and throughout its watershed have created problems. Many of the major tributaries to the two main rivers have been dammed to control flooding, create hydropower, and supply water for agriculture and large urban populations in both northern and southern parts of the state. Levees were constructed in the delta itself to create farmland. Major highways cross through the delta and the large metropolitan areas of San Francisco, Oakland, Sacramento, and Stockton border on this fragile area. Water from north valley dams is channeled through the delta on its way to provide water in southern metropolitan areas. The area has been fundamentally altered from how it looked 150 years ago.

One issue confronting the delta region is the potential of a catastrophic failure in its levee system: As the levee system slowly deteriorates, rising sea level has resulted in much of the dry land of the delta being below sea level.[9] One failed in 2004. Another issue is that the delta is home to endangered species. Continued demand for water for agriculture and consumers, along with a series of droughts in the past ten years, has reduced inflows of fresh water, harming water quality, harming endangered species, and possibly threatening the viability of the transport of water through the delta.

Fixing the problems of the delta has not been easy. First, there is a lack of consensus on how to meet the conflicting demands of water users, residents (the delta is a major source of tourism and recreation revenues), and environmentalists. Second, there is a problem of paying for improvements, which could potentially cost billions of dollars.

such as coastal wetlands, is vital for the protection of communities.[6] It is not a luxury, but must be funded so as to be effective. A corollary lesson is that although building and maintaining an effective infrastructure is very expensive, to not do so may be more costly.

Inadequate Communication. Part of the tragedy of the hurricane was the way people were left waiting for help in the days after the disaster struck. Even as much of the world was transfixed by media images of people stuck on rooftops or in evacuation gathering centers, some of those responsible for getting help to these people seemed to be unaware of what was occurring. Again, this is a situation that should be anticipated and planned for. A major trait of disaster planning must be securing alternative ways of communicating during the height of the problems of the disaster.[7]

The effort to protect vital areas from hurricanes must begin far in advance of an approaching storm. Infrastructure must be properly engineered and maintained if areas are to be preserved. Communications systems must be tested, emergency plans practiced, and potential problems anticipated. In addition, building codes and code enforcement must be part of these preparatory efforts.

Floods

Flooding from all sources, high storm waters, rising streams, and so on, is a major cause of property damage as well as of deaths. In general, planners and engineers tend to focus on what is known as the hundred-year flood. This is based on historical records of what was the maximum high water level in a given area. There are two problems with this. One is that as development patterns change and impervious surfaces increase, the risk of flooding in a given area may also increase. The other problem is that due to global climate change, the frequency of large-scale and extreme weather events is increasing; thus, interpretations of what areas might be at risk of flooding based upon what has flooded in the past few decades may not be a good predictor of future risks.[10] Local communities tend to rely on maps of potential flooding areas produced by the Federal Emergency Management Agency (FEMA). These FEMA maps represent the best official estimate of flooding potential across the United States. Governments, insurers, and individuals often turn to these maps to gauge the amount of potential flooding risks in an area. They are not 100% accurate; just because the area is not identified as being in a potential flood zone does not mean that the flooding risk there is minimal.

A major problem in many, if not all, floods is that floodwaters are often contaminated with chemicals, pesticides, and sewage. As floodwaters rise, they can take in all the various toxins that are in the environment, such as chemicals stored in warehouses, worksites, and houses or pesticides and other chemicals that are used in agriculture. The floodwaters can spread these potential contaminants widely across the environment and may affect the health of people who are caught in floodwaters, those who go out to rescue stranded persons, people engaged in flood cleanup, and those who occupy the buildings after the floodwaters recede.[11]

Contamination from sewage may be one of the greatest problems arising from floods because a small amount of sewage can contaminate a large amount of floodwaters. While it is unlikely that a flood in the United States would pose a risk of cholera because that disease is not normally present in this country at any given time, there are many other waterborne diseases that can cause very uncomfortable illnesses. Though the risk of death from these diseases for most healthy people is fairly remote, the problem of water contamination during flooding is serious.[12]

Another problem is that flooding can often lead to a buildup of mold, which can create health problems for those cleaning up after the flood or for those living in these buildings after the floodwaters have receded, sometimes becoming so widespread that entire interiors need to be replaced or buildings become contaminated beyond repair. Mold can be very costly and time-consuming to remove safely. In any case, the safe removal and disposal of mold-covered debris must be carefully monitored and the public made to understand that unsafe removal of mold can create health problems.[13]

Because floods can often happen quickly it is essential that local governments develop a warning system so that the number of lives lost is kept as low as possible. Infrastructure can help reduce the risk of flooding, but as time has gone on it is increasingly recognized that there are limits to the ability to stop floods by erecting structures such as levees. Unfortunately, levees can often serve to simply move the location of the flood upstream or downstream or they can become particularly problematic if they fail. They may be essential in some places, but in other areas it may be better to limit the construction in floodplains or other flood-prone areas. (See the discussion on restricting building in vulnerable areas).

Earthquakes

Many parts of the United States and other countries are at particular risk for earthquakes. These include not only California, which is well known for its earthquakes, but also areas as far distant as Missouri and other states. The major way in which earthquakes kill and injure is the failure of buildings and other structures that can be caused by either the shaking of the structures themselves or through the failure of the land underlying these structures. An earthquake may cause a number of stresses on structures as the force of the shaking causes acceleration that can displace buildings off their foundations, causes walls to collapse, or dislodges objects in the building that can strike people.[14] Some buildings are more vulnerable than others. For example, unreinforced masonry buildings or buildings in which the ground floor has been opened up for windows or parking are more likely to fail during an earthquake.[15]

Ground or soil failure is also a major problem during an earthquake and causes some of the most severe damage. Many soils may lack the strength to sufficiently hold up the weight of a building above them during an earthquake leading to the building sinking or even resulting in its total collapse. Some soils, particularly those that are made up of fine clays or poorly consolidated fills in areas with high water tables can undergo a process known as **liquefaction**. In simple terms, shaking causes soil particles to become suspended in water and lose all ability to support any kind of structure on top of them, including foundations or even roads and water pipes.[16]

The most vulnerable places during an earthquake are those communities with unreinforced masonry buildings on landfill. It was this type of neighborhood that was the scene of some of the worst destruction during the 1989 Loma Prieta earthquake: though the Marina District of San Francisco was distant from the earthquake's epicenter, the neighborhood had many unreinforced masonry buildings and was built on landfill. Buildings collapsed; gas pipelines exploded.[17]

Planning for earthquakes must begin decades before they strike. Though the exact day, year, or even decade of a major earthquake cannot be predicted given our present technology, the fact that an earthquake will strike at some point should not be a surprise to those who live in earthquake country. The first step to prepare for earthquakes is the adoption of strong protective building codes. Though the technology of building earthquake-safe buildings is evolving and is modified over time, some of the most vulnerable building practices should be prohibited and buildings that predate these more restrictive codes need to be retrofitted and brought up to current safety standards. It is often the case that low-income property owners may not have the resources to upgrade their homes and funding mechanisms to assist these owners may be necessary. Codes should be continually reevaluated and updated based on new information from quakes in other parts of the world. For example, studies of building failures in the Long Beach earthquake of 1931 prompted changes in school construction codes in California[18] and it was after a series of earthquakes in the Los Angeles area in the 1990s that engineers identified a problem with buildings that have opened first floors (walls removed to accommodate parking or storefronts). Efforts are now being made to reduce the risk of collapses of such buildings.

As in the other natural disasters described in this chapter, disaster plans must be put in place in advance of the earthquake itself. One very important factor regarding earthquake planning is that an earthquake can put at risk the various facilities that emergency responses may need during the disaster. Hospitals can collapse, highways and major roads that emergency vehicles need may fail, the buildings that house emergency services may be knocked out, and water and power supplies disrupted. The potential for failure of these facilities must be assessed and mitigated. Another important factor regarding earthquake preparedness planning is the very large scale of seismic-related disasters. A major earthquake in a large metropolitan area could leave millions without electricity, access to emergency medical services, or even access to food and water. Thus it is very important that individuals be educated on how to prepare for an earthquake or similar large-scale disaster. However, it should be recognized that simply telling households they should stockpile food, water, and extra medications for emergency will still leave some people vulnerable. For example, many poor households cannot afford food to meet immediate needs, much less pay for food they may not use for many months or years. Low-income households often move frequently, which makes it even harder to stockpile food and water. Many poor households, those with inadequate insurance, or even those who may have insurance but whose insurance companies do not allow for the stockpiling of extra medications may not be able to maintain a supply of critical medicines that they would need in the event of a disruption of transportation infrastructure. Again these problems need to be anticipated in advance of the disaster itself.[19]

Extreme Temperature Events

Extreme weather events, particularly heat waves, are important health problems. The elderly may be most at risk during these events because of preexisting conditions, medications they are taking, fear of crime and personal safety issues, and because of social isolation. Again, the solution to protecting elderly people is planning and identifying those elderly who are most at risk, advanced structuring of services and emergency responses, and practicing these plans well before an actual emergency.

There have been several major events regarding extreme heat or extreme cold across the developed world in the last two decades that have severe impacts on health. One of the most dramatic of these was the Chicago heat wave of 1995, when over 600 people died. In 2003, a heat wave across Europe killed over 35,000, over a third of them in France.[20] Heat waves are not uncommon and it is not that these temperatures are not regularly seen in more tropical places, but humans in temperate areas have a special sensitivity to heat events. Again, the most vulnerable people in Chicago and Europe were the elderly, the poor, and the socially isolated. Low-income African American elderly were at particular risk in the Chicago heat wave.[21]

The elderly appear to have a special physiological vulnerability to heat. As people age, they lose their ability to regulate their body so that ambient temperatures can leave them at risk for heat-related illnesses. In addition, many of the medications that are used to treat conditions prevalent among the elderly can exacerbate their vulnerabilities to heat and lessen their ability to meet heat problems. The elderly may not be aware that their health is at risk or may not be able to seek medical attention.[22]

The social vulnerability of the elderly may also be very important. Many elderly people are poor and may not be able to afford air-conditioning, or they may live in older buildings that may not be well sealed against leaks, making cooling costs higher. In addition, some elderly live in neighborhoods where they may be reluctant to leave their homes because they fear for their physical safety or worry that their homes may be burglarized or vandalized. They may be afraid to open windows to take advantage of natural ventilation, further increasing interior room temperatures. The elderly may be so isolated that there is no one to take care of them or check up on them during the event, and no one to summon help from authorities.[23]

Again, these vulnerabilities must be anticipated and planned for in advance of a heat wave emergency.[24] Addressing the underlying social and economic vulnerabilities of the elderly is important. In addition, procedures must be planned, responsibilities assigned, and procedures tested. The first step is to identify at-risk elderly in advance of a heat emergency so that they can be monitored while the heat wave is happening. Some cities have used voting lists, elder service providers, health outreach workers, or door-to-door surveys to identify at-risk persons. Once the heat emergency is declared, the action plan needs to be implemented. This may include periodic visits to at-risk persons in their homes, setting up special cooling centers (places with air-conditioning that can accommodate the numbers of people who might need to go to such a place), setting up emergency response teams so that those who have a heat-related medical event can be quickly brought in for treatment, and other similar kinds of community-based actions. Again, any plan must include provisions for evaluation so that future events can be better addressed.[25]

Wildfires

Strategies to reduce the impact of household fires are discussed in the chapter on housing. Many parts of the western United States are arid or semiarid, or are subject to periodic dry spells so that they are prone to forest or grassland fires that can affect thousands of acres or more. Aside from the effects of natural environments, these fires could be catastrophic to neighborhoods or other human-built structures in their path. The 1991 fire in the Oakland Hills in California, for example, destroyed 3,500 housing units and killed 25 people.[26]

It appears that these wildfires can be periodic events in many parts of the arid west, but there are many ways that built environments can be modified so as to reduce their impact on people and property. These actions, often required by state or local law, can include special building codes that prohibit certain types of materials such as wood-shingled roofs and encourage the use of nonflammable building materials; creation and maintenance of buffer zones around buildings so that fires cannot reach up to the edge of structures; development of emergency procedures to inform residents in at-risk areas in the event of a fire and to create plans for evacuating places very quickly; and other similar measures. These efforts require enforcement, which can be expensive or politically difficult to achieve, but if carefully adhered to, these measures can reduce property damage and protect lives.[27]

Mudslides and Landslides

Another problem that often strikes semiarid areas on the edge of metropolitan areas is mudslides. These are common in Southern California, where there appears to be a pattern of a dry weather series of fires followed by problems with mudslides once wet weather returns. One of the first indications that there may be a mudslide problem is geologic evidence of past mudslides in an area or a fire the summer before. Some committees have tried to prevent the potential for mudslides by creating barriers and some areas have tried to develop procedures to warn of mudslides and evacuate residents when one occurs. Strategies to reduce the effects of mudslides include prohibiting construction in mudslide-prone areas, the building of special retaining walls and other protective infrastructure, the prohibition of using unconsolidated fill on hillsides, and so forth. Again, these efforts may be expensive and politically difficult to achieve.

Natural Disaster Response

Responsibility for responding to natural disasters depends upon the magnitude of the disaster and the relationship between local, state, and federal government in the United States.[28] The federal agency that usually takes the lead during an emergency is the Federal Emergency Management Agency (FEMA). In general, FEMA only acts after a state requests assistance and a disaster is declared.[29] This explains some of the lack of coordination between local officials in New Orleans and FEMA during Hurricane Katrina.[30] Many states have agencies that parallel FEMA to provide for state resources during the disaster. Local governments, which may be cities or counties, tend to rely on police, fire, and public health agencies to respond to an emergency but may have emergency coordinators to plan and coordinate emergency responses. However, these local organizations themselves may be adversely affected by the disaster.[31] There is also a network of nongovernment agencies such as Red Cross, who have the training and ability to assist during and immediately after a disaster.[32] In general, utilities are responsible for restoring local electrical and water services.

During an emergency and immediately afterwards, disaster response may include search and rescue operations, responding to immediate threats to loss of life or property, and other similar activities.[33] Once the emergency itself is past these agencies may also coordinate cleanups and distribution of supplies to people in the affected area.[34] The community may need water, food, electricity, and shelter. Again, all this takes advance planning and coordination to minimize loss of life and property and assist the community to meet the needs of the disaster and its immediate aftermath.[35]

There may be immediate and long-term health consequences to a disaster, which, depending on the disaster, may include injuries, heat- and smoke-related issues, reactions to contact with mold or sewage, and post-traumatic stress disorders or longer-term mental health issues.[36] People with preexisting chronic illnesses such as cardiovascular disease and diabetes may also need medical assistance.[37] Local medical resources may be strained.[38]

Again, as demonstrated by Hurricane Katrina, Hurricane Andrew, and the floods in Grand Forks, North Dakota caused by the Red River of the North in 1997, and many other disasters, recovery from a disaster can take years.[39] Many people do not have flood insurance or they may not have sufficient financial resources on the road to pay to rebuild and restore homes and businesses.[40] Local governments may be overwhelmed by a sudden surge in building permits, a lack of building materials, and a shortage of skilled labor. And the economic uncertainty that can follow a disaster can further slow down rebuilding.[41] Thus, in 2011, six years after Hurricane Katrina flooded large parts of New Orleans, some parts of the city have recovered and other neighborhoods remained very much in distress.[42]

Often, the declaration of a disaster makes local communities eligible for federal and state loans to assist rebuilding. Sometimes grants are secured for restoring infrastructure and some states have provided tax credits and other incentives for reinvestment in destroyed neighborhoods.[43] Private donations and volunteer labor may also be important in bringing community back to what it once was.

Brownfield Restoration

A major problem in many communities that have suffered from disinvestment and deindustrialization are abandoned or underutilized sites that may have some type of contamination that could affect the health of the environment. These sites where there are known or suspected contamination are also called

Brownfields.[44] The U.S. General Accounting Office estimates there are 425,000 Brownfield sites across the United States, though others have suggested there may be as many as 5,000,000 abandoned industrial sites.[45]

Brownfields have a negative impact on the neighborhoods around them in several ways. They may release their contamination into the surrounding environment, or people and animals may come in contact with pollution on site.[46] There is often a special fear that children may be exposed to toxins if they visit the sites to explore or play. The sites also have a negative economic effect, as they can reduce property values or create eyesores. There are environmental justice concerns in that they may exist disproportionately in low-income neighborhoods and communities of color.[47]

Often there are barriers to redeveloping the sites. Environmental laws of the United States tend to place liability for contamination on any person or entity who ever owned the site even if they were not responsible for the pollution or contamination. Therefore many investors may be reluctant to get involved in redeveloping a Brownfield site because of this fear of liability.[48] Furthermore, the cost of identifying the full extent of contamination and the cost of remediation may be so high that it makes redevelopment plans uneconomical. These may all contribute to these sites continuing to be unused or underutilized.[49]

Addressing Brownfields has developed into a major program in many states along with the federal government. Some of the programs that have been developed to encourage redevelopment include:

- Grants to pay for site assessment
- Low-cost loans to pay for cleanups
- Agreements to limit liability in exchange for site remediation[50]

Though some sites have been cleaned up under Brownfields programs, many sites remain contaminated. One problem is that there have tended to be limited dollar amounts for assisting with Brownfields redevelopment while the potential need for the program is very large. Another is continuing fears about liability. Often, neighbors and communities can oppose redevelopment plans particularly if the remediation plan does not result in a full cleanup of the site (sometimes pollution sources are capped and left in place rather than removed) or there may be concerns with the proposed redevelopment use.[51]

Restricting Building in Vulnerable Areas Versus Building Protective Barriers

Even before Katrina, major floods from rivers and high tides associated with storms in coastal areas prompted a reexamination of policies to protect people and property from floods. Rebuilding flooded homes and businesses or buildings along coastlines is expensive. It is very difficult to get flood insurance for these properties and many have come to rely on flood insurance provided by grouped pools administered by state and federal governments or assistance from FEMA to rebuild. But even these institutions have reached the limits of their ability to provide funds for rebuilding.

Increasingly, public agencies,—city and town planning boards, state coastal management agencies, and FEMA—are requiring that areas most prone to floods not be built on. In particular, these programs and policies are enforced after an event that has destroyed buildings. This can be unpopular with property owners, who often want to keep or replace their homes in these areas, but there are several arguments against rebuilding. It is expensive to protect these areas and the problem is made worse because the forces that are responsible for making these areas at risk can be expected to continue and future floods or destruction may be inevitable. There is an equity issue resulting from the use of public funds, often collected from poorer taxpayers or those who do not enjoy the serenity and views of these properties, to pay for the protection of at-risk properties or for subsidizing insurance costs. And there is the fact that by preserving natural places—flood plains, wetlands, seaside dunes—areas further

---

FOCUS ON

Moving a Town to Prevent Flooding

Sometimes, the potential for flooding can be so great that it is easier to move a town rather than try to construct sufficient levees to protect it. Such was the case of Valmeyer, Illinois. The 1993 flood in the upper Mississippi River basin was one of the worst in recent history. Despite billions of dollars in flood control, there was substantial flooding along the Missouri, the Mississippi, and many important tributaries. The winter before had seen heavy snowfall, followed by above-normal spring rains. The result was that much of the flood plain of these rivers and beyond was underwater for much of late spring and the summer.

Valmeyer was built in the flood plain of the Mississippi, north of St. Louis. The town was inundated and was faced with two options: (1) rebuilding, which was strongly discouraged by the providers of flood insurance and would have meant that the town would eventually flood again, or (2) the entire town could move to higher ground. This was the option agreed to by town residents and the new town was built three miles east. There hasn't been a major flood event since the town was moved, but the new location may well prove to be less flood-prone than the old site.[53]

inland are protected from flooding and the undeveloped habitats provide a resource for wildlife. The issue of whether to rebuild or to protect these areas is controversial and present in almost all at-risk areas. Furthermore, purchasing properties is expensive and may require subsidies from state or federal programs and successfully implementing these programs is not easy. Areas at risk must be identified and the public educated regarding the need for such a program.[52]

River Restoration

In the mid-twentieth century, the standard way to prevent a river from flooding and protect surrounding property often included substantial channelization and reconstruction of once untouched waterways. Channels were straightened and any barriers to water flow were removed. Often these projects resulted in rivers being lined with concrete floors and walls, eliminating all vegetation along the banks and eventually killing most of the wildlife and fish in the river. As a result, these waterways were often little more than concrete-lined ditches, unsuitable for any use except drainage, and the channelized streams deprived communities along these rivers of a potential recreational resource. In addition, these measures sometimes proved to be ineffective. Channelization increases the speed and volume of runoff, potentially making floods more extreme.[54]

By the end of the twentieth century, environmentalists and the communities along rivers were demanding a rethinking of how urban rivers and streams were managed. In response, current ideas about how to manage these streams have changed. Natural channels, which can include rocks and other barriers, can slow down the speed of currents, increase the absorption of water into aquifers, and provide places for fish and wildlife to thrive. Similarly, maintaining the natural curve of rivers is also better for water management because these slow down the velocity of flood waters, lessening their destructive impacts. Another alternative is to restrict buildings so that rather than build up levees, the flood plain is left as open space. The result is that floods spread out and dissipate without destroying property and the surrounding areas can be used as farms or parkland. There is also a new understanding that trees along waterways can cool the water and help maintain the vitality of natural ecosystems. These efforts are a nationwide phenomenon, but perhaps the most famous is the effort to restore the Los Angeles River in California. In the past, it was such a smooth concrete wasteland that it was used in several movies as the site for car races, and though many parts remain channelized, more and more stretches of the river have been restored to a more natural environment and the river is becoming a resource for many of the poor neighborhoods along its course.[55] The restoration also promises to promote health by increasing access to recreation and improving social capital.[56] There are a number of barriers to these types of programs: expense, public opposition, jurisdictional difficulties, and so on.

Reducing Impervious Surfaces

One feature associated with the built environment is that large amounts of land become paved over with concrete or asphalt or become occupied by buildings. The problem is that these types of surfaces do not absorb water and thus can add to the volume of runoff from storms. This can lead to an increase in overall storm volumes, which increases the risk of flooding. There are a number of ways that these effects can be mitigated, including using pervious rather than impervious surfaces for sidewalks and parking areas, amending codes so that the percentage of land that can be covered by pervious services on a given lot is limited, relying on site storage of storm waters, and other similar factors.[57]

Decaying Infrastructure

A major problem in the United States is that the infrastructure to protect against floods, deliver clean water, clean up or eliminate sewage discharges, facilitate transportation, and provide other vital services has not been well maintained. There is also a lack of capital investments for new infrastructure to keep up with population increases or to address an evolving understanding of what is needed to protect human health and the environment. As a result, there are periodic well-publicized failures of infrastructure such as the collapse of the I-35W Mississippi River bridge in Minneapolis in 2007 as well as less publicized failures that resulted in problems with pollution or threats to human health.

The cost of maintaining and improving infrastructure in the United States is very large. The Congressional Budget Office estimated that in fiscal year 2007, federal, state, and local expenditures on transportation and water infrastructure alone totaled $356 billion. But the Environmental Protection Agency estimated a need of between $300 and $500 billion for water improvements alone between 2006 and 2010.[58] And the American Society of Civil Engineers estimated a need for $1.6 trillion for total infrastructure maintenance and improvements during that same time.[59]

Financing Infrastructure

Protecting the public from natural disasters and building and maintaining infrastructure is clearly very expensive.[60] Municipal finance, capital planning, and public bonds are a specialty beyond the scope of this book, but there are some important aspects of this process that should be kept in mind here. In general, public works are built by local entities, either state or local government or special districts set up under state law to build and/or manage infrastructure. For example, the Massachusetts Water Resources Authority (MWRA), a quasi-state agency, built the large-scale treatment plant to clean up Boston Harbor. In Houston, the Public Works and Engineering Department of the city provides water and manages the infrastructure for delivering water to homes and businesses. Sometimes the federal government, such as the Army Corp of Engineers, builds public works.[61] The Army Corp of Engineers operates an extensive system of dams and facilities to reduce the risk of flooding along the Ohio River, for example.

The financing of public works is also often subject to state and local regulation and laws and, in general, there are important constraints on the ability of these governments and agencies to borrow money for capital projects.[62] Projects funded by the federal government are very different because the federal government does not directly borrow to pay for these infrastructure projects (beyond the amount to pay for the entire federal budget deficit); instead they are counted as expenditures from the annual budget. Though occasionally state and local government will pay for some type of infrastructure out of its annual operating budget, this is rare and, in general, improvements are paid for out of a state or local entity's capital budget. Furthermore, the usual way these are financed is by borrowing money, usually by issuing bonds.

There are two kinds of bonds: general obligation bonds and special issue bonds. General obligation bonds are backed by the full financial power of the issuing entity; all tax dollars and user fees collected by the entity can be used by the entity to pay back the bonds. Special issue bonds are backed by certain types of revenues. These can include fees paid by the customers of a water district or tolls paid by users of a bridge.

The ability to float bonds to pay for infrastructure is subject to many potential limitations. Some states place caps on the bonded indebtedness of cities, and agencies and localities must apply to float a new bond issue. Other states require a vote of the taxpayers, or the total electorate, to approve a new bond project. Sometimes these votes are subject to supermajorities rather than just more than 50% of those voting. Most important, states and local governments and agencies are limited in how much they can borrow by the amount of income they can rely on to repay the bonds. If the bond sellers (the underwriters) think an entity already owes too much money relative to its projected revenues, the interest cost of the bond can rise or there could be no buyers for the bonds. Thus there are limits to these kinds of financing.

Many types of infrastructure are funded by state and city government. Police and fire facilities usually are central municipal functions. Though there may be a targeted tax, such as a development impact fee to pay for these improvements, the funding of these projects is fairly straightforward. But parks, waters, sewers, and transit are often planned, funded, built, and managed by special districts that rely on special taxes. A flood protection district may use a parcel tax or a property tax to pay for levees and flood protection or a transit district may use a sales tax, along with fare box revenue, to pay for a new light rail line. Again, local ability to pay for improvements is limited by the amount of revenue they can raise.[63]

Maintenance

Just as important as the financing of infrastructure improvements is their long-term maintenance. Unfortunately, because maintenance is usually an operating rather than a capital expense, sometimes maintenance is cut back to reduce expenditures and deficits, or because maintenance often has less political support than new capital spending. But maintenance is critical and without proper and long-term maintenance the useful life and effectiveness of infrastructure can degrade. It's hard to establish constituencies for maintenance but doing so may be as important to protecting health and property as is the construction of infrastructure itself.

Parks and Playgrounds

The role of infrastructure is greater than simply protecting health; it can have a positive impact as well. The infrastructure of streets, neighborhoods, and metropolitan areas is described in previous chapters, but the positive role of parks and playgrounds will be discussed briefly here. There are a wide range of recreational open spaces from national parks to local playgrounds, and though the national, state, and regional open spaces are important, the role of local infrastructure to support physical activity should not be overlooked.[64]

Parks and playgrounds are important for providing opportunities for physical activity and may also play a role in improving the cognitive skills of young children.[65] Studies suggest that most users of parks and playgrounds come from a very local area, usually not much more than a quarter mile.[66] In particular, low-income and minority populations are most dependent on having access to free, accessible, quality open spaces for recreation.

Well-maintained playgrounds and parks can be assets for the neighborhood around them.[67] They may increase the livability of a community and contribute to residential stability and increased property values.[68] Parks have been associated with increased social capital and provide an opportunity for community members to interact.[69]

Some parks may have issues with crime, drug use, or other problematic behaviors.[70] If neighborhoods don't perceive a park as being a safe place, they may not use it.[71] Park maintenance is critical if parks are to be perceived and used as community assets.[72]

These facilities should be designed to have age-appropriate equipment, accommodate different groups, and have equipment that meets current safety standards. Our understanding of what constitutes a safe playground is evolving, but organizations such as the Consumer Product Safety Commission publish guidelines for safe playgrounds.[73] In addition, these spaces must be well-maintained and if necessary, should be sensitive to issues of crime and safety.

Summary

People in the United States are vulnerable to a variety of natural disasters including hurricanes, floods, earthquakes, heat waves, and fires. Planning to prevent death and injuries is crucial and should include the preservation of natural buffers, sound infrastructure planning and maintenance, strict building codes and enforcement, identification of at-risk populations, and advance practicing of emergency procedures. Infrastructure can also promote health; for example, parks and playgrounds can be important for physical activity.

Key Terms

Brownfields

Liquefaction

Storm surge

Discussion Questions

1. Name the ways hurricanes destroy property and injure people.
2. Describe how wetland preservation might help protect urban areas from tidal surges.
3. What is the role of a building code in protecting people from earthquakes?
4. Why is advance planning important for preventing injuries from natural disasters?
5. Who is most at risk from natural disasters such as heat waves?
6. What are Brownfields?

7. Why is maintenance of infrastructure important?
8. How can parks improve and protect health?

For More Information

Hooke, W. H., & Rogers, P. G. (Eds.) (2005). *Public health risks of disasters: Communication, infrastructure, and preparedness —workshop summary*. Washington, DC: National Academies Press.

Klinenberg, E. (2003). *Heat wave: A social autopsy of disaster in Chicago*. Chicago: University of Chicago Press.

National Research Council. (2003). *Preventing earthquake disasters: The grand challenge in earthquake engineering*. Washington, DC: National Academies Press.

Pan American Health Organization. (2000). *Natural disasters: Protecting the public's health*. Pan American Health Organization. http://www.paho.org/english/ped/sp575.htm.

Prevention Web. *Serving the infrastructure needs of the disaster preparedness community*. www.preventionweb.net.

ENVIRONMENTAL MEDIA

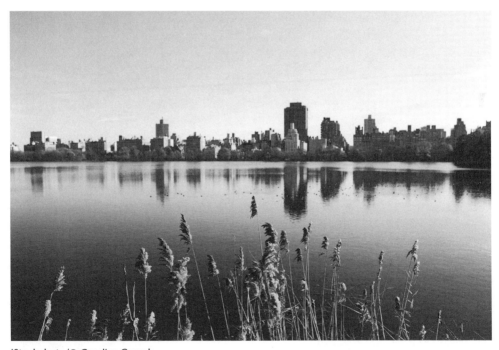

iStockphoto/© Candice Cusack

CHAPTER 7

INDOOR AND OUTDOOR AIR QUALITY

LEARNING OBJECTIVES

- Describe major trends in outdoor air quality.
- Discuss the association between land use and air quality.
- Describe the federal-state framework for maintaining air quality.
- Evaluate the ability of government regulation to ensure indoor air quality.
- Explain the different regulatory frameworks between criteria and noncriteria air pollutants.
- Discuss the biological pathway between particulate exposures and cardiovascular disease.
- Identify the strategy of preventing indoor air quality issues through ventilation, securing of building envelopes, and reducing use of hazardous building materials.

Take a deep breath and let it out. Do you ever worry about the air quality where you live? Does anyone you know have a problem with asthma or heart disease that gives you concerns about pollution levels near where they live? Furthermore, what can you do about it? What laws and regulations are there to protect you and your family's health? In this chapter, we will not just talk about federal policies to enhance air quality; we will explore ways in which the built environment influences patterns of pollution.

Overview

The pollutants in both indoor and outdoor air can have a substantial impact on health. Traditionally, environmental health scientists have described three main pathways that chemicals can enter the body: absorption, ingestion, and inhalation, and thus air exposures are an important pathway between toxins and health.[1] Because oxygen is vital to human life, the lungs have a tremendous surface area and have a very large capacity to absorb oxygen and pollutants. To protect health, the respiratory system has a system to defend itself from negative chemicals and compounds in the air. As will be seen, however, these protections can fail and the lungs, as well as the entire body, can be at risk from air pollution.

The built environment plays an important role in shaping the risks inherent in poor-quality air. Certain features may result in an increased production of pollutants. For example, land use patterns may encourage the use of cars and therefore contribute to the concentrations of volatile organic compounds and oxides of nitrogen in ambient air.[2] Other features of the built environment may play a role in concentrating pollutants or facilitating exposures as in the case of radon gas accumulating in certain dwelling units that are poorly ventilated and prone to the seepage of radon-containing groundwater. The role and implications of these factors varies from pollutant to pollutant. For an additional discussion on the effects of transportation-related air pollution, see Chapter Four.

Air Pollution Trends

With important exceptions, the outdoor air in many parts of the United States is cleaner that it was in the 1970s when the major anti–air pollution programs were first enacted. Overall levels of sulfur dioxide and oxides of nitrogen have been reduced, volatile organic compounds' concentrations are declining, and there are generally lower levels of particulates. Most of these reductions have come from restrictions on emissions from factories and power plants, the requirement of catalytic converters in cars, higher fuel efficiency standards, and other similar large-scale regulatory practices implemented on the federal level but sometimes administered by states and local authorities.[3] However, ozone levels in many parts of the country continue to be above standards set by the U.S. Environmental Protection Agency (EPA) and it may be that the improvements in particulate levels may not have been sufficient to protect health. In addition, ambient air may still have concentrations of toxics that may place significant health burdens on the general population as well as on susceptible populations. Another issue is that exposures to air pollution are not evenly or randomly distributed across the population. In general, Hispanics and blacks are more likely to live in areas with higher levels of air pollution than whites.[4] Furthermore, the Clean Air Act, as interpreted for most of the past twenty years, has not covered carbon dioxide emissions, which are a major threat because of global climate change; however, there have been recent efforts to bring the production of greenhouse gases into the purview of the act.[5] Though the overall air in the United States is cleaner, it may still not be clean enough to protect the public's health.

It is not clear how indoor air quality has changed over time because there has been no systematic monitoring of it. Some of the most dangerous contaminants, such as asbestos, are now banned, and education and mitigation efforts may have reduced some exposures to such dangers as radon gas. But the use of solvents and problematic building materials has continued and may have even increased. New design and construction methods, aimed to reduce energy and environmental impacts by sealing building leaks and reducing the amount of infiltration of outdoor air, may be contributing to a decline in indoor air quality because they can reduce the rate of exchange of outdoor air. Because the relative impacts and magnitude of these trends are not known, it is not possible to assess the change in the overall quality of indoor air in this country at this time.[6]

Land Use, the Built Environment, and Air Quality

As discussed in other chapters, there are close links between land use and health on both the local and regional level that operate through many pathways. These linkages represent one of the most important ways that the built environment affects health and can reinforce inequities in exposures and health between various demographic groups.

At the local level, highways and sources of air pollution can increase exposures in neighboring residential areas. As noted elsewhere, there is evidence that these land uses are disproportionately likely to be in low-income neighborhoods and communities of color. Low-density land use patterns associated with sprawl can also produce more automobile use, further burdening some communities and metropolitan areas.

Sprawl's effects on driving behavior help produce many of the regional impacts of the built environment on air quality. As noted elsewhere in this book, sprawl increases daily vehicle miles traveled, which then creates more of the pollutants associated with driving.

Regulatory Framework

There is a complex regulatory framework for both indoor and outdoor air. In general, the EPA has established air quality standards for a number of substances known as **criteria air pollutants**. These include carbon monoxide, particulates, volatile organic compounds, sulfur dioxide, ozone, and oxides of nitrogen.[7] Lead was on this list but as lead in gasoline has been phased out, it has become less of an air pollution issue except in certain locations near smelters and other similar local features. The federal government sets a standard for ambient air for these criteria air pollutants and requires states to meet these standards. Though many parts of the country remain out of compliance, especially for particulates and ozone, in general a locality has to make progress toward meeting the standards or it may face the loss of certain types of federal funds. To meet their obligations under the Clean Air Act, states and their local air quality authorities have used their permitting system and regulatory authority to reduce factory emissions, have addressed mobile sources such as ports and highways, and have even limited the use of wood burning in certain urban areas during certain weather conditions.[8] It should be noted that these permits and regulations may not result in what the neighbors of facilities believe to be adequate protection; in addition, many permitted heavy emitters of pollutants, such as oil refineries and smelters, continue to affect conditions in their surrounding communities. The distribution of these facilities has been questioned by environmental justice activists, who have concerns that they may be disproportionately burdened by them. In addition, large power plants have also been accused of spreading pollutants over a large geographic area.[9]

Indoor air is much less highly regulated and, with the exception of radon, there are few guidelines as to what would be clean and healthy indoor air.[10] Furthermore, states and the federal government are reluctant to monitor homes or assist homeowners in maintaining healthy indoor air quality because of concerns about privacy and the great expense it would take to test and mitigate these problems. In general, building codes provide some guidance as to allowable building materials, proper installation procedures, recommended rates of air exchange, and so forth, but these may not always be helpful to occupants of older buildings, single-family homes, or buildings that have significant health problems. There are standards for some occupational exposures to indoor air pollutants, but these are not necessarily relevant for office workers and residential exposures. For one thing, these standards are set for healthy workers and are not designed to take into account susceptible populations such as infants, children, and the elderly. Another problem is that they may be set to prevent acute effects, which often occur at different levels than what may be needed to prevent chronic effects. So a maximum eight-hour exposure standard for a workplace pollutant is not meant to address what would be a safe exposure over a lifetime for a population. As pointed out in other chapters, mold and indoor air are a particular issue in many low-income and minority households.

Health departments, with the exception of indoor tobacco use at worksites, generally do not become involved in air issues unless they are called in to investigate a problem in an individual building; ambient air is usually a responsibility of other municipal, county, or regional authorities.[11] This does not mean there is not a role for public health practitioners in combating air pollution issues. Most important, they can take the lead in educating the public about issues and how to reduce exposures. Urban planners can have a role in permitting local land uses (such as factories) or in establishing land use policies that might reduce ambient pollution levels, but they do not always make these decisions while taking air emissions into consideration.

Air Pollutants

As noted above, the built environment can affect both indoor and outdoor air. The effects in any given place are dependent upon the nature of the pollutants themselves. Some of the most important air pollutants are discussed below.

Particulates

A major problem with air quality is particulates (see Table 7.1). These go by various names including soot, smoke, and a taxonomy based on size (PM10, which is particulate matter less than 10 μ in size, PM2.5, and so on). Over time, science has increasingly concentrated on the health effects of smaller and smaller particles. To some extent, this is the result of the ability of the respiratory system to block or trap larger particles. The upper respiratory tract ensures that

Table 7.1 Source of Particulate Matter Pollution (PM2.5) 2005

Source Sector	Percent of Total Emissions
Electricity Generation	11.5%
Fertilizer & Livestock	0.0%
Fires	9.2%
Fossil Fuel Combustion	4.8%
Industrial Processes	12.1%
Miscellaneous	17.0%
Non Road Equipment	6.0%
On Road Vehicles	3.0%
Residential Wood Combustion	8.5%
Road Dust	21.5%
Solvent Use	0.2%
Waste Disposal	6.2%

Source: EPA

larger particles do not make it down to the alveoli where they can be absorbed or where they can cause inflammation. However, smaller particles, particularly those now known as ultrafine particles (PM2.5 or smaller), are not trapped in the nose, mouth, or upper respiratory system, and can go very deep into the lungs.[12] Particulates themselves are heterogeneous. In general, they tend to be predominantly carbon, with or without other chemicals absorbed by or on the surface of these particles; metals, silicates or other rock-based particulates; or very fine threads such as those composed of asbestos or the result of textile manufacturing. All of these can have profound health implications.[13]

Particulates can harm health in a number of ways.[14] They can cause inflammation, setting off a cascade of effects in the lungs that can result in asthma or other breathing problems. Over time, chronic inflammation can lead to other problems as lung tissues become damaged or modified. These can include asbestosis, chronic obstructive pulmonary disease, and other similar problems. Sometimes, inhalation exposures can lead to cancers, such as the case of the association between asbestos exposure and mesothelioma. Other problems occur when particulates and the chemicals associated with them are absorbed in the alveoli and then transmitted by the bloodstream to other organs. This can result in inflammation, tissue damage, or cancer in other organ systems.[15] As will be

FOCUS ON

Anti-Idling Campaigns

Bus depots and bus stations represent important sources of air pollution for surrounding communities. Though diesel fuels are cleaner than they once were and many buses now run on natural gas or other less polluting sources, these facilities continue to pose burdens in many communities, particularly those with high rates of asthma and other respiratory diseases. One factor exacerbating the health effects of buses is that many sit running while waiting to pick up passengers. Though some states have laws in place to prohibit idling, these are often ignored.

One response to the problem has been anti-idling campaigns, concerted efforts on the part of students or community members to educate bus drivers and operators about the health consequences of idling and the need to reduce idling in at-risk communities. Residents have distributed brochures, given out mock tickets, and called in the media to attract attention to this issue. The goal is to increase awareness among residents, empower youth and other community residents to work to make their environment cleaner, and reduce exposures to diesel particulates.[18]

discussed, the transport of particulates from the lungs to the heart can lead to severe cardiovascular problems.

Many particulates are produced by power plants or by diesel-burning engines. Increasing concerns about the health impacts of particulates has led to changes in the formulations of diesel fuels and changes in the design of diesel engines. These have reduced the amount of sulfur emissions as well as the amount of particulates produced.[16]

Exposures to particulates can be heavily affected by features of the built environment. For example, exhaust from ports and bus depots may have important health impacts on communities downwind from these facilities. Some communities, such as West Harlem in New York and neighborhoods near the Port of Los Angeles or along the highways serving the port, have argued that the use of diesel has negatively affected their health, and neighborhoods across the country have complained about diesel exhaust from highways.[17] Many of these issues are related to environmental justice concerns in that it has been suggested that these problems disproportionately impact low-income and minority communities.

Radon

Radon is a colorless and odorless gas that is naturally occurring in the Earth's crust, particularly in certain rocks such as granites. It is a radioactive gas that results from the decay of uranium that in the lungs can lead to increased risk of cancer, perhaps second only to tobacco as a cause of lung cancer. Because of the underlying geology and common types of building practices, certain parts of the country have a higher risk of exposure to radon gas than others and certain types of housing, such as units with basements, are more likely to have higher levels of radon in the air.[19]

The solution to a radon problem is to reduce exposures. In general, this is done by sealing leaks in basements because water can carry dissolved radon gas from source rocks into the building; and by ventilation, airing out basements so that the radon is dispersed into the ambient air rather than seeping into living areas.[20] The federal government sets standards as to how much radon in the air is safe, though it does not directly intervene in housing itself.[21] For the most part, it is up to individual property owners to measure how much radon they may have in their indoor air and to remedy any problems that are thus identified.[22] Because the primary effort against radon exposure is prevention, programs to reduce the impacts of radon should work to identify geographic areas that are at risk for radon exposure and to educate owners to test the air in the basements and living areas for radon in these communities. If unsafe levels are found, then it is important to work with property owners to take actions to mitigate the problem.[23]

Volatile Organic Compounds and Household Chemicals

A major class of air pollutants in ambient air as well as in indoor air in homes, schools, offices, and other buildings is volatile organic compounds (VOCs). These are a set of chemicals that have a wide range of sources and have a wide range of potential health effects. Outdoor sources of volatile organic compounds include gas stations, factories, and hazardous waste handlers. Indoors, they can include chemicals that off-gas from new carpets, furniture, and other consumer products; chemicals purposely brought into a building such as cleaning supplies and pesticides; or personal care products such as hairsprays and other similar products. Many of these result from solvents that are used in manufacturing processes or are used as vehicles for delivering a chemical or service.[24]

In outdoor air, volatile organic compounds are considered to be major air pollutants; releases are subject to regulatory processes and overall levels in the air are monitored. Indoor air, however, is typically not monitored and for many years the general consensus was that these indoor exposures did not have any important health consequences. However, research in the past few decades has produced evidence that these chemicals can lead to health problems, particularly for those who are sensitive to these chemicals and compounds.[25] For example, people with asthma may have an acute attack if they inhale commonly used cleaning products. Also important, biomonitoring of the population has revealed that many substances are ubiquitous in the U.S. population.[26] Sometimes, the presence of these chemicals that can lead to publicized problems such as **sick building syndrome** (discussed later in this chapter). The health effects of VOC off-gassing from construction materials can be mitigated by the proper phasing of construction (installation of these products before buildings are enclosed and sealed) or by temporary use of air filters immediately after installation. Ensuring adequate ventilation to prevent buildup of VOCs may assist as well.

In the absence of a regulatory framework to address these chemicals in indoor air and the statutory power to intervene when problems are identified, the primary tools to address the problems associated with exposures to volatile organic compounds in indoor air is to educate consumers, building designers, and building operations and maintenance staff regarding these issues with the goal of reducing exposures. Designers and construction personnel can be taught to consider less toxic alternatives to, and installation processes for, building materials that may have high toxic content such as certain types of furniture, carpeting, and finishes.[27] Manufacturers' guidelines for installation and use must be strictly followed—something very difficult to monitor—though it may also be worthwhile to enforce standards during the building process. Operations staff can be educated to understand the need for proper ventilation and less toxic cleaning materials. Consumers can also be targeted for education and the use of nontoxic alternatives stressed.

Asbestos

A major problem in many buildings constructed in the mid-twentieth century is asbestos. When it first became commonly used in buildings, asbestos appeared to solve many problems. It was cheap, easily mined, and easily manufactured into a wide range of products that included insulation and building materials.[28] It was a great insulator and, wrapped around pipes from air conditioning or heating units, it could prevent the loss of heat or cooling, reducing energy use and the cost of operating systems. It helped make central air and central heating possible and affordable. Very important, asbestos is nonflammable, does not burn or conduct heat, and thus served to reduce the danger of fire or burns. To make buildings safer, it was added to flooring, ceiling tiles, and other surfaces that might be at risk for fires.[29]

These advantages were eventually found to be accompanied by severe health risks. By the 1970s, the health problems of mesothelioma and asbestosis were well known and the accepted premise by the 1980s was that there is no safe level of exposure to asbestos (though only certain types of asbestos appear to be responsible for most of the health risks).[30] Touching or even ingesting asbestos is not a problem; it is the inhalation of these fibers that is problematic and thus well-sealed asbestos may not pose a health risk. But when pipe coverings or floor tiles are cut or worn, they have the potential to release fibers into the environment, harming health.[31]

The use of asbestos has been banned in most products and most exposures now result from exposures to older, decaying legacies of the asbestos era.[32] Public health solutions include monitoring of products that may have asbestos in them, insuring that these products are properly maintained, training of workers in how to safely remove asbestos, monitoring that safe removal practices are being followed, and safely disposing of asbestos-contaminated products. Asbestos should only be removed by trained professionals using approved methods and wearing appropriate protective equipment and it must be carefully disposed of in an authorized landfill. If asbestos is intact and covered, it should not be disturbed. But if it does pose a threat, safety precautions must be observed.[33] Though most of the public is not currently at risk of asbestos-related disease, its large-scale past use means that there will ultimately be billions of dollars spent on its removal and thousands of workers who remove and manage the disposal of asbestos will continue to be at risk of asbestos-related health problem.

Lead

The elimination of lead in gasoline and the resulting reduction in concentrations of lead in the air and in the bodies of most of the U.S. population represents one of the greatest public health triumphs in the last hundred years. Lead was added to gasoline to improve engine performance, but even at the time of its introduction it was known that lead was a serious health problem; several prominent deaths among gasoline refinery workers led to some of the earliest laws regulating lead in the United States. But well into the 1970s it was common practice to use leaded gasoline and it was almost impossible to find alternatives.[34]

The elimination of lead from gasoline was the by-product of another environmental policy, the requirement of catalytic converters. There was a pollution trade-off in the engines of cars. Running the engine hotter reduced the production of carbon monoxide and volatile organic compounds, but it increased the amount of ozone and oxides of nitrogen. Running the engine cooler reduced the amount of ozone and oxides of nitrogen but increased the production of carbon monoxide and volatile organic compounds. The solution was a catalytic converter, which allowed engines to run at a higher temperature but without pollution by-products. But lead interfered with the operation of the converters and destroyed them.[35] The solution was to eliminate lead from gas, which was no longer technically necessary anyway because of the discovery of alternative methods to improve engine performance.

The effects of taking lead out of gas have been dramatic. Blood lead levels in the general population dropped from a median level that was just under what would be seen to be actionable by our current standards to undetectable levels for the majority of the population. By 2000, most people had near zero levels of lead exposures unless they lived near a lead smelter or other source of lead, or drank water contaminated with lead. A major exception to this population-wide improvement in heath is inner-city children exposed to lead paint—another legacy of past uses (see Chapter Five).[36] The health consequences are great and because there is no safe exposure to lead, systematic reduction of blood lead levels probably has resulted in important increases in cognitive abilities throughout the U.S. population.

Carbon Monoxide

Ambient air levels of carbon monoxide are regulated because it is one of the criteria air pollutants. At the levels often found in outdoor air, carbon monoxide may cause cardiovascular or neurological problems and has been associated with increased hospital admission and higher mortality risks.[37] The primary sources of carbon monoxide in ambient air are motor vehicles and power plants. There has also been increasing awareness that carbon monoxide is a major threat in indoor air, but the federal government does not provide oversight of indoor air levels. Carbon monoxide is the result of incomplete combustion; instead of two oxygen atoms combining with each carbon atom that produces carbon dioxide, only one oxygen atom combines with each carbon atom. In indoor air this is usually the result of poorly operating or poorly vented heaters. Carbon monoxide is an odorless and colorless gas; occupants of buildings where there has been a buildup of carbon monoxide have no idea that their health is threatened. Carbon monoxide kills because it is selectively taken up by hemoglobin in the blood rather than oxygen, in effect suffocating its victims.

There are several ways to reduce the threat of carbon monoxide. One is to have properly functioning, properly vented heating equipment; ensuring this should include periodic inspections and testing of furnaces. Another way to protect health is to discourage the use of indoor combustion sources such as grills and space heaters. Many states and communities ban these indoor combustion sources, but many consumers continue to use them anyway. Thus there is a need for education, enforcement, and in the case of space heaters, making sure that there are alternative, safer methods of keeping people warm during the winter time. The third way to reduce the risks of carbon monoxide is to use carbon monoxide monitors and alarms.[38] These constantly monitor the amount of carbon dioxide in the air and they sound an alarm, alerting inhabitants if the amount of carbon monoxide rises above an unsafe level. These can be highly effective if they are properly maintained and serviced, but a major problem is that many people fail to install carbon monoxide alarms or they fail to keep them properly functioning.[39] Many communities require carbon monoxide alarms in all housing and checking that the alarms are properly functioning is a standard part of a housing inspection. In addition, many state and local jurisdictions are requiring that carbon monoxide monitors be hardwired into new residential construction rather than allowing the use of battery-powered detectors.

Hazardous Air Pollutants

In addition to the criteria air pollutants, there are other problematic contaminants in outdoor air that are present in concentrations that can potentially impact public health. Collectively called Hazardous Air Pollutants (HAPS) or air toxics, these include solvents such as benzene and toluene, metals including chromium, and complex mixtures. The federal government estimates that only about 20%

of the total concentration of HAPs results from large stationary sources such as factories and refineries. Just over 40% of the total concentration is the result of small local sources including pesticides applied to lawns, painting of cars and buildings, dry cleaners, and other similar types of operations and household uses. Just under 40% comes from mobile sources which include cars, buses, trucks, planes, and trains.[40] As with other air pollutants, HAPS are not randomly distributed. Exposures are greater in low-income and minority communities.[41]

Taken as individual pollutants, these HAPs may have a substantial impact on the public's health, particularly in urban areas and near places where there are concentrations of these contaminants. They may have important significance for cancer, respiratory effects, and neurological effects. Less well characterized are the combined effects of these very different pollutants. It is not known if collectively these pollutants increase the risks in synergistic manner or if they cancel each other out.[42] Little research has been done in this area.

These HAPs are regulated in a different manner than the criteria air pollutants. The federal government does not set a limit on these pollutants nor does it require monitoring at the local level. There are several types of solutions to reduce exposures to HAPs. One is through the federal and state permitting process that regulates the amount of chemicals that can be released into the air. Another strategy is to promote the use of alternatives so that industries reduce the quantity of chemicals they consume and thus limit their releases. This is part of a growing toxics use reduction movement. Similarly, educating the public so that they understand that their use of chemicals contributes to the overall burden of chemical exposure for everybody is important. Finally, there have been calls for increasing regulation of mobile sources, which include greater fuel efficiency for cars so that the release of toxics per mile driven declines, new regulations on buses and trucks to reduce their contribution to the air pollution, and similar programs.[43]

School Indoor Air

Children are particularly vulnerable to air quality problems because of their relatively high respiration rates, their ratio of lung capacity to body weight, and the vulnerability of developing respiratory systems. Second only to the time spent at home, time at school represents a large percentage of indoor hours, so the potential for problems related to school indoor air quality is important. School air quality varies greatly from location to location and school to school and may even vary by classroom within the school.[44] Many older schools lack proper ventilation systems, many schools have mold and volatile organic compound problems, and many schools may be close to highways or have classrooms close to places where buses idle.[45]

Given the special vulnerability of children to air contaminants and the necessity that they spend large amounts of time indoors at school, the U.S. EPA has developed a major program to assist local communities to address indoor air quality known as Tools for Schools. The program is voluntary, but it has been adopted by thousands of local communities who wish to improve their schools and protect the health of children. The program has identified several important steps, which include: organizing, assessing, creating a plan, taking actions, evaluating, and communicating.[46] Note that this program relies on local parental involvement in conjunction with the support of school personnel.

Environmental Tobacco Smoke

Environmental tobacco smoke is related to the built environment because most secondhand smoke exposures occur inside buildings, particularly residential and commercial buildings that lack proper ventilation. Smoking rates have declined substantially in the United States over the past several decades so that only about 20% of the U.S. adult population smokes today. One consequence of this improvement in smoking is that exposure to environmental tobacco smoke has substantially decreased as well.[47] These exposures can be measured by biomonitoring the county's population. For example, the National Health and Nutrition Examination Survey (NHANES) measures the amount of cotinine, a metabolite associated with exposure to tobacco smoke, in the blood. It found that the number of people with detectable cotinine levels has substantially dropped, but the percentage of nonsmokers who are exposed to tobacco smoke is not zero, which indicates there is an ongoing problem with exposure to tobacco smoke. One strategy to reduce exposures has been the banning of smoking in workplaces, particularly bars and restaurants. Data show that this substantially reduces exposures for nonsmokers (as well as reducing the prevalence of smoking itself).[48] An additional strategy has been to change social norms so that it is no longer acceptable to smoke near children or inside homes.[49] Again, there have been benefits of both reduced exposure of nonsmokers to tobacco smoke and the reduction in smoking itself.

Air Pollution–Associated Health Conditions

Some of the strongest links between the built environment and health are related to issues around air quality. The research in these areas is ongoing, but the health impacts associated with cardiovascular disease, asthma, and sick building syndrome are illustrative of how the built environment can shape health outcomes of air exposures.

Cardiovascular Disease

There has been growing concern that there is an association between exposure to air pollution and the risk of cardiovascular disease and sudden death. At first the evidence was only found in ecologic and time series studies that compared the overall levels of pollutants, particularly particulates, and mortality data from public data sources. The association also seemed to lack biological plausibility; it was not known how exposures in the lungs could lead to problems in the heart or the brain. Since that time, experiments on volunteers and other research have shown that very fine particulates can pass into the bloodstream to the lungs and travel throughout the body.[50] In the heart, for example, this can create inflammation, which can lead to malfunctions that can result in the health problems that were seen in epidemiological studies.[51] These findings are being used to call for greater controls on the sources of particulates, particularly power plants and diesel buses and trucks.[52] This also raises concerns about exposures for people living near highways and other major roadways.

The cardiovascular health consequences of particulates, ozone, and other air pollutants are profound. It has been suggested that particulates may be responsible for thousands of hospitalizations and deaths each year.[53] Exposure to air pollutants may also be a factor in infant mortality.[54] The economic cost of this is high as well. To the extent that exposure to particulates reflects features of the built environment (highways, ports, truck depots, and so on), this may be one of the essential ways in which the built environment affects health.[55] Similarly, the unequal exposure to air pollution based on race and income may be a factor that contributes to disparities in health.[56]

Asthma

A major disease for both children and adults with strong associations to the built environment and the pollutants found in substandard housing and areas with high levels of contaminants in the air, asthma is a complex disease with a poorly understood causation. Although the disease was described in ancient times, it was relatively rare until the past few decades and only reached epidemic proportions in the United States in the 1990s. It is important to consider that asthma is a chronic condition that affects people even when they are not displaying symptoms. A person with asthma tends to have ongoing sensitization, which is often symptomless but which can result in an acute episode. During an asthma attack, the lungs constrict and swell and a person with asthma has the characteristic symptoms of the disease: wheezing, coughing, and shortness of breath. Thus asthma causation is a combination of factors that are associated with this underlying chronic sensitivity and factors that set off acute episodes.

Separating out these factors is very difficult and therefore our understanding of asthma is still incomplete.[57] Among the factors that are associated with either increased sensitivity or an acute attack (or both) are tobacco smoke, certain chemical exposures, cockroach antigens, cat and other pet dander, mold, and air pollution. Many of these factors are associated with the built environment and the air quality both inside and outside of buildings. Poor housing is more likely to be infested with roaches and to have leaks from windows, roofs, or plumbing that can lead to mold. Many urban at-risk populations live near highways and other sources of ozone and particulates, two of the air pollutants most associated with asthma.[58] A major problem with asthma prevention is that these factors are ubiquitous in the lower-income inner-city neighborhoods that have the highest prevalence and greatest rates of hospitalization. This makes it difficult for people with asthma to avoid asthma triggers.

Asthma has a profound impact on health and is a major cause of hospitalization of children and a major cause of death. Though it can be controlled by medication, there is no cure. Modifying aspects of the built environment such as moving or closing bus depots, truck routes, and other sources of pollution may be one community-level intervention that can reduce the impact of asthma, but these tend to be political decisions. Also associated with asthma are poor housing quality and problems with indoor air in schools and day-care centers, particularly water leaks that can lead to mold or housing infested by roaches and other vermin.[59] Therefore, programs that address housing quality, including housing subsidies, integrated pest management, and code enforcement aimed at assisting low-income tenants reduce their exposure to known asthma triggers, can also reduce the threat of asthma. Finally, there can be education for individuals with asthma and their families, helping them to avoid exposure to tobacco and modify their personal environments (to the extent possible) to reduce asthma exacerbations.[60] Care must be taken, however, not to rely on these individual and family interventions while ignoring the potential large-scale contribution of housing and neighborhood factors that are beyond an individual's control.[61]

Community coalitions to address asthma issues at the neighborhood level have been implemented in a number of places. Through these programs there has been success in raising asthma awareness, addressing local pollution sources, and increasing the ability of communities to address multiple health threats. These coalitions can help individuals meet the burden of asthma.[62]

Sick Building Syndrome

In the past few decades, there has been an increasing recognition of a problem that at its most severe levels is known as sick building syndrome. People who live or work in certain buildings are afflicted with headaches, itchy watery eyes, upper respiratory symptoms, or other health problems. These problems have proved very difficult to study and remedy, but in general, they seem to be related to newer buildings that have inadequate ventilation and highly effective barriers against air infiltration along with building materials that contain solvents, adhesives, and other chemicals that are released into the air. They are also associated with older buildings that have issues with moisture and associated mold.[63]

Investigating structures that may have sick building syndrome is not easy because the range of potential indoor air pollutants is very large and often monitoring devices are very substance-specific and are not designed to measure the very many chemicals that may exist in indoor air. Which agency has jurisdiction over indoor air is often not clear. Sometimes the local health department will investigate, but in other situations, it is the local agency responsible for workplace health and safety that will have responsibility for office building issues (these agencies may not have the authority to assess residential problems). For the people living and working in these buildings, simply finding an expert to investigate the health problems can be frustrating.

Even if a problem is identified, it can be difficult to find a solution. Often the cause of the building users' symptoms is only hypothesized and it is not certain what is causing the health problems. Moving people out while the offending part of the structure is sealed or removed is expensive and may not be covered by insurance. Fixing the ventilation system to increase the amount of clean air or replacing building systems or building materials can be very expensive and time-consuming. Worse, there is no guarantee that these repairs or replacements will solve the problem.[64]

Ultimately, the solution to sick building syndrome is prevention: designing and constructing buildings so that they are not susceptible to a buildup of problematic chemicals and ensuring that the building envelope is waterproof. These are mandated by standard building codes and thus careful attention to these provisions may reduce the risk of problems. This may mean that the capacity of the ventilation system, particularly the amount of outside air that is drawn into the building, must be carefully calibrated. Though bringing in outside air can be expensive, particularly if it has to be heated or cooled, it is vitally necessary for the health and comfort of occupants, especially if the building has a higher grade of insulation, windows, and entry systems which reduce leaks.[65] Another part of prevention lies in the proper training of contractors in how to safely use potentially problematic chemicals so that they are not released into the environment. Finally, it is very important that hazardous chemicals be avoided. This may be difficult as designers and consumers may not have any choice in the products that are used in the construction and furnishing of a building or they may not have any knowledge of the chemicals used in these products. But ultimately the solution to the indoor air quality problem, as it is in many other environmental problems, is to reduce the reliance on problematic chemicals and products to begin with.[66] Proper maintenance is also essential.

Summary

Air quality in the United States is generally improving, but there are important exceptions including problems with radon, particulates, and air pollution associated with living near highways. Outdoor air is generally the responsibility of states, which are charged with complying with the mandates of the federal Clean Air Act. Indoor air is less well regulated and remains a major health concern, and both indoor and outdoor air have been associated with cardiovascular disease, asthma, and sick building syndrome.

Key Terms

Criteria air pollutants

Sick building syndrome

Discussion Questions

1. Describe some of the ways that land use is related to air quality.
2. Who regulates indoor air quality?
3. How do particulates impact human health?
4. What are the advantages of asbestos? What are its potential health effects?
5. Why was lead banned from gasoline? What were the health impacts of this ban?
6. How does radon get into indoor air? How might this be prevented?
7. What is asthma? How might air pollution exacerbate asthma problems?
8. What is sick building syndrome? How might it be prevented?

For More Information

California Air Resources Board. www.arb.ca.gov.
Environmental Protection Agency—Air and Radiation. www.epa.gov/air.

Environmental Protection Agency—Indoor Air. www.epa.gov/iaq/.
Health Effects Institute. www.healtheffects.org.
Indoor Air Quality—Tools for Schools. www.epa.gov/iaq/schools/.
Indoor Air Quality Association (IAQA). www.iaqa.org.
National Clearinghouse for Educational Facilities. www.edfacilities.org.

WATER

In a sense, water is democratic—everyone uses it, everyone depends on it. But that does not mean that everyone feels safe about the water they drink. Do you trust the water that comes out of the tap where you live? Any idea where that water comes from or whether there are chemical or biological agents in that water that might make you sick? Maybe you buy bottled water instead. Is that water any better? Think about the many ways people use water. Not only is it used for drinking, but also for cleaning, bathing, cooking, and landscaping. Many communities face threats to supply and quality, but what are some of the ways we can reduce the amount of water we consume?

Impact of Water on Health

Water and water quality have profound public health impacts because in addition to being essential for sustaining life, water is an important medium through which diseases are transmitted. Historically, waterborne diseases have been major killers and in many parts of the globe they remain so. These waterborne diseases can kill directly, as when cholera causes massive dehydration, or they can kill indirectly, as in the case of chronic diarrheal diseases that can weaken children and make them more vulnerable to other infections.[1] Clean and abundant water supplies have other important functions, including providing irrigation for agriculture and water to fight fires.

The growth of cities that began in the nineteenth century propelled extensive efforts to secure clean water supplies, cumulating in large-scale aqueduct projects moving water hundreds of miles. In our time, increasing understanding of the many ways diseases can slip through purification processes have prompted ever stricter methods to manage and process water. We are also becoming more aware of how chemical contamination can travel through the water system and affect health. As science has refined our knowledge of water and disease, and as we have grown to understand how our need for water can affect the environment, how we use and manage water has changed.[2]

Access to water is closely linked to the built environment. As noted in Chapter Two, developing clean water sources and providing sewer services posed large challenges well into the twentieth century.[3] Despite this progress, water and sewer infrastructure continues to have major impacts on health. In addition, water access can shape urban development and it has been posited that one reason that development patterns in the West differ from those in the South is that the former area is dry and water must be provided in order for land to be developable; the resulting need for piped-in water makes large lots uneconomical for services. In the latter area, new development can rely on wells, larger lot sizes are feasible, and sprawl can increase.[4]

This chapter begins with a discussion of the regulatory framework for clean water and clean drinking water. It then describes current standards for drinking water and sewer systems, followed by issues related to the safe drinking water and environmentally sensitive sewage discharge. The chapter concludes with two alternatives to conventional water and sewer system supplies: xeriscaping and composting toilets.

Regulatory Framework

The federal laws overseeing water and similar state laws reflect the history of water regulation in this country. In general, the Clean Drinking Water Act regulates water from the source to the consumer while the Clean Water Act regulates water that is discharged out to destination water bodies.[5] Though the federal government sets the standards for drinking water and the water quality of rivers, lakes, and near shore ocean waters, it is up to state and local governments to provide strategies for meeting these standards. To a certain extent this is effective, allowing municipal water providers to better comply with regulations and enabling sewage treatment facilities to concentrate on fulfilling

Table 8.1   Drinking Water—Selected Characteristics of Suppliers

Type of System	Number of Systems	Number of Customers (Millions)
Community Systems	11,671	204.1
Small or Very Small Systems	9,103	61.3
NonTransient Non-Community Systems (Schools, Office Buildings, etc.)	18,742	6.3
Transient Non-Community Water System (Gas Stations, Campgrounds, etc.)	84,159	13.6

Source: EPA

their responsibilities under the law.[6] But this is also an inefficient and confusing system because in many places one authority provides the drinking water, another authority is responsible for the collection and treatment of sewage and then discharges this treated water, while still another authority downstream then has to re-treat the water before sending it off to consumers (see Table 8.1). Furthermore, private companies may be responsible for distributing water from public water supplies, or an independent but publicly owned authority may be responsible for water delivery. More confusing, these patterns vary from place to place. This fragmented system is difficult to regulate and though in general water quality is high, important disease outbreaks can still occur.[7] In general, the Clean Drinking Water Act only applies to what are known as public water suppliers, companies or utilities that have more than a specified minimum number of customers.[8]

Infrastructure

A major goal of urban reform movements in the nineteenth century was to find ways to import clean and safe water into cities and get this water into the dwelling units of the poor. Some of the first efforts to purposely modify the built environment were laws passed in London that mandated that the private companies supplying water to the public had to access sources upriver from London because downstream water tended to be more polluted.[9] As the nineteenth century progressed, city after city began to implement large-scale public works projects that brought in water from distant secure reservoirs and connected buildings to these new supplies and to sewers.[10] By the mid-twentieth century, large-scale movement of water such as the California Water Project, which connected reservoirs in the northern part of the state with urban centers in the south, became common. The era of these large projects came to an end as more accessible water supplies became scarce, the environmental impacts of these water projects became clear, and the financial costs to tap distant water sources rose. Today, many localities rely on reducing local demand and reducing waste rather than trying to overcome the barriers posed by moving large amounts of water over large distances.

Just as important as the vision of clean water for drinking and other uses has been the treatment of sewage. Up until the nineteenth century, human wastes were often simply dumped into city streets where they remained until they were washed away by the rain or blown away by the wind. Though the Romans were famous for their sewers, much of this engineering skill had been lost by the Middle Ages. But with the growth of cities and the demand for better sanitation by the middle and upper classes, by the nineteenth century there was a renewed effort to build sewers. Part of this demand resulted from the introduction of running water into (upper-income) homes that resulted in a need to dispose of this contaminated water. London and similar cities had deployed storm sewers to drain away rainwater and homeowners with running water wanted to connect with the storm sewers rather than draining their waste into their backyards—which often resulted in contamination of lower floors in the building. But these new connections quickly overwhelmed the storm sewers, causing severe backups, which helped lead to the building of sanitary sewers that collected the waste from homes and businesses.[11] But the resulting systems then discharged untreated sewage into local surface water bodies, causing algae blooms, foul-smelling water, fish kills, and other small- and large-scale adverse environmental impacts. This was the situation in much of the developed world until well past the mid-twentieth century when regulations for the treatment of sewage became the norm. Today, few developed countries allow untreated sewage waste to be dumped directly into rivers, lakes, and bays, though it's quite common for rural areas to rely on septic systems that can leak sewage out into aquifers and beyond. In addition, many local areas remain out of compliance, resulting in ongoing water quality issues.

As with other types of infrastructure, the state of the water and sewer systems in the United States has been negatively affected by delayed maintenance, aging components, and difficulty in keeping up with increased demand and evolving standards. Despite the fact that almost all systems charge users fees and most receive public funding, the overall ability to meet the fiscal challenge of infrastructure remains constrained.[12]

The provision of clean water and the treatment of sewage represents an enormous health and environmental improvement and it has become a fundamental service of developed societies.[13] But as will be seen, the risks posed by contaminants in water continue. Despite these shortcomings, water and sewer systems represent a fundamental example of how the built environment has been used to promote health.

Drinking Water

The introduction of clean water for drinking has had a dramatic impact on the health of people in cities and the burden of infectious diseases has eventually receded so that most people in the United States do not worry about microbial contamination of their drinking water.[14] Along with rising incomes, clean water helped to dramatically improve longevity and reduce mortality. The improvements began even before chlorination became common and it was demonstrated that even the simple act of filtering the water was a major health advance. Over time, however, it has become clear that there are a large range of threats present in partially treated water and even in the last few decades, the standard set of practices used to ensure water cleanliness has become stricter.[15]

At first, public water supplies simply brought in untreated water from a relatively pristine source. This by itself helped to increase cleanliness and promote health improvements. Then filtration was introduced and disease rates plummeted. The next innovation was chlorination, the adding of chlorine gas to the water. Chlorination kills many, but not all, of the microorganisms that can cause disease and it has the advantage that its disinfection properties persist through the water distribution system so that if contamination occurs after the water leaves the purification plant, it remains safe to drink. However, after an outbreak of Cryptosporidium in Milwaukee in 1993 that sickened over 400,000 and may have killed dozens, it was clear that some disease-causing organisms could make it through the basic filtration and chlorination system.[16] Another process began to be adopted—**ozonation**, the forcing of ozone through water—because it had the advantage of killing other organisms that chlorination could not eliminate. However, ozonation has the drawback that it does not provide protection downpipe from the treatment plant; that is, the ozone quickly disperses and dissipates so that any downpipe contamination is not addressed. Therefore, it cannot totally replace chlorination by itself. The Milwaukee incident also demonstrated that it was vitally important to protect water supplies from contamination because it was found that the source of contamination of Milwaukee's water was farm animals who were pastured above the aquifer that fed the city's water supply; subsequently, new federal regulations called for preventing development around water sources and the covering of water supplies whenever possible. The goal is to prevent human and animal wastes and pollution from contaminating water.[17] Today, an ideal system is one that begins with the protection of the water source itself, uses a combination of ozonation and chlorination along with filtration to remove pathogens from the water, and provides continuous protection between the treatment plant and the consumer. The goal is that by providing multiple barriers and treatments, the risk of disease is reduced.

FOCUS ON

Bottled Water

In the 1990s, the United States saw a dramatic increase in the amount of bottled water consumed. The advantages of bottled water can be that it is convenient, safe, and relatively healthier than sugared soft drinks. Many consumers use bottled water at home because they do not trust the water that comes out of their faucets or their tap water may not taste good.[18] But over time, there have been some concerns about bottled water. For one thing, the water often comes from public water supplies and thus it is seen as an unnecessary alternative to public water. In response to this criticism, regulations now require that the source of the water be displayed on each bottle. However, it is not clear if this has been sufficient for consumers to know where their water has come from. Another criticism is that this water is very expensive, particularly when compared to the cost of public water, which is usually provided at the cost of pennies per gallon or less. In contrast, bottled water can cost several dollars per gallon.[19]

The past decade has also seen concerns about the environmental effects of bottled water. The plastic bottles themselves take energy to produce, the plastics involve the use of chemicals which may then leach into the water, the bottles are often exempt from recycling requirements and thus contribute to the solid waste stream, and the energy needed to move water from sources to consumers is wasteful.[20] There is also concern that the water is not fluoridated and thus lacks some of the benefits of drinking regular tap water.[21] In response, some environmental organizations and consumer groups have launched public relations campaigns against bottled water.[22] This issue is evolving.

Water Quality Monitoring

Just as critical as the engineering components of a safe drinking water supply system is the monitoring of water systems and the regulation of the providers.[23] The federal government mostly relies on states, local governments, and water providers themselves to monitor and maintain the safety of their systems. Much of the safety of the water supply rests on self-regulation, and this reliance grew in the first decade of the twenty-first century because of budget cutbacks and the thought that the private sector could adequately police itself. In looking back at the water system in the past decade, however, there are serious gaps in the regulatory system of our drinking water.[24] For one thing, many violations go unreported or if they are reported, a simple promise to remedy the situation is all that may be required of a water provider. The regulations themselves do not mandate continuous monitoring of every potential contaminant and a problem may go unidentified for quite some time. It should be noted that the 1993 Milwaukee outbreak was only identified after public health authorities noticed that local pharmacies had run out of antidiarrheal medicines.[25] The records of the water provider did indicate that there had been an increase in turbidity about the time of the outbreak, but the response at that time was simply to temporarily increase the amount of chlorine added to the water. Unfortunately, chlorine is ineffective against the Cryptosporidium oocysts and the epidemic grew.[26] The failure of monitoring protocols, along with inadequate infrastructure to prevent disease, can result in outbreaks.[27]

In addition, some systems seem to be in constant violation and yet the regulatory bodies have been unable to bring them into compliance. As a result, millions of U.S. residents have been drinking water that did not meet current standards for at least some time during the past decade.[28] Although there may have not been a widespread serious outbreak of disease since 2000 that we know about, some public water supply systems may be vulnerable.[29]

Water Recycling

Given the high cost of securing new water supplies, some cities, particularly those in arid areas, are turning their attention toward water recycling.[30] San Jose, California, has created a second water distribution system, called **graywater**, which takes water from its sewage treatment plant and delivers it to golf courses, college campuses, and parks. The water is used for irrigation, but not for drinking.[31] Orange County, California, has gone a step farther and is using what is referred to as toilet-to-tap water recycling with the water outflows from a sewage treatment plant added to other water sources and then delivered to consumers for drinking and other household uses. Both of these types of water recycling have raised concerns. The development of the parallel water distribution system may result in consumers unknowingly using recycled water for drinking. Though the local sewage treatment authorities maintain that the water is safe for drinking, there may still be a fear of drinking such water.[32] There is a similar problem for the toilet-to-tap system. Is the water safe to drink? And even if the water is safe, will consumers be willing to drink it? In either case, are there contaminants such as metals and pharmaceuticals that are passing through the treatment and drinking water systems and ending up being consumed by people? These are major questions as yet not fully answered.[33] However, it should be pointed out that water is already being recycled as communities downstream from the water discharge of one metropolitan area draw that water into their own water system.

Desalination

In certain areas it is so difficult to find freshwater sources that local water providers have turned to desalination to create a water source. Given the vast amounts of saltwater on this planet and the fact that a large percentage of humanity lives less than a hundred miles from an ocean or sea, saltwater is a very abundant potential source of drinking water.[34] However, the salts must be removed before the water is drinkable. A number of processes, such as reverse osmosis, have been developed to desalinize water. Unfortunately, these processes require a large amount of energy and thus have great environmental impacts and can be very expensive.[35] In the United States, only the Santa Barbara area of California relies on desalinization for its water supply.

Wastewater Treatment

The treatment of wastewater has evolved over time as well. In the past, wastewater was simply discharged untreated into rivers, lakes, or bays. This sometimes produced heavily polluted surface water bodies where fish and wildlife disappeared, recreation became impossible, and any downstream uses became problematic. The biological contaminants resulted in algae blooms, eutrophication, and the depletion of oxygen in the water that resulted in only anaerobic bacteria being able to survive. The water turned green, fish died, and the air reeked of hydrogen sulfide (the smell of rotten eggs).[36] Other consumer products such as detergents, particularly those that used phosphates, contaminated water bodies, often resulting in their being covered with foam.[37] Since there were no laws prohibiting the dumping of industrial wastes into the water, it was standard practice for industry to release heavy metals (such as lead, mercury, and cadmium), solvents (for example, trichloroethylene), and other hazardous chemicals (for example, PCBs) into the environment. Not only did these contaminate the water column, they also contaminated sediments (potentially leading to decades if not centuries of potential health risks) and could easily move up the food chain and threaten ecosystems and human health.[38]

At first, there was little regulation of what could be discharged into open waters, but the growing environmental movement that began in the 1960s produced calls for greater restrictions on sewage discharges. In the beginning, raw sewage was simply dumped into any convenient water body. The first stage of treatment is to use screens and filtration to eliminate larger contaminants in wastewater. Although this is effective in reducing some of the contaminants, the water is still substantially polluted with both organic matter and inorganic contaminants. It is now standard practice to provide secondary treatment, usually using microorganisms to consume organic matter in the wastewater. This reduces the risks of algae blooms and eutrophication, but because the wastewater can still have important amounts of nutrients, some wastewater treatment systems now use tertiary treatment methods that further eliminate nitrogen and phosphates from the water. Accompanying all of these treatments have been new regulations to reduce the inflow of contaminants into wastewater. Though some discharges of chemicals are still allowed under the current federal and state permit process, the release of many of the most dangerous chemicals and metals is now prohibited. Some of these regulations have been the result of findings that some pollutants can harm the microorganisms that are used for secondary treatment. Other regulations were implemented because of the serious environmental and health effects of the chemicals themselves.

There is a continuing problem in many areas with **combined sewer overflows**, situations where untreated sewage is diverted into the storm drain system during and just after heavy rains. Similarly, some sewer systems receive large influxes of rainwater which can stress their ability to treat effluent, sometimes leading to untreated discharges. Both of these situations can lead to contaminated surface and groundwater. The ultimate solution to this problem is costly: the complete separation of storm waters from waste streams along with special infrastructure to capture and store storm waters when necessary.[39] In the context of aging infrastructure and revenue limitations, these situations may be difficult to implement.

Sludge

A by-product of the sewage treatment process is sludge, the accumulated biological debris produced by the bacteria working on organic matter in the water; a well-functioning treatment system produces a fair amount of sludge which must be disposed of.[40] Some treatment authorities simply dump the sludge into landfills, but this adds to the burden on landfills and can be expensive. Some authorities heat the sludge to reduce its water content and thus reduce its bulk and weight, but this has led to concerns that this can produce air pollution as some chemicals in the sludge volatilize. Still other authorities have tried to sell sterilized sludge as fertilizer, but this raises concerns that there may be metals present in the sludge that can contaminate soils and food supplies.[41] Although there may be environmental benefits for the reuse of sludge, these concerns need to be addressed.

Chlorination By-Products

One of the benefits of using chlorination to purify water supplies is that the protective actions of chlorination persist. Chlorine is added at the drinking water treatment plant and it stays in the water and remains chemically active for several days. Thus the safety of the water persists as well. But there is a downside to this positive feature of chlorination. The chlorine can react with organic matter in the water and form what are known as chlorination by-products. These by-products have been implicated in certain cancers, such as those of the colon and bladder, and with increased risk of adverse pregnancy outcomes.[42] There is a trade-off: the more chlorine added to the water, the more effective it is in reducing the amount of disease-causing organisms, but the amount of chlorination by-products is increased. Reduce the chlorine and the amount of chlorination by-products is decreased, but the chance that biologically active pathogens can remain in the water increases. There are two ways that this trade-off can be reduced. One is to reduce the amount of organic matter in the water supply. This is done by protecting water sources, reducing the amount of animal and human waste that flow into reservoirs, and so forth. This results in less organic matter that can react with the chlorine. The second way this trade-off can be reduced is by the introduction of ozonation, which decreases the need for large amounts of chlorine. Chlorine is still necessary because ozonation does not persist and thus cannot protect downpipe contamination, but the lower chlorine levels result in a reduced amount of chlorine by-products as well.[43]

Lead in Drinking Water

For most of history, and until very recently in the United States, it was common to use lead to make pipes or to use it in solder; the word *plumbing* comes from the Latin word for lead. The result is that for many U.S. residents, one of the few remaining potential sources of lead in their household environment—now that leaded paint and gasoline have been banned—is the tap water that they use for drinking and cooking, and there have been instances where exposures from drinking water have been associated with elevated blood lead levels.[44] The U.S. EPA sets a maximum standard for the amount of lead allowable in water and local public water suppliers are required to annually sample a certain number of homes in their service area to help determine how much exposure to lead may be in the area. The results of the surveys must be reported to customers.[45]

Given that there is no safe exposure to lead, there are a number of ways to reduce exposures through this route. Water providers often manipulate the pH levels of their water system so as to reduce its corrosiveness and its ability to absorb lead from pipes and solder. Consumers can protect themselves by simply running tap water for a minute before using so that water that has accumulated in the pipes is replaced by fresh water, by never using hot water directly from the faucet for drinking or cooking, or by using filters.[46] All of these efforts may require education if they are to be effective.[47]

Pharmaceuticals in Drinking Water

Water treatment has many limitations and rarely does it produce an end product that is pristine and completely free from all contamination; most utilities don't take a final step of using a process such as reverse osmosis that can actually remove chemical contaminates from water. In most systems, the nonbiological contaminants in the water remain. One issue that has recently come to the attention of environmental health scientists has been the contamination of drinking water, and water in aquifers, rivers, streams, and lakes, with pharmaceuticals that have been excreted or disposed of by people and have then passed through the treated wastewater stream out into the environment. This is a recent problem because only in the past few years have scientists had the ability to detect these contaminants at the low levels at which they are typically found in water, but they probably have been there as long as the use of antibiotics and drugs themselves. Of particular concern is chemicals that have estrogenic properties, such as birth control pills and other similar hormone-mimicking chemicals. It is not known if the small amounts of these chemicals, which now have been found in at least trace amounts in almost all drinking water, have a biologically active presence. If they do, this could present a serious health threat. But at the present, the effects of pharmaceuticals in water supplies are unknown.[48]

There are several programs that could potentially reduce the amount of pharmaceuticals in water and the environment. One of the most important might be to educate consumers not to dispose of extra, unused, or no longer needed drugs down toilets or drains. It is not known to what extent this is a common practice but it is hypothesized that this is a major source of contamination. It could also be that the alternative of disposing of drugs in garbage might ultimately result in contamination of water supplies if these landfills leak. Public relations campaigns to educate consumers about the environmental effects of these practices may be one way to reduce them. Of course, changing consumer behavior also means providing alternatives and some have proposed that pharmacies should be required to accept discarded drugs so that they do not end up in the water supply. This most likely will necessitate regulation on either the state or federal level and also will take time and education to become fully effective.[49]

Overuse and Contamination of Aquifers

A serious problem in many places has been the overuse of **aquifers** either for drinking water or for irrigation. The water in many aquifers is the result of the accumulation of thousands of years of rainfall that has slowly produced a buildup of underground water and, in some places, current underground water supplies represent water stored during the ice ages. One problem for some aquifers is that the groundwater may be contaminated. Aquifers are very susceptible to pollution because almost any hazardous chemical used at the surface or charging area of the aquifer can percolate into the underground water supply or be moved there via rivers or long-range transport of chemicals. These chemicals can persist for many years in an aquifer because of the stable temperatures and lack of sunlight underground, or because of the stability of the contaminants themselves. When this water is then pumped up for use or the water from the aquifer is discharged into a surface water body, these contaminates can harm human or ecosystem health.[50] Another problem is that land can subside as water is pumped out of the underlying aquifer. This is the particular problem in places such as Mexico City where depleted aquifers have resulted in land subsiding ten feet or more.[51] As the land subsides, buildings can collapse and pipes break. Even if the land does not subside, if water tables fall, there can be serious effects on the buildings above them. Boston, Massachusetts, has seen buildings in several historical neighborhoods become at risk as falling water tables have exposed wooden pilings which then rot, a very expensive condition to remedy.[52] A final problem with the overuse of aquifers is that the aquifer could become so depleted that it becomes unable to provide water for farming and urban residents. For example, there have been concerns that the overpumped Ogallala aquifer, which parallels the Rocky Mountains under the Great Plains, could eventually cease to be a source of agricultural water because it is so heavily used.[53] This would threaten the agricultural viability of hundreds of thousands of acres over the aquifer.[54]

The solutions to these problems rely on the protection of the aquifer itself and careful monitoring and regulation of the amount of withdrawals from the aquifer. Protecting the aquifer means carefully regulating and limiting the use of chemicals at the land surface.[55] This includes monitoring chemical users so that leaks are avoided, educating consumers that they should avoid the use of pesticides and other harmful chemicals so that these do not leach down into the aquifer, and limiting the pumping of groundwater so that it is not depleted. This may even involve the importation of water and using it to recharge aquifers.

Reducing Residential Water Use

The ever-increasing cost of providing clean water has prompted communities to examine how they use water and to work with households to reduce water consumption.[56] One of the most important ways this is done has been to address all the various ways a typical household uses water (see Figure 8.1). In general, water is used for drinking, cooking, cleaning, sanitation, and landscaping.[57] One way that water use can be decreased is by requiring high-efficiency plumbing fixtures. These can include aeration devices on faucets and shower heads that provide strong water pressure even as they reduce the amount of water flow. There has been some consumer resistance against these devices because many of them are not as effective as they have promised. Also drinking and cooking often require a certain amount of water and thus consumers react to volume reductions by simply running the faucet longer. Another innovation has been low-flow toilets. Some of these have also proved to be ineffective, but in general they have been adopted in most parts of the United States and are now a standard part of the building code. Other efforts to reduce water consumption can include changing how water is priced. Many consumers do not see a bill or are not aware of their water consumption, but if they are informed of the cost of their water, consumption can decline.[58]

Outdoor watering is a major use of water and many communities have taken steps to limit either short- or long-term landscape watering. It is quite common during times of drought for local authorities to limit the amount of water

FIGURE 8.1   U.S. Indoor Water Use—1999

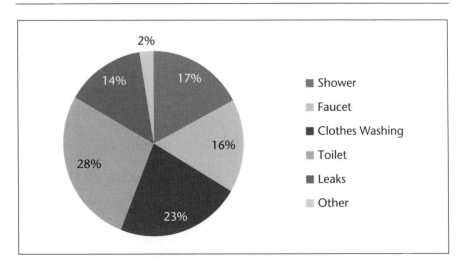

Source: American Water Works Association

households consume, specify the time of day that outdoor watering is allowed, or even prohibit all outdoor watering. The time-of-day restrictions are reflective of the fact that some of the water that is used to irrigate yards evaporates before it reaches plants and the amount of this evaporation can be reduced if watering is prohibited during the warmest parts of the day. These restrictions may not be well received by communities even if they are in the middle of a severe drought.[59]

Rather than waiting until a drought begins or lengthens, some communities have become proactive and are now requiring homeowners to put in landscaping that needs less water to maintain. Often called **xeriscaping**, this practice relies on groundcovers, such as cacti and succulents and other, often native, plants that simply do not need to be watered as much and can resist a dry spell.[60] The success of these requirements is often dependent upon educating consumers about the benefits of these alternatives.[61] See Chapter Sixteen for further discussion of this issue.

Reducing Leaks

Many water distribution systems are now approaching a century or more in age and are beginning to show the effects of time. Past installation practices may not have been as effective as they are today or many pipes may simply be approaching the end of their effective life span.[62] Some communities have found that a way to reduce waste in the system is to systematically look for and repair leaks.[63] Given that the consumption of water by end users is carefully metered and that the amount of water going into the system is also easy to know, it is fairly easy to identify how much water is going out versus how much water is being used, and it can be assumed that the difference is being lost to leaks. New technologies, including acoustic sensing, may detect leaks as well.[64] The ability to maintain the systems is predicated on the ability to have sufficient water rates to pay for a leak identification and repair system, but the benefits in reducing waste are great.[65]

Nonpoint Pollution

Though the disposal of raw sewage into water bodies is no longer permitted under the Clean Water Act, there are ongoing problems with sewage discharged from what are known as **nonpoint pollution sources**. Point pollution sources include the large outflow pipes from municipal systems and water treatment plants. Potential nonpoint sources include millions of septic systems that are spread across the rural and suburban landscape. Nonpoint sources include agriculture runoff, urban street runoff, and other sources that can pose potentially important environmental impact.[66] Many septic systems have been poorly maintained or poorly sited and over time they can allow raw sewage to seep through soils into aquifers, lakes, rivers, and bays. This can cause algae blooms, microbial contamination, and other problems.

The solutions to the problems posed by nonpoint pollution are not easy. Many septic systems are not regulated by existing federal and state law and the owners of these systems have little incentive to spend the money it takes to maintain or improve them. Some states, such as Massachusetts, have decided to bring certain of these systems into a regulatory system and property owners along waterways have been forced to spend tens of thousands of dollars either to connect to sewer systems or to substantially upgrade their septic systems. There have been some grants to make the process less financially painful, but improvements to water quality can come at the cost of great expense to property owners. Other areas have taken an educational approach, explaining to property owners how to maintain their systems and the consequences of a system failure.[67] Collectively, pollution from nonpoint sources continues to be a major national issue even though it often originates on a very local geographic scope.[68]

Composting Toilets

Rather than depend on expensive large-scale infrastructure projects, some have suggested that the way to address the waste disposal problem is to use small-scale technologies and have proposed innovations that include what are known as composting toilets. These are different from the traditional septic/leaching field systems that have been found to cause problems associated with nonpoint water pollution. Instead, these self-contained units accept a variety of organic waste, including wood scraps, discarded food, grass clippings, and other similar household wastes and promote the use of aerobic bacteria to convert this waste into benign compost.[69] They tend to need careful monitoring of their temperature and air supply to maximize the ability of the bacteria to consume the waste and minimize the potential for foul odors or accidental discharges.[70] The resulting compost is as clean as, if not cleaner than, what is produced by conventional waste systems and can be used to fertilize gardens and lawns.[71] There are number of composting toilets now on the market and there has been some thought that these might ultimately and collectively replace the need for expensive large-scale sewer projects.

The acceptance of these alternatives has been uneven, however. Some localities prohibit them and require that all buildings be connected to the available sewer system.[72] There has been some greater acceptance of these systems in places where sewers do not exist. But even in these locations, it may be necessary to convince the local building and health department that composting toilets are an acceptable alternative. It may be that there is a need for consumer education to make these alternatives more highly used.

Summary

Water quality falls under the federal Clean Drinking Water and Clean Water Acts, but its maintenance is mostly the responsibility of local water providers. A well-designed water system includes the protection of water supplies and aquifers, filtration, chlorination, ozonation, and constant vigilance and monitoring. Given the scarcity of water in many areas, some communities have turned to desalinization and water recycling. Others are trying to reduce water use through programs to address leaks and promote xeriscaping.

Key Terms

Aquifer

Combined sewer overflow

Graywater

Nonpoint pollution sources

Ozonation

Xeriscaping

Discussion Questions

1. What are the two main federal laws governing water?
2. Name the features of a state-of-the-art drinking water system.
3. Who is responsible for the day-to-day monitoring of water quality?
4. What are the concerns with water recycling and desalinization?
5. What are chlorination byproducts? Why are they public health concerns?
6. How do pharmaceuticals end up in drinking water? What can be done to protect drinking water?
7. Name some of the problems associated with overuse of aquifers.
8. What are composting toilets? What are some of the barriers to their being used more?

For More Information

American Rivers. www.americanrivers.org.
Clean Water Action. www.cleanwateraction.org.
Environmental Protection Agency—Water. www.water.epa.gov.
National Association of Clean Water Agencies. www.nacwa.org.
National Resources Defense Council. www.nrdc.org/water.
Xeriscaping: Creative Landscaping. www.ext.colostate.edu/pubs/garden/07228.html.

CHAPTER 9

FOOD, NUTRITION, AND FOOD SECURITY

LEARNING OBJECTIVES

- Describe the role of the built environment in food safety.
- Define food insecurity.
- Describe the major programs and policies to assist households and individuals to access food.
- Define a food desert.
- List the health and environmental impacts of factory farming and large-scale livestock operations.
- Explain how locavorism may have environmental benefits.
- Discuss the impacts of urban gardening.

Let's think about where you get the food you eat. Consider all the places you buy food, including restaurants, school, work, and the stores where you purchase groceries. Can you buy the elements of a healthy diet in the neighborhood you live in? How far would you have to travel to buy fresh produce? In addition, do you know anything about where and how your food was grown or how far it traveled to get to your plate? As we will discuss, these questions are all associated with the environment. The built environment helps shape what you eat and contributes to your health.

Because of the influence of physical activity on obesity, many researchers of the health impacts of the built environment have focused on this side of the food consumption: the physical activity and energy balance equation. Many of the built environment's effects on physical activity are discussed in other chapters in this book, but weight gain is a function of both calories expended and calories consumed; a comprehensive program to address obesity must also include the food we eat.[1] In this chapter we will discuss how the built environment affects food consumption. It will cover topics ranging from the built environment's influences on food quality and the food distribution system to concerns regarding some communities' lack of access to nutritious food. This chapter also discusses food assistance programs because of how they help make food more affordable.

The initial focus on the consumption side of the obesity equation had been on how to get people to eat less and make healthier food choices. Toward that end, there have been studies of diets and the design of individual-level interventions that explore or attempt to modify how people consume calories. But an environmental perspective on nutrition looks at how the built and social environment may support or hinder healthy eating or assist consumers to limit themselves to the appropriate number of calories to maintain a healthy weight.[2] Eventually, this interest has expanded to include the environmental impacts of food production itself and the impacts of promoting food production inside urban areas. Thus the study of the built environment includes issues of production, safety, distribution, sources, and the types of food that are available to consumers. Many of the efforts to modify the built environment to address food issues and obesity center on increasing access to nutritional food, reducing the environmental impacts of food production and distribution, and improving the affordability of food.

A major success of the global food system at the beginning of the twenty-first century is that for the most part, we have reduced the risk of famine in the developed world, at least as it relates to large-scale, acute episodes of life-threatening hunger.[3] With the exception of countries that are undergoing large-scale disruption from war, repression, and unrest, the kind of famines seen throughout much of recorded history, and in many places in the nineteenth and twentieth centuries, have been eliminated. But even as large-scale agriculture and food production and the long-distance movement of foodstuffs have solved the problem of famine, it has exposed continuing problems of hunger and food insecurity that have profound impacts on people's lives and health. In addition, there are ongoing concerns about the environmental effects of food production and the quality and safety of the food supply.

Foodborne Illnesses

A major ongoing health problem in the United States is that of foodborne illnesses. Because of a food infrastructure that can move foodstuffs across thousands of miles, foodborne illnesses are not local to any one place or time but can strike anywhere, at almost anyone. Thus foodborne illnesses are relevant to the subject of this book because many of the sources of contamination are associated with features of the built environment: contamination from point and nonpoint pollution sources, a distribution system that uses packing plants and processing centers, and local food environments that are dependent on national and international movement of food supplies. Each of these parts of the food-producing infrastructure can introduce contamination and disease. Indeed, the very large-scale movement of food has made it possible for a single incident to sicken people thousands of miles away.[4] In the United States, there have been periodic outbreaks of disease associated with *E. coli*, salmonella, and other organisms in the food supply. At first, it was thought that these illnesses were only related to meat consumption, particularly chicken and hamburger and other highly processed meat and poultry products.[5] There have been repeated outbreaks of illnesses and deaths caused by contaminated meat from individual processing plants that, because of a widespread distribution system, can affect multiple states.[6] In the past ten years it has also been revealed that outbreaks could arise from produce as well as meat; for example, contamination of spinach from a grower in California resulting in deaths across a dozen states.[7] The CDC estimates that there are 76 million annual cases of foodborne illnesses, resulting in 325,000 hospitalizations and 5,000 deaths, though the percentage attributable to food production and distribution practices is not clear.[8]

Most food-related illnesses are not reported because if an individual becomes sick they may not seek medical attention or the doctor may not diagnose illness in such a way that the food supply is suspected. Perhaps it is only the most extreme cases and outbreaks, when vulnerable populations such as children are affected or when otherwise healthy people become very ill and become hospitalized, that these problems come to light.

Efforts to prevent these outbreaks have not been totally effective.[9] For example, it is extremely hard for consumers to protect themselves because these organisms can be in food yet be undetectable by the naked eye. Even so, many do not even take precautions that are within their power that might prevent some illnesses. For example, consumers are advised to cook hamburger and poultry until internal temperatures are sufficiently high that microorganisms are destroyed, but surveys suggest that these recommendations are not always followed.[10] Nor would these recommendations protect consumers against infected produce that is consumed raw. Perhaps if consumer demand for greater protection of the food supply could be translated into political action and programmatic and legal policies to change how food is produced and distributed, this problem might be reduced. Local and state health departments can do little more than monitor outbreaks and issue warnings once an outbreak is detected, thus providing little primary prevention to the public.

The federal government, which ultimately has the greatest potential power to protect the food supply because of its ability to regulate interstate commerce, lacks the resources to closely monitor the hundreds of thousands or more farmers, producers, distributors, and retailers of food so that outbreaks can be prevented or identified in advance of serious illness. The testing of samples is limited and may not be sufficient to protect the food supply and tightening regulations can be politically difficult and expensive to comply with.[11] Though the frequency of disease outbreaks could be reduced by more effective regulation, it is not certain that they could be entirely eliminated.[12] As will be seen, although there are alternatives to the current global system of large-scale agriculture, these alternatives are not yet capable of replacing the industrialized food system on which most developed nations and particularly the United States rely. Built environment–related solutions include better sanitation in rural and semirural communities, cleaner processing plant standards, creating linkages between communities and local food producers, facilitating community gardens, and so on.

Food Insecurity

Even though the risk of famine has been substantially eliminated in the world, there is still the ongoing problem of food affordability and insecurity. In other countries, particularly developing nations, there are billions of people who are extremely poor and for whom securing food is an ongoing struggle. But even in the United States there are many who cannot afford to purchase food. In an effort to meet the challenges of household budgets and the cost of food, parents may go without food to provide for their children, meals may be reduced in size, or cheaper, less nutritious but high-calorie foods may be substituted for healthy foods.[13]

This food insecurity results from the inability of households to meet other costs and still purchase food.[14] Over the past several decades, the relative cost of food has declined from what once represented approximately 25% of household income in the 1960s to what is now usually less than 10% even for many of those who have lower incomes. However, other expenses have risen so greatly that households are sometimes forced to reduce their purchases of food. One of these rising costs is that of renting or owning a home.[15] In the 1960s, it was thought that a household should spend no more than 25% of its income on rent or home ownership costs. By the beginning of the twenty-first century, however, it was not uncommon for households, particularly low- and middle-income households, to spend more than 50% of their total income on housing. As a result of the scarcity of low-income housing, health can be affected by the inability to afford food. The high rate of inflation in medical costs has also put stresses on families' ability to afford food (see Figure 9.1). Data from national surveys suggest that

FIGURE 9.1   Percentage of Households with Food Insecurity
Among Children

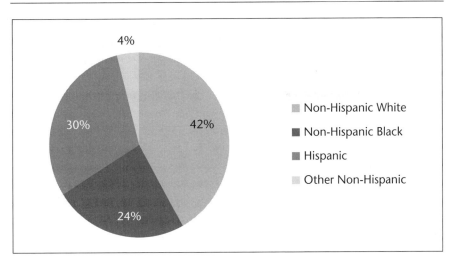

Source: USDA

as many as 10% of U.S. households may experience food insecurity at some point during a given year. Low-income, under- and unemployed persons, and persons of color are the most likely to report being food insecure. These are also the groups most likely to suffer from obesity. Communities with elevated rates of food insecurity tend to be those facing other health and environmental issues: inner-city neighborhoods and rural areas.[16]

The health effects of food insecurity are becoming increasingly clear. Individuals and households that are food insecure are at higher risk for obesity, poor diet, hypertension, and other illnesses.[17] This may be a result of a complex set of behaviors and perhaps physiological changes that can accompany hunger. Addressing food security and its underlying social and economic issues is vital if we are to address obesity.[18] Some of the food-insecurity solutions related to the built environment include creating more affordable food options in at-risk neighborhoods, addressing unaffordable housing, and developing connections between high-risk communities and food sources.

Nutritional Subsidy Programs

The main U.S. program to meet the challenges of food insecurity has been the federally funded food stamp program, formally called the Supplemental

Nutritional Assistance Program (SNAP).[19] SNAP is administered by the states and each state has its own application process. Eligibility guidelines are set by the federal government and include an assessment of household assets, total household income and size, and any special circumstances that may affect the ability to purchase food. A major problem with this program has been getting those eligible to receive food stamps to actually apply for and use them. Many are not aware of the program and many are reluctant to use the program because of the associated stigma or because they fear government scrutiny.[20] States have tried publicizing the programs, linking applications for food stamps to applications for other assistance programs, and streamlining the use of the program at food stores by replacing the old stamp system with a system that resembles a credit card. The program has also been extended so that it can be used at farmers markets.[21]

Another major program to assist those in need of adequate nutritious food is the women, infant, and children program known as WIC.[22] It is open to women during pregnancy and for up to one more year if breast-feeding, to infants up to their first birthday and children under the age of five. Again there are income-based and situation-based eligibility requirements and the program is administered by the states and funded by the federal government.[23] There are similar problems in encouraging those eligible for the program to sign up for it.

Food Pantries and Emergency Food Assistance

Despite public funding of nutritional programs and outreach efforts to those who are in need and eligible to participate in these programs, many families still find themselves without food.[24] To help alleviate this problem, a private nonprofit network of food pantries and emergency food assistance programs has been established across the country.[25] Many of these are based in churches and other faith-based institutions, and others have been established to serve special populations such as those who do not speak English. In many metropolitan areas, there are special organizations that work to receive donations of food and money to channel to the individual food pantries.[26] These local, regional, and national networks of food pantries are now a critical part of the United States' food infrastructure and represent one way the built environment has been modified by nongovernmental organizations to meet the needs of at-risk people.

Collectively, these organizations and the many volunteers and donors who support them have done major work to address the problem of poverty and food insecurity in this country. However, during times of recession or economic problems, it is not clear that they can entirely help the communities most at risk, and even during good times such organizations can only supplement but not eliminate the need for WIC, SNAP, and other food assistance programs.[27]

Subsidized and Free Student Lunches

Poverty in the United States is strongly associated with age, and children are much more likely to be poor than any other age group. Therefore, one way to meet the challenges posed by poverty was to use the country's public school system to improve the diets and health of children. Beginning in the 1960s, the United States Department of Agriculture introduced the subsidized lunch program, which by the year 2006 provided free or subsidized lunches to over 30,000,000 students in over 100,000 schools each day and in many districts has been extended into the summer vacation period so that students do not suffer from hunger or malnutrition when school is out.[28]

Children, particularly elementary students, are highly dependent on what their schools offer for meals and snacks. In a sense, school food offerings represent a significant part of a child's food environment and the quality of school-based meals is therefore critical to health. The program has been criticized for the low nutritional quality of its offerings that too often are high in sugar, salt, and fat, and low in vegetables and fruits.[29] There has been a movement to require school districts to provide more nutritious servings and reduce their nonnutritious offerings, and over time it appears that the nutritional quality of the offerings has improved, though there is much work yet to be done.

One of the problems with the program is that it can be difficult for parents to influence the offerings in school meals. Some schools do not believe it is their responsibility to promote healthy eating behaviors, for example.[30] At other schools, though school personnel might be interested in improving the quality of menus, the schools themselves are under tremendous pressure to improve academic performance, create safe environments for learning, and address other educational and social issues so that they may lack the ability to respond to parent requests for improvements in menus. Another problem is that the subsidies that go to schools to provide meals are not generous and nutritious foods may be more expensive and beyond the budgets available for school lunches. A final problem may be simply that no one is monitoring the situation and thus no one is aware of the nutritional status of a school menus.[31]

Rather than address issues regarding the quality of school meal offerings on a school-by-school or district-by-district basis, some advocates have begun to press for change by targeting state and federal governments. The federal government has the ability to regulate school offerings because it subsidizes much of the cost of these meals and there may be some movement at the federal level to require better offerings at schools. State governments have traditionally set education policy; thus they have a long-established ability to set guidelines for local schools. Promoting new state or federal regulations requires coalition building and partnerships between health professionals, education advocates, and parents.[32] See Chapter Fifteen for a discussion of additional school-based anti-obesity efforts.

Farm to School Programs

One way to improve nutritional offerings and boost local economies at the same time is to require the purchase of locally grown produce for use in school cafeterias. This has the advantage of providing fresher produce, supporting local farmers, and strengthening ties between communities and schools. These programs link local providers of produce directly to school food providers and are an alternative to cafeterias serving food grown and processed elsewhere. Farmers benefit from having local, secure contracts, and the built environment benefits from the way these programs might stabilize farming on metropolitan peripheries.

These programs are designed to connect schools with local farmers and have the goals of providing more nutritious offerings in the schools as well as promoting local agriculture.[33] Preliminary results of the programs suggest that they are having profound effects on school diets, as students like these new, more nutritious offerings. Such programs may also have positive benefits for the local economy.[34]

School Vending Machines

Given the high rate of childhood obesity in the United States, attention has turned to how young people purchase food and the kinds and quality of food offerings that are available to them.[35] Accompanying this reassessment has been a major focus on changing the school food environment for young people. This has led to a concern regarding the offerings in vending machines in many schools. Too often these are limited to chips, candy, sugared sodas, and other unhealthy snacks.[36] Thus there have been efforts in many places to change what is available in these machines so that students are provided with nutritional alternatives alongside the traditional offerings, or more effectively, so that the non-nutritious offerings are eliminated altogether.[37] The underlying goal is to modify the in-school food environment, that is, removing vending machines to promote healthier eating.

One problem that has emerged is that many schools depend on the income from these vending machines to support both day-to-day and extracurricular activities and many schools have signed long-term contracts with vending machine companies that may limit the ability of schools to modify the offerings.[38] However, experience has shown that when the offerings in these machines are changed or limited to nutritious items such as granola and fruit juices, sales volumes are maintained. The mechanics of how to implement such programs are still being perfected and there is debate as to whether the nutrition offerings in school vending machines should be addressed at the school, district, state, or federal level.[39] Public health departments on the state and local level have often taken the lead in implementing these programs to modify what is offered in school vending machines. It is important that such efforts educate children, involve parents, engage school authorities, enlist the support of politicians, and work with vending machine suppliers.[40]

School Gardens

Another growing movement in the United States is an effort to establish gardens in schools. Among the benefits of these programs are that students can learn how food is produced, gardening-related activities can be used to teach other subjects such as math and writing, the programs are an effective way to renovate outdoor spaces at schools, and the produce grown in the school garden can be used to make school lunches and breakfasts more nutritious.[41] It appears that these programs are very popular, as they improve the overall school environment and can help connect schools with their surrounding neighborhoods.[42]

Food Deserts

The food offerings available in a community represent one of the major pathways that the built environment affects obesity risk and health.[43] Consumers reside at the long end of a distribution chain that begins at farms possibly thousands of miles away, utilizes a large number of intermediary companies to package and process food, and finally ends at the places where consumers buy the food itself. But the kinds of food available for purchase in any given locale are highly varied. Some communities, particularly those in affluent suburbs, have a wide variety of food-buying choices that include large supermarkets and specialty food stores, all accessible to anyone with sufficient income and a car. Other communities, particularly minority and low-income inner-city neighborhoods and low-density rural areas, do not have either of these food options.[44] In fact, some communities appear to have almost no sources from which an individual or family can assemble a healthy meal. Surveying the food landscape of fast-food restaurants, corner convenience stores, and a dearth of supermarkets, some have called these areas *food deserts*.[45] In other words, there is no nutritious food to be had.[46]

It should be noted that the very existence of these food deserts has been debated. Their definition is dependent on assumptions of how far a person will travel to purchase food and also on the assumption that if there is a supermarket or other source of quality food in a community, local residents can afford to purchase higher-quality diets.[47] These are also most likely a function of access to automobiles and the walkability of a neighborhood, which can vary from place to place. For example, in a high-density community such as New York City, the assumption is that a supermarket should be within 5–10 blocks of a person's home if it is to be accessible.[48] Other less dense communities may use a metric that is much larger, again being highly related to whether or not a household has access to a car. In certain communities, the problem of food deserts is quite clear: in Detroit, a city of nearly a million people, there is not a single chain grocery store in the city.[49] In other communities the grocery stores exist, but they are in locations on the edge of neighborhoods, not inside them. There is no standard definition of a food desert; it must be defined based on local conditions and local assessments as to what constitutes an accessible quality food source.

The existence of a food desert is critical because without a source of healthy food, residents often turn to fast food or highly processed foods purchased in liquor stores and convenience stores, which provide calories but relatively little nutrition; in addition, patronizing such places is highly associated with weight gain and obesity. It is very difficult for small stores to provide fresh produce, for example, because they may lack the space for the proper refrigeration of produce and their volumes may be small so that their prices are high and the quality is low. Thus residents of food deserts have no alternative sources and may have no ability to eat healthy meals, control their weight, and protect their health. In such communities, many people may be at increased risk for obesity, diabetes, and hypertension. So the health effects of living in a food desert may be severe. For example, a study of adults in eastern Massachusetts found that having a supermarket in one's zip code was associated with a 10% decrease in obesity risk after controlling for individual factors including age, sex, smoking, income, education, and other neighborhood factors such as median income and the percentage of black residents.[50]

Communities have tried a variety of programs to address food deserts. One model that dates back to the 1960s is to subsidize the development of supermarkets by local but inexperienced entrepreneurs. There have been mixed results. Many stores were severely undercapitalized or managed by inexperienced operators, which led to problems. Eventually, maintenance and quality suffered, setting the store into a downward spiral that eventually led to the store closing. Somewhat more successful has been the Boston experience of working with large chain grocery stores. These chains have management experience, have the ability to negotiate for low prices from suppliers, and can find profits in their high volume of sales.[51] Although the problem of location has not been totally solved by this strategy, the program has resulted in a number of large grocery stores opening across the city. There has been legislation proposed at the federal level to provide subsidies to promote the development of supermarkets in at-risk communities.

Another strategy, an alternative to programs that rely on attracting big corporate chains into cities, has been to work with small stores to get them to improve the quality of their offerings.[52] Many small corner stores offer little more than snack foods, canned goods, soft drinks, and candy. They tend to sell cigarettes and foods that are high in calories and salt, two items that communities with high rates of obesity and hypertension do not need. To address this problem, communities have tried to work with small store owners to help them develop strategies that will enable them to provide healthier options.[53] These programs include education to the store owners and subsidies for buying equipment they may need to store and sell fruits and vegetables.

A related idea is to work with consumers, particularly young people, who often patronize these places. By teaching consumers about the health and weight consequences of buying certain items such as chips and sodas, the goal is to make participants healthier and to help shape the offerings in small stores by influencing demand. In a sense, these programs aim to help people cope with a built environment that is posing problems for healthy living. A subset of these programs rely on peer education, using young people to engage and educate other young people. Empowering young people to use their own words to educate each other may lead to greater understanding of health issues that affect them and a willingness to change their behaviors to protect their health. These programs also have the benefit of providing skills to peer educators and increasing social capital.

Still another approach, famously proposed in South Central Los Angeles, has been to ban fast-food restaurants. The rationale behind this effort is that given the tremendous health and obesity problems associated with the offerings of fast-food restaurants, these restaurants establishments are as bad for human health as hazardous waste facilities or noxious factories. Thus it would be an appropriate use of zoning power to ban them altogether.[54] There is some evidence that low-income and minority communities are more likely to house these kinds of restaurants, that these restaurants are more likely to be near schools, and that people who patronize fast-food restaurants have higher rates of obesity.[55] Hence the movement to ban or limit them; however, implementing such ordinances may not be easy. For example, these restaurants are often the only ones available in a community and they are particularly attractive to residents who are working long hours at multiple jobs or to young people traveling to and from school. It is not certain that the public health underpinning of the zoning code provides the legal justification for banning fast-food restaurants, nor is it yet known if these bans actually result in better eating habits and reduce obesity rates. It is also not clear how the public will react to such programs. Decisions must weigh the goal

FOCUS ON

Detroit and Urban Agriculture

The large-scale population decline in Detroit, Michigan, which has seen its population decrease by 50% since its peak in the 1950s, has created large tracts of vacant land. A critical issue for residents and government officials in the city is how to manage this land and how to plan for its eventually reuse. Vacant urban properties are at risk of becoming crime magnets and their lack of economic activity means that these parcels do not generate tax revenues to the city. Many of these parcels are now owned by the city because their owners have stopped paying property taxes.

One proposal has been to consolidate vacant parcels and lease or sell them to farmers who could grow produce for local consumption, or use the land for commercial agriculture ventures. Detroit is a classic food desert with no large grocery chains in the city and relatively few options for residents to access healthy food choices in the city. By encouraging agriculture, the city might help address this problem.

There are several concerns. One is that much of the land might be contaminated by lead from abandoned or demolished housing or unknown materials left by illegal dumpers. Another problem is that abandonment has not been clustered (though some neighborhoods have been more severely affected than others) and creating large parcels would require relocation of some residents. Another issue is that land tenure may not be certain for every parcel, as some lots are still in the foreclosure process and others are still privately owned.

Despite these problems, a network of community advocates, environmentalists, and those concerned with the nutritional needs of the city have emerged as advocates for the encouragement of agriculture in Detroit.

of improving health with the concern of infringing on local property rights. See Chapter Fifteen for an additional discussion of this issue.

Environmental Effects of Farming and Food Production

Farming can be characterized as a human activity that can have large-scale impacts on the environment and on the health of residents near farmland. With the rise of industrial agriculture, large-scale farming practices that are heavily reliant on the use of chemicals, genetically modified organisms, and the long-range transport of foods, there has been a reaction that focuses on how to reduce the energy and environmental impacts of farming and food consumption.

The environmental case against this industrialized method of food production has been well laid out. The chemicals that are used on land and crops, the pharmaceuticals that are given to livestock, and the vast amounts of energy it takes to produce, process, and transport food has created concerns that such production is neither safe nor sustainable. The quality of food has declined as producers have prioritized the ability of foodstuffs to survive long-range transport over the taste and nutritional value of the food itself. Therefore, a number of alternatives have now been proposed, most tending to have the goal of promoting higher-quality food with fewer environmental impacts.[56]

Large-Scale Livestock Operations

A particularly problematic built environment feature of contemporary food production has been the development of large-scale livestock operations. In particular, the environmental consequences of hog and chicken production have been extensively documented and the humaneness of this type of livestock production has been criticized. Placing livestock into extremely cramped conditions and feeding them combinations of highly processed grains, supplements, and pharmaceuticals can result in conditions that are bad for the animals, who can exhibit symptoms of mental stress and physical illnesses.

These operations can also have a negative effect on people who live near them, and at least one study found an association between the density of these operations and infant mortality.[57] The operations are often heavy polluters because of the odors, vapors, gas emissions, and other air pollutants associated with them and because the manure they produce is often stored on site in open-air lagoons.[58] These lagoons can leak, which may lead to contamination of aquifers and water bodies, and they have been associated with eutrophication, a large-scale blooming of algae and other microorganisms that can deplete the oxygen in the water and lead to fish kills or can render drinking water supplies unusable.[59] Furthermore, a study in North Carolina shows that in at least one state, these operations are not randomly distributed but are concentrated in low-income African American communities, raising environmental justice considerations.[60] The problems have led to requests that state and federal government regulation of these facilities include monitoring operations, requiring minimum standards for the housing of livestock, inspecting or covering lagoons, limiting the odors from these operations, addressing accidental and routine runoff of contaminated wastes, and other similar policies. Others have questioned the appropriateness of large-scale livestock operations and have called for them to be banned altogether.[61] Though there have been some efforts made to regulate such operations, there are still concerns that they are bad for the animals in these facilities, that they produce inferior quality food, and continue to create problems for their neighbors.

Organic Foods

One alternative to conventional factory-farmed food that has been around for several decades and has continued to increase in popularity is organic foods. Encouraging the use of lower-impact farming practices can result in safer food supplies, reduced pollution from farming and other positive food and environment effects. Rather than rely on foods that are heavily dosed with pesticides and other chemicals, many of which have never been thoroughly safety tested, consumers have turned to organic foods. In general, these foods are thought to be more humane on the environment and to have higher nutritional value.[62] There have been concerns about organic food, however. Some have criticized organically produced foods because they may be still exploiting low-wage farm workers and others point out that the high cost of these foods places them beyond the reach of low-income consumers.[63]

In addition to the large private-sector interest in organic foods, local actions to increase access to organically produced food include programs creating direct connections between farmers and consumers, establishing standards for labeling organic foods (mostly adapted on the state or federal level), promoting education campaigns aimed at consumers that identify the health and environmental concerns connected to conventional farming methods, encouraging the use of organic products in school cafeterias, reducing or banning the use of certain chemicals and pharmaceuticals in agriculture, and other similar actions.[64] Some of these policies are only legally possible on the federal level. Others, such as the campaigns to eliminate the use of growth hormones in the dairy industry, can work at the local level with consumers, individual stores, and others.

Locavore Movement

Recently there has been a growing movement to eat more locally produced foods. The advantages of what is now known as locavorism is that it promotes local economies, it is easier to monitor the environmental and labor practices of local farmers, the food tastes better and is more nutritious, and locally grown foods are more environmentally friendly because less energy is used for transportation.[65] Locavorism can result in improvements in the local built environment by keeping local farms profitable, thus preserving open space and reducing sprawl. A center of the U.S. locavore movement has been the San Francisco Bay Area, where a combination of a large number of environmental progressives, a benevolent climate, and a thriving produce industry have combined to make locavorism a viable alternative. There have been concerns that to eat locally in other places is neither as practical nor as environmentally friendly as it is in Northern California. These concerns include the possibility that the energy costs associated with locally grown produce may exceed those contributed by long-range transport and that local climates may necessitate substantial changes in diet that consumers may not be willing to accept.[66] The movement is in its infancy, though it is growing, and its impact on health and the environment has still not been totally assessed. One way that locavorism has been operationalized is by the concept of "food miles," metrics that aim to measure how far food has traveled from farmer to consumer. Food stuffs that have more food miles may have higher transportation-associated energy use and lower nutritional quality, and are less supportive of local farming infrastructure.[67]

Farmers Markets

Given that the offerings in many communities may be limited to a few nationally marketed vegetables and fruits that have been produced by large-scale conventional farm operations, or that other neighborhoods may not have access to fruits and vegetables at all, a major effort to change the local food environment in cities and low-income neighborhoods has been the establishment of farmers markets.[68] These have several advantages. Typically, the food is locally produced, reducing transportation costs and supporting local agriculture. The costs are often only slightly higher than what is available in grocery stores and often lower than what can be found in local convenience stores. In addition, the food offerings tend to be more nutritious and more highly focused on what the neighborhood wants.[69] The program has not been without problems, however. Some areas may lack a sufficient number of farmers who are ready and able to participate in a farmers market, resulting in shortages of produce and higher prices. These can be addressed by working with local farming communities to increase the number of suppliers. Another issue early on was that sellers of farmers markets were not able to process the new credit card–like food stamp system used by households receiving assistance. These issues have been addressed by subsidies and programs to provide card readers. Some states subsidize farmers markets, providing funds to maintain, operate, and publicize them. Others make grants to communities that work to organize a farmers market, particularly in areas that are suffering from a lack of nutritious food.[70] There is now a large network of markets across the country and many sources of information on how to organize a farmers market.[71]

Community-Supported Agriculture

Another growing movement to improve food options and the quality of diets is what is known as community-supported agriculture. Through these programs, consumers contract to purchase a season's or year's worth of produce from an individual farm and the produce is delivered weekly to participating households. The farmer receives a guaranteed steady income stream and the consumers can chose their farm supplier so that they can be sure the produce is organic or otherwise fills their desired attributes. This can make farming on the fringe of urban areas more sustainable and it can make diets easier to plan.[72]

Farm-Residential Interface

The continued expansion of metropolitan areas and the growing popularity of development in many rural areas have created conflicts between residential users and farmers. Conventional farmers use herbicides, pesticides, and other chemicals that neighbors fear may harm their health and the drifting of sprayed chemicals can be problematic. Even organic farmers can come into conflict with neighbors because of the odors associated with farming and the production and application of manure for fertilizer. This has prompted some communities to pass laws preserving the rights of farmers to carry out their tasks, known as right-to-farm legislation.[73] Other communities have focused on the rights of neighbors to not be exposed to chemicals or offensive smells. Many of these have targeted the application of pesticides near schools. Some farm communities in California, for example, have seen extensive actions on managing the conflict between its schools and neighboring farms.[74] These conflicts have not yet been fully resolved.

FOCUS ON

Hartford, Connecticut: Community Food Advocacy

For over thirty years, the Hartford Food System (HFS) has been working to improve the food environment in that city. Through community gardens, public education, advocacy, and coalition building, the HFS has sought to address the underlying causes of hunger in that city. It also provides training and technical assistance to organizations throughout Connecticut and elsewhere.

HFS helps staff City of Hartford Advisory Commission on Food Policy, an entity that has helped the city government and others address hunger and food insecurity issues in the community. HFS also participates in the Connecticut Food Policy Council. Its Grow Hartford program works with young people and others to promote advocacy around food issues and to teach about healthy eating. HFS also works with retailers to promote healthy offerings in stores and helps sponsor a farmers market.

For more information, see www.hartfordfood.org.

Urban Gardening

The United States has a long history of individuals growing their own food, even in cities. During times of war these "victory gardens" have been promoted as a patriotic way that those on the home front can support the war effort. But even during times of peace, and particularly during economic downturns, urban gardening has been popular. In low-income neighborhoods there is the added benefits that urban gardening can preserve and protect open space that may otherwise be possibly subject to illegal dumping and other illicit activities.[75] There are also numerous advantages for the gardeners that include increased social capital, more physical activity, and better nutrition.[76] Studies of urban gardeners suggest that gardens provide multiple opportunities for interaction and can help the elderly keep from becoming isolated. A major concern with gardening has been preexisting contamination of urban soils, particularly lead, on land that was formerly used for residential purposes; oils, lead, petroleum products, and solvents on land that was once used for parking; metals and other contaminants if the site was previously used for industry; and of the various unknown contaminants that may be found on any land that was once abandoned.[77] To address these concerns, organizations that own and develop urban gardens in conjunction with local groups often will extensively test the soils and remediate them if they are found to be contaminated.

The community benefits of gardening include the potential for managing vacant and abandoned land, their ability to bring neighbors together and thus promote increased social capital, strengthening of the local food environment, contributions to open space preservation and reductions in the amount of impermeable surfaces in the city, and positive psychological effects on neighbors and communities for having attractive, well-maintained open space. These gardens can also be significant locations of physical activity.[78]

A major issue in some communities has been land tenure, or who owns an urban garden site. Many gardens are located in areas that have seen large-scale disinvestment and thus the parcels have been abandoned. If the city has foreclosed on these parcels and transferred title to a local nonprofit organization, the long-term ownership of the site can be more certain. But often these gardens are located on parcels whose ownership has not been established or ownership of which a city may be reluctant to relinquish permanently to a local organization—and when values begin to rise because of gentrification or competing demands for the land, the city or other landowner may try to eject the gardeners and use the land for other purposes. This was a major issue in New York City when the city administration decided it wanted to use land that had been gardened for new housing construction. It was only ultimately resolved after long negotiations and the intervention of benefactors who helped fund local groups' purchase of the land.[79]

One solution to this problem of ownership and community control is the land trust, a community-based and/or nonprofit organization created specifically to own and manage land for gardening purposes. These organizations, which often need grant support to function, can hold on to the title of the land under gardens. They can provide support to local gardeners, assist gardening groups to administer and manage gardens, serve as an interface between local gardening groups and city administrations, and work to ensure harmonious relationships between gardeners and the neighbors.[80]

There have been objections to gardens. Some neighbors have expressed concerns about the establishment of gardens because they fear that criminals may hide in the gardens, they do not like the way the gardens look, they fear that there may be decreased land values around the gardens, or other similar reasons. The solutions to these problems with the neighbors include education, so that neighbors understand the value added by a garden, neighborhood involvement so that problems do not become a conflict between insiders and outsiders, and fencing of gardens so that they look attractive from the street. All these actions may require resources that some gardens may not have.

Summary

In the United States, there are continuing problems associated with food contamination, affordability, and accessibility. Many contamination issues are related to food production and distribution factors. There are a variety of programs that aim to address affordability. But some communities have no local places to buy nutritious food, a situation that results in what is known as food deserts. Environmental-based strategies to improve nutrition include locavorism, farm-to-school programs, community-supported agriculture, and community gardens.

Key Terms

Community-supported agriculture   Food miles

Food desert   Locavorism

Food insecurity

Discussion Questions

1. Discuss the advantages and disadvantages of our global system of food production.
2. How can we reduce the incidence of foodborne illnesses?

3. What is food insecurity? Who is at risk?
4. Describe some of the factors that make up the school food environment.
5. What is a food desert? What does living in a food desert do to the ability to achieve a healthy diet?
6. How do large-scale livestock operations impact the environment?
7. What is locavorism? What are the potential health and environmental benefits of eating locally grown foods?
8. Name some of the benefits of urban gardening.

For More Information

Food Research and Action Center. www.frac.org.

Hynes, H. P. (1996). *A patch of Eden: America's inner city gardens*. White River Junction, VT: Chelsea Green.

Local Harvest. www.localharvest.org.

National Association of School Nurses. www.nasn.org.

National Farm to School Network. www.farmtoschool.org.

Nutrition.gov www.nutrition.gov.

Robert Wood Johnson Foundation Center to Prevent Childhood Obesity. www.reversechildhoodobesity.org.

PART
IV

POPULATION HEALTH

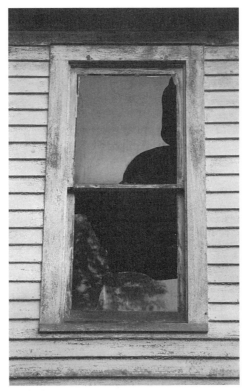

iStockphoto/© andydidyk

VULNERABLE POPULATIONS

As we begin this chapter, consider the concept of vulnerability. What does it mean to be vulnerable? Can you think of ways that some people are more sensitive to the environment around them? Are some people more dependent on their local environment to protect their health? Let's think about why this may be so. Perhaps some people are more liable to suffer injury or fall ill than others, while others may have less exposure to risks. If you have a moment, develop a list of the many ways in which the built, social, and physical environments contribute to vulnerability.

It has been long known that certain people are more susceptible to health risks than others. Even in the early nineteenth century, for example, it was seen that risks of disease and mortality were greater among the poor than among the well-off.[1] In our time, despite a stated goal of many environmental laws and regulations to protect those who are especially vulnerable, there is an increasing realization that certain populations face a cluster of risks. They are more vulnerable to a variety of environmental threats and we have not yet created a regulatory and policy framework to address these vulnerabilities.

Partly, this is a result of a growing understanding about the interrelationships of environmental vulnerabilities and social and economic inequalities. We may know more about these issues than we used to, but we have yet to fully put this knowledge into practice.[2]

Today we know that there are many different kinds of vulnerabilities and that they can arise from causes as diverse as underlying genetic susceptibility to social factors and features of the built environment. Among the various descriptive categories that appear to be associated with different degrees of vulnerability are race/ethnicity, income, age, sex, sexual preference, and immigration/citizenship status. This is not an all-inclusive list of potential vulnerabilities and it should be noted that people's levels of vulnerability change over time. Consider that many of these vulnerabilities are socially constructed and features of the built environment can often either increase or diminish their potential impacts.[3]

Vulnerability may work in many different ways which have been defined using different methodologies. For example, one way of thinking about vulnerability is that because of a range of causative factors, certain people may have unequal exposures to risk, unequal access to environmental benefits, preexisting health conditions, problematic infrastructure, and a lack of political power to remedy these situations. Any one of these factors may increase vulnerabilities and in combination, their negative impacts may be heightened. Another way of thinking about vulnerabilities is the concept of **cumulative risk** or the idea that there are a series of factors that together are responsible for some people having worse health status than others. These can include increased risk of exposure to environmental hazards, increased possibility of becoming ill given a certain level of exposure, decreased ability to secure proper medical attention for that condition, and decreased ability to fully recover from disease.[4] This may place individuals and groups at increased risk for recurring problems and may be one way that vulnerabilities in one generation can translate into increased vulnerabilities for the next. For example, vulnerability may lead to an inability to work, forcing a family to live in poor-quality housing. If the children in this family are then exposed to lead paint, they may have lower cognitive abilities as they reach school age. These reduced cognitive abilities could harm school performance, which may lead to lower incomes during their adult years. The vulnerability has thus been transmitted across generations.

There is a concept known as **weathering**. Low-income and minority persons are burdened by a variety of acute and chronic stresses that, over time, result in premature aging or a lifelong decrease in health status.[5] This heightens their vulnerability at any one point in time and contributes to ongoing disparities in health outcomes.[6]

In terms of the built environment, among the most defining types of vulnerabilities are those based on race. In general, certain groups, including African Americans and Latinos, are more likely to live in places that are heavily polluted or near hazardous waste facilities, and less likely to be able to prevent the building of new environmental threats in their communities. This has led to what is known as the environmental justice movement, which we will discuss in Chapter Thirteen. In this chapter, we will consider some of the many kinds of health and environmental disparities that help frame the geography of risk that one researcher has called "the riskscape."[7]

The Built Environment and Vulnerability

There are a number of ways that the built environment can have an impact on vulnerability.[8] In some cases, the built environment concentrates disadvantages in communities that have high percentages of vulnerable populations.[9] Thus, in the chapter on environmental justice we will see how low-income communities have been disproportionately burdened by environmental problems and have a systemic lack of access to environmental amenities.[10] Sometimes the built environment itself can foster the vulnerability. For example, as noted in previous chapters, difficult street crossings and sidewalk designs can turn problems with mobility and sensory perceptions into major barriers for senior citizens and others.[11]

The distribution of problems posed by the built environment are related to inequalities along racial, economic, and other lines.[12] This may imply that addressing these issues will involve both mitigating the impacts of problematic environments and working so that everyone has equal access to high-quality places to live, work, go to school, and play.

Four types of vulnerabilities are discussed here: race, income, age, and disability status.

The Definition of Race

One of the long-standing factors that have been known to be associated with differing levels of risk and differing levels of health outcomes in the United States is **race**. It is important to stress that race is not a biological construct. There are no absolute genetic markers that allow scientists or others to define racial classifications or to identify who is of one race and who is of another. There are only probabilities that certain polymorphisms of individual genes can be found more often in one group than another.[13] This lack of biological certitude is one of the reasons why definitions of race can vary over time and place.[14]

Rather than being biologically determined, race is socially determined. That is, the race of an individual is set by the society that person is living in along with the reactions of that person to the social situation around them. In other words, race is determined and defined through a complex set of social factors.[15] This does not mean that race does not have a profound impact on health or that it does not contribute to biological mechanisms that affect disease prevalence and outcomes. On the contrary, the continuing importance of race to health is evidence that social processes underlie many health-related vulnerabilities. The high degree of correlation between self-identified race and health status found in many health outcomes and in a variety of mortality risks illustrates the impact of social factors on health.[16] To be of one race or another in this country, as in many others, can ultimately mean that people may have a legacy of past exposures, an increased probability of certain current exposures, and a high likelihood of potential future exposures.[17]

At one time defining an individual's race was left to government officials or doctors. But today, race in the United States is defined based on self-report using the federal Office of Management and Budget's (OMB) guidelines in a two-part process.[18] In one question, individuals are asked to identify themselves as one of several racial categories provided to them, including black, white, Asian, Pacific Islander, Native American, and so on. In a second question, individuals are asked to identify themselves as being of Hispanic origin or not. According to the official definition as put forth by OMB, Hispanic origin is not a race but an ethnicity. Again this is a social distinction, not a biological one. In addition, individuals are allowed to choose multiple race categories to identify themselves. Because of the great influence of federal programs on the collection of data that identifies by race, these guidelines shape how most health research regarding race and ethnicity is conducted in this country and are responsible for how most government agencies collect data on race and ethnicity. Note that these definitions of procedures have changed over time. Until fairly recently, for example, individuals were only allowed to report a single race and multiple race reporting was not possible.[19]

Pathways Between Racism, Discrimination, and Health

It should be noted that racism is not the same as discrimination and that they both can work in multiple pathways to affect health.[20] Racism, or racial prejudice, is a thought or way of thinking but does not necessarily imply action; that is, a person can hold racist thoughts without necessarily acting upon them. Discrimination is an actual act in which one treats a member of one group differently than another. Furthermore, in terms of the built environment, one of the most important ways that discrimination acts upon health is by its contribution to racial residential segregation, or the race-based tendency for one group to live in particular areas against its will.[21] In this case it could describe how African Americans typically are restricted by housing discrimination to live in certain neighborhoods and have problems moving outside of these neighborhoods even if they have the economic resources to do so.[22] Because pollutants are not randomly distributed but are often higher in communities of color, the exposure to environmental toxins is greater among certain populations, potentially increasing the burden of environmentally related disease.[23] Discrimination can act upon health in many other ways. These can include stress, particularly the physiological reactions that are associated with chronic stress and are known as allostatic load, or the inability of one group to access current standards of care even though they may have health insurance.[24]

Racial Disparities in Health

However defined, there are profound differences in the health status of different racial groups. Note that this is a comment about the overall health status of groups, not individuals; in all population groups, there is a wide variation in health status and outcomes. For the most part, whites have a better overall health status as a group than blacks or Latinos. When considered as a whole, Asians tend to have a health status closer to that of whites, but when considered as people with backgrounds from individual countries, this group's overall health status masks important differences among country-of-origin groups.[25] For African Americans, the disparities in health begin at birth where there are much higher infant mortality rates among black infants (see Figure 10.1) born in this country, as compared to non-black infants.[26] These health inequities continue throughout childhood, with African American children more likely to suffer from asthma, lead poisoning, and other childhood illnesses.[27] Mortality differentials exist throughout almost the entire lifespan of African American men and women until the very oldest ages are reached. For Latinos, the situation is more complex.[28] Puerto Rican women, for example, have child-bearing experiences closer to those of African Americans and have similarly high infant mortality rates. Women of Mexican ancestry, whether they were born in the United States or in Mexico, appear to have better than expected rates of infant mortality.[29] Latinos who self-identify as black tend to have morbidity and mortality profiles similar to African Americans. Latinos who self-identify as white tend to have better morbidity or mortality profiles. However, there may be evidence that this Latino health

FIGURE 10.1   U.S. Infant Mortality—2006

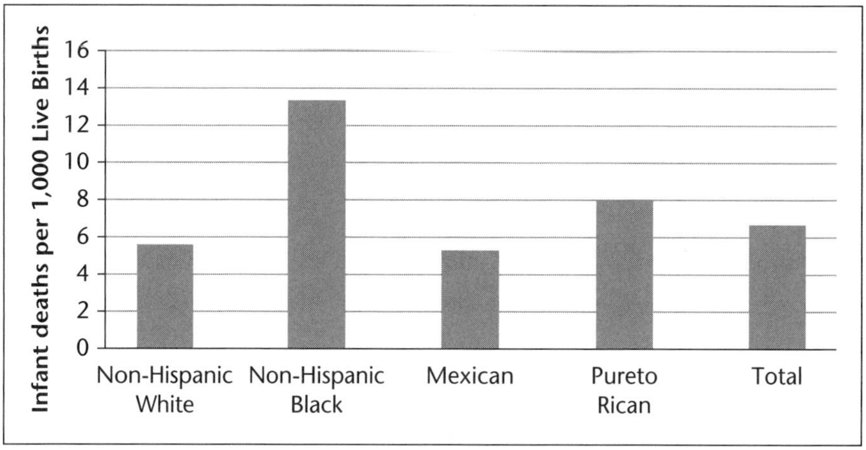

Source: CDC—National Center for Health Statistics

advantage disappears over time as Mexican immigrants become assimilated or increase their amount of time in the United States. Furthermore, Latinos of Cuban ancestry tend to have better health outcomes than Latinos as a whole. These differences are highly related to, but not entirely explained by, differences in education, income, social status, and reported racial background.[30]

Race and the Built Environment

In general, there are important differences in where different racial groups live across United States and some of these differences can result in different patterns of exposures to built environment issues. African Americans tend to be concentrated in inner cities and close-in suburbs as well as in parts of the rural South.[31] Inner-city communities are more likely to have problems with air pollution, abandoned industrial sites, hazardous waste facilities, and problems accessing supermarkets.[32] Some parts of the rural South have problems with hazardous waste sites, lack of access to health care, and water quality issues.[33]

Hispanic people tend to live in large metropolitan areas and smaller communities that often have a concentration of industrial facilities.[34] These populations are thus more likely to have issues with access to parks, air quality problems, and other similar issues.[35] There are many differences in distributions of various Asian populations and some communities have problems with air quality in substandard housing, whereas other populations have issues that are more similar to the problems posed by contemporary suburbs.[36]

The distribution of these problems cannot be understood unless there is an acknowledgment of the underlying features of racial discrimination and historical immigration and settlement patterns.[37] However, concentrating on overall patterns of distribution may lead to overlooking problems affecting small populations.

Throughout this book we have looked at how race, income, age, and other factors affect exposure to environmental hazards. It must be stressed that these hazards are not randomly distributed across the landscape but appear to be concentrated in communities that have preexisting disadvantages.[38] Similarly, environmental amenities also are distributed along the lines that are reflective of underlying inequalities of race and income.[39]

Interventions to Reduce Racial Disparities in Health

There are two levels of intervention that should be considered when trying to address racial disparities in health. At the individual level, where most health care providers operate and where many interventions focus, efforts are often focused on helping individuals understand the social forces affecting their health and on helping them work to mitigate the impact of these forces through behavior changes or by avoiding the stressors associated with being a member of a minority group.[40] These types of interventions may include smoking cessation programs, alcohol and drug counseling, healthy baby initiatives, and the like. However, simply emphasizing individual risks may result in shifting the responsibility away from the social factors that are responsible for the poor health of many members of ethnic minorities in this country.[41] Therefore, interventions also may be needed to address the social and environmental forces that drive racial disparities in health; only by addressing the factors ultimately responsible for poor health can the health of communities be improved.[42] Addressing racial disparities in health must include efforts to address such issues as disparate exposure to environmental contamination, the proliferation of tobacco or alcohol advertising in certain neighborhoods, the availability of illegal firearms, and other similar factors. Improving the built and social environments can provide opportunities for addressing racial disparities in health.

Segregation and Health Disparities

As famously stated in the 1968 Kerner Commission report, "Our nation is moving toward two societies, one black, one white—separate and unequal."[43] Segregation levels have decreased since 1968 (they peaked in 1950), but African American communities remain very highly segregated in the United States.[44] Overall, the segregation of Latinos and Asians in this country is moderately high.[45] This matters because segregation is associated with poorer health outcomes such as increased infant mortality, higher overall mortality, and a wide range of health problems.[46] Segregation frames how certain people live across the metropolitan landscape and exposures to risks are highly associated with this distribution.[47]

Evidence suggests that segregation is associated with higher levels of pollution for everyone and a greater degree of inequality of exposures to pollution between groups.[48] Other problems associated with segregation include the probability that certain features are more or less likely to be found in neighborhoods with large percentages of people of color. For example, tobacco and alcohol advertising is more likely to be found in African American communities than elsewhere.[49] Minority neighborhoods are less likely to have hospitals, parks and playgrounds, supermarkets, and other amenities that reinforce healthy behaviors and provide vital services.[50] One reason that behavioral risk factors may cluster in certain neighborhoods is that these areas are less supportive of healthy lifestyles. The lack of amenities in many minority neighborhoods suggests that programs to address infrastructure and economic development in these communities are necessary.

Poverty

An extremely large number of studies have documented the association of low incomes with poorer health outcomes and increased risk behaviors. Poorer is riskier.[51] Low incomes appear to be highly associated with risk behaviors such as smoking, poor diets, physical inactivity, and almost every other studied risk behavior. Poverty has been associated with such health outcomes as infant mortality, obesity, diabetes, cardiovascular disease, cancer, HIV infections, and others.[52] Also, unfortunately, low-income status in childhood can have lifelong health implications.[53]

Addressing the vulnerabilities of the poor may be difficult because there are a large number of potential risks that might be concentrated among a group or locality at one time.[54] Low-income people are less likely to have access to jobs, education, nutritious food, health care, environmental amenities, social support; in addition, basic government services such as fire, police, schools, and so on may be worse in low-income communities.[55] They may have increased exposure to violence, environmental toxins, fast-food restaurants, smoking and tobacco advertising, poor housing, and other factors that may directly or indirectly lead to health risk behaviors or poor health outcomes. Much of the focus of public health has been how to help people who are in these types of situations.[56]

It is not just a person's absolute income but also income relative to the rest of the population that is important. Thus higher levels of income inequality are also associated with poor health. Also called the relative income hypothesis, it appears that as inequality increases so do poor health behaviors and poor health.[57] Studies have found, for example, that as income inequality increases on the national, state, or local level so does the risk of fair or poor health.[58] Some evidence suggests that overall mortality increases as income inequality increases.[59] This may explain part of the reason why the United States does not enjoy the best health outcomes in the developed world: even though this country's median income is among the highest, its level of income inequality is also among the greatest of all developed countries. This inequality may be harming the health of U.S. citizens, but the high degree of income inequality is difficult to address. The solutions proposed to reduce income inequality—education, tax policies, and so on—are often beyond the agendas of public health practitioners and urban planners. Furthermore, increased income inequality may result in part from a political climate that reduces funding for social programs that might mitigate its impacts.[60]

Poverty, Income Inequality, and the Built Environment

Levels of poverty and income inequality have been associated with a number of problems related to the built environment.[61] For example, poor communities often have residents living in households that do not have cars. To the extent that the only way to access supermarkets, jobs, parks, schools, and other amenities is by car, those households who cannot afford a car are effectively denied access.[62] There have also been issues with access to health care in low-income communities.[63] Some of these areas lack doctors, others do not have hospitals and emergency services, others may not have pharmacies, or the neighborhood pharmacies may not stock critical drugs such as opiates and other drugs that address pain.[64]

Low-income communities are more likely to have abandoned buildings, vacant lots, streets in disrepair, and the overall quality of the built environment may be so low as to hinder physical activity.[65] Thus, even though these neighborhoods might be dense and have strong street conductivity, they may ultimately fail to adequately protect health.

Poverty and Access to Environmental Amenities

As noted in this chapter and elsewhere in this book, there have been concerns that low-income communities and households living in poverty have a decreased likelihood of being able to access supermarkets, parks, health clinics, and other features of the built environment that can promote health.[66] Potentially exacerbating these problems of access is that low-income households may be more dependent on having access to these amenities than others. For example, low-income people may have to rely upon parks and public open spaces for physical activity because they cannot afford gym memberships and other alternatives.[67]

Many low-income communities suffer from a related problem of a lack of a tax base from which to support the development and maintenance of amenities. There may be fewer parks and the parks that are available in these neighborhoods may not be as well maintained as they need to be. To the extent that local governments rely on local tax bases to provide amenities, such situations can reinforce the health inequities that result from problems of the built environment.[68]

Concentrated Poverty

One potential problem is that certain communities have high rates of poverty and overall low incomes that may end up concentrating and exacerbating the problems associated with poverty.[69] These **concentrated poverty** areas may result in increased crime rates and lower quality of public services.[70] There is also concern that concentrated poverty can end up reducing access to employment opportunities for residents or may promote unhealthy risk behaviors.[71]

Addressing concentrated poverty can involve community organizing efforts to bring in economic opportunities or to address some of the environmental problems that affect the community.[72] More controversial have been efforts to break up populations and distribute people outside of traditionally low-income communities.[73]

Spatial Mismatch

In the 1960s, it became increasingly clear that many low-income and minority communities faced a challenge: they did not have enough jobs to meet residents' demand for work. At the same time, it appeared that many of the jobs, particularly those that typically hired people with lower levels of education and work skills, were in the suburbs. Areas of high growth were located on the urban periphery; poor areas with high need were in the inner city. The term **spatial mismatch** was coined to describe this geographical disconnect between supply of jobs and supply of labor.[74]

It has not been easy to address the issues of spatial mismatch. The social factors underlying barriers to employment have generally been addressed by job training; economic problems are usually addressed by efforts to promote development in low-income communities; and the built environment solution has often been to look at ways to connect impoverished neighborhoods with job centers through transportation. The record has been mixed. It is difficult and expensive to build transportation, which has traditionally been focused on moving suburban residents to center-city jobs. Many suburban employment centers are very decentralized and it is expensive to build sufficient numbers of high-quality transit options. Some suburban communities have opposed transit extensions into their neighborhoods as well.[75]

FOCUS ON

Addressing Spatial Mismatch: Buying Cars for the Poor

The problem of spatial mismatch—the fact that most jobs are being created in suburban locations while the areas with highest unemployment tend to be inside center cities—has been discussed several times in this book. The problem is made worse by the fact that many poor urban households do not own cars. One proposed solution is to build more transit or to encourage the opening of bus lines between inner cities and suburban locations.

Others have proposed that it would be cheaper to buy used cars for the poor than to build transit; they suggest that giving cars away would also allow more mobility for the urban poor and assist them to access health care and healthy food as well.

Others have criticized this proposal, pointing out that the cost comparisons did not consider the costs of insurance, maintenance, and gas, or the cost of expanding road capacity. Other concerns are the environmental impacts (older cars tend to be higher polluters) and the health impacts of encouraging more driving. No city or state has implemented such a program at this time.

Children and Environmental Health

Vulnerabilities are not static across an individual's lifespan. On the contrary, they are greater at both the beginning and the end of life. There are a number of ways that children are affected by aspects of the built environment that can increase or decrease their vulnerabilities.[76] Children are considered to be a vulnerable population for a number of reasons. For example, because their bodies are still developing, they may have special physiological vulnerabilities if an environmental stressor or toxin is encountered at the wrong time. Developing organ systems may be altered by pollutants.[77] The developmental effects of toxics including lead and estrogenic chemicals are well documented; there is evidence that there can be lasting neurological damage, sexual organ changes, or age of sexual maturation impacts to children exposed to these toxins.[78] Other potential health risks have not been as well studied but that does not mean that they do not exist. Another problem that highlights the vulnerability of children is that they are unable to respond to threats as adults may respond. For example, children do not decide where they are going to live, nor are they allowed to vote. So they can neither move away from environmental threats nor influence environmental policy. Because they spend more time outside and are less likely to be able to drive, children are also more sensitive to barriers in the built environment to physical activity. They may also have a great need for safe local parks and playgrounds.[79]

There may be different ideal environments for children as opposed to adults. For example, for older children and adults, cul-de-sacs are major barriers to walking and biking because they make destinations beyond the cul-de-sacs virtually impossible to access except by car. But for young children who are at an age where they can play outside with minimal supervision but are not old enough to access further destinations on their own, the traffic-free streets of a cul-de-sac might be ideal in terms of maximizing their physical activity. There should be no assumption that an environment that is helpful for one group is helpful for all.

As we discussed in Chapter Five, young children are particularly at risk for lead exposures because it is natural behavior for children to put their hands and other objects into their mouths just at the same time as they are beginning to crawl and walk, and they are most likely to come in contact with lead-contaminated dust. This is also a key moment in their neurological development. Thus housing with lead paint is a particular problem for very young children.[80] Children are also increasingly at risk for obesity and have a particularly high need for physical activity, which means they are dependent on living in an environment which fosters their ability to be active. Asthma is also a major health issue for children and they may be very vulnerable to problems with indoor and outdoor air quality.[81] Asthma represents the single largest cause of hospital admissions in the United States and one of the major causes of missed school days. Its economic burden is large.

Creating Healthy Environments for Children

It has long been a given in environmental health theory that children are not merely miniature adults with the same vulnerabilities and needs as people who have reached maturity. Addressing the special needs of children is not going to be easy.[82] Part of the solution would involve special attention to improving well-known issues in contemporary environments including contaminated housing, poor air quality, and similar factors that are supposed to be regulated by the array of environmental laws that have been established since the 1970s. From our built environment perspective, there is a need to develop design strategies that separate children from traffic, allow for safe walking to and from school, create access to parks and other opportunities for physical recreation, and other measures that may well provide a healthy environment not only for children but for everyone.[83]

The Elderly and the Built Environment

There are also increased environmental vulnerabilities at the end of life spans. The elderly are vulnerable to environmental threats for a number of reasons: they may be in poor health; they may be taking medications that increase sensitivity to heat waves and other environmental stressors; they may suffer from respiratory and other organ system declines due to natural aging processes, which may make it difficult for them to overcome exposures. Many seniors may be socially isolated, placing them at particular risk during times of extreme weather events, and many have difficulty finding support from family and friends (reduced social capital). Others may be suffering the consequences of earlier exposures, such as women with osteoporosis who find that their blood lead levels have increased because, as their bones decalcify they also release lead stored from past exposures.[84]

The built environment may exacerbate these vulnerabilities by creating additional barriers to reaching destinations outside the home.[85] Busy streets, areas with poor lighting, unwalkable streets, and destinations only accessible by car may pose particular problems for individuals experiencing increased difficulty with eyesight, walking, and other issues. Many elderly no longer drive; living in environments that are not supportive of walking, or that do not have adequate public transportation, may be particularly problematic. Many elderly move to live in more supportive environments; however, for a variety of reasons, many cannot or do not move, despite limitations in the built environment around them.[86]

There is also much interaction between age, race, and income when it comes to vulnerabilities. Many of the most vulnerable among the elderly have been poor for long periods of their lives or may have had a lifetime of exposure to discrimination or the effects of a segregated society.[87]

Assisting the elderly to meet these burdens is challenging but crucial. Some actions must be ongoing such as working to ensure that elderly are getting proper nutrition or have access to the medical services they need. Some programs may be episodic, such as a response to a heat emergency, but they must be planned well in advance so they can be implemented quickly. As discussed in Chapter Four and elsewhere, care should be taken so that the built environment does not contribute to the social and physical isolation of the elderly.

Housing Needs of the Elderly

The conventional suburban development patterns identified in Chapter Three may not meet the needs of elderly populations.[88] As people age, they tend to have less access to automobiles, may not be able to drive, and are more sensitive to barriers posed by improper street designs.[89] Housing itself may become a problem if people cannot use the stairs in their homes or if disability and other issues prevent them from using cars to access supermarkets, friends and families, and health care.[90]

Many elderly prefer to stay in their long-term homes and communities, a concept known as aging in place. Facilitating this may be a challenge in some places.[91] Some elderly may need assistance in adapting their homes to meet their physical needs.[92] Other communities may not have sufficient resources that are within reach of people who cannot drive. Many communities have responded to this problem by promoting the development of special housing for senior citizens.[93] These units are often specially designed to meet potential problems. They should be sited so as to be close to the amenities that seniors need and they should be affordable for people on fixed incomes; however, not every community has such facilities. There are programs to assist seniors to continue living in their long-term homes, but these programs may not be able to help those who have the lowest incomes or greatest physical limitations.[94]

FOCUS ON

Aging in Place

The U.S. population, like that of many other countries, is slowly growing older. The number of people over the age of 65 is increasing faster than the population under 18. But many suburban locations and homes, the location of the bulk of development activity for the past several decades, were built for people who could drive or had the physical ability to walk up and down stairs. As the population ages, the number of people who will not be able to perform these activities will increase.

At the same time, the majority of the elderly population does not want to move, preferring instead to age in place near where they have lived most of their lives. To make this possible, there are several potential strategies. These may include education and technical assistance to older persons to assist them in retrofitting their homes to accommodate decreased mobility and perception abilities, retrofitting streets to make them safer for the elderly, or building affordable and appropriate options in communities so that as people age, they can move to more supportive living situations.

Persons with Disabilities

People with disabilities may face major problems in their interactions with the built environment. Some people have mobility issues that may make it difficult for them to access destinations, and features of the built environment may reinforce these problems.[95] For example, people in wheelchairs or who have difficulty walking may have problems with stairs or curbs. People with sensory issues may face challenges crossing streets or in finding their way across neighborhoods. A well-designed built environment should aim to reduce or eliminate its contribution to these issues rather than reinforce them.[96] Research suggests that many people with disabilities, particularly those with the most limitations, are very sensitive to problems with street designs and barriers to mobility.[97] People with disabilities are also more at risk of isolation if they live in communities that rely solely on automobile transportation.[98]

The 1990 Americans with Disability Act was a major milestone in the effort to foster the inclusion of people with disabilities into broader society. The act helped establish guidelines for how the built environment should be modified in ways large and small so that the participation of all people may be maximized. Another major way that the built environment has been reengineered to assist persons with disabilities has been the movement known as universal design. Universal design assists in making the environment more supportive for all persons, and an environment that incorporates universal design principles is often a place that promotes walking and other healthy activities.[99] Its principles include: equitable use; flexibility in use; simple and intuitive; perceptible information; tolerance for error; low physical effort; and size and space for approach and use.[100]

There are a number of ways that a house can be redesigned to promote safer living for people with disabilities.[101] This may mean equipment to help those who have sensory issues. For example, emergency warning systems for fires might include flashing lights as well as alarms for those whose hearing is impaired. Physical mobility issues can be addressed through special fixtures such as grab bars for the elderly in bathrooms and kitchen cabinets that are accessible for those in wheelchairs. The designing of housing for the elderly is a long-established architectural discipline and as this population grows, the modifications that can help people stay in homes are becoming more widespread.[102]

Summary

Many population groups are at increased risk of environmental-related illnesses and all of us experience these vulnerabilities at some point in our lives. Many of these issues are related to the built environment even though they may arise from social or other causes. For example, segregation and other problems may increase the problems associated with race. Income may play a similar role. Addressing these issues may require addressing underlying social inequalities as well as problems in the built environment.

Key Terms

Concentrated poverty

Weathering

Cumulative risk

Spatial mismatch

Race

Discussion Questions

1. Name some of the groups that have increased vulnerability.
2. Define cumulative risk.
3. What is race? What do we mean when we say race is a social rather than a biological construct?
4. What is the difference between prejudice and discrimination?
5. How does poverty affect the built environment?
6. Describe some of the ways that children are more susceptible to environmental hazards?
7. Why are the elderly at risk for environmental problems?
8. What is universal design?

For More Information

Berkman, L. F., & Kwachi, I. (2000). *Social epidemiology*. New York: Oxford University Press.
Center for Universal Design — North Carolina State University. www.design.ncsu.edu/cud/.
Children's Environmental Health Network. www.cehn.org.
Institute for Children's Environmental Health. www.iceh.org.
Massey, D., & Denton, N. (1993). *American apartheid: Segregation and the making of the underclass*. Cambridge, MA: Harvard University Press.
Polednak, A. (1997). *Segregation, poverty, and mortality in urban African Americans*. New York: Oxford University Press.
Wilkinson, R. G., & Marmot, M. G. (2003). *Social determinants of health: The solid facts*. Geneva: World Health Organization.

CHAPTER 11

MENTAL HEALTH, STRESSORS, AND HEALTH CARE ENVIRONMENTS

LEARNING OBJECTIVES

- Describe the role of the developing field of sociology in the early twentieth century in understanding how cities might affect mental health.
- Discuss the association between immigration and health.
- Define biophilia.
- Compare the relative health impacts of urban versus rural living.
- Assess the contribution of density to health.
- Describe the concept of defensible space.
- Define evidence-based design.
- Identify the potential impacts of gentrification on health.

Let's think about how you feel when you get home from work or school. Do you feel relief? Or are there issues in your home, apartment, or dorm, large and small, that make you feel anxious, stressed out, or tired? When you visit a park, do you feel calm or energized? Does the crime, litter, and graffiti in your neighborhood make it seem less safe? Or does the amount of disorder in the environment make you feel that the neighborhood is abandoned? These questions relate to how the built environment might be affecting your levels of stress and contribute to your mental health.

From the very beginning of large-scale urbanization in the nineteenth century, there were concerns that cities and city living were bad for mental health. Even before the rise of modern psychology and diagnostic procedures, it was noted that social pathologies seemed to cluster in urban slums and that cities appeared to promote self-destructive behaviors. These observations led to an effort to understand how the built environment influenced mental health status.

It is interesting to note how some concepts have stayed constant over the last century and others have changed over time. In addition, we should note that these observations from the nineteenth century helped lead to the modern professions of sociology and social work.

This chapter begins with early sociologists' ideas about the influence of the environment on the health of immigrants and traces how this area of theory has changed over time. Then we discuss biophilia and issues related to access to nature. We proceed to a consideration of rural versus urban environments and health, and of density, high-rise housing, and what is known as defensible space. We will talk about stress and allostatic load and the effects of displacement. Next there is a discussion of the effects of open space on children with attention deficit hyperactivity disorder. We conclude with a focus on health facility design and a discussion of the emerging field of evidence-based design.

The Beginnings

At the beginning of the twentieth century, in an effort to understand rapidly urbanizing communities, a group of researchers at the University of Chicago, including Robert Park and Ernest Burgess, began to systematically observe and study immigrant neighborhoods in that city.[1] Building upon the work of European researchers such as Emile Durkheim, these researchers were to systematically catalogue problems in urban areas and propose ways in which these issues could be addressed.[2] Some of the techniques and practices are still used today and can help inform current issues. For example, one of the most important techniques they employed was to take detailed observations of the communities they were studying. These observations can then lead to generalized theories, policies, and interventions. One idea they pioneered is that universities can take advantage of local opportunities to study social and environmental problems and that in return, academic researchers can assist communities in need. Another result of these efforts that have continued to influence policy well into the twentieth century is that these researchers documented underlying strengths even in the poorest neighborhoods: connections between neighbors, community institutions, and shared experiences and histories. Another fundamental lesson is that environmental context helps shape behaviors for both better and worse.

Perhaps one of the longest-persisting ideas that came out of sociology at the beginning of the twentieth century was the concept of **anomie**. It was based on the observation that immigrants were coming from small villages in rural parts of Europe (and later, African Americans from the rural South) and as their lives shifted from constant contact with a few well-known individuals and family members to a situation where they were continually being forced to interact with countless strangers and very new situations, it was thought that this led to a psychological dislocation, a form of alienation called *anomie*.[3]

Part of the theory of anomie was that alienation contributed to the breakdown of social norms and internal self-controls that ultimately resulted in the various observed pathological behaviors of that era, including prostitution, drunkenness, and abandonment. Based upon this, one goal of social workers and settlement house workers at the time was to assist newcomers to cope with the dislocating effects of city living and to reestablish the social connections and internal controls that once guided their behavior. A major priority of the settlement house movement was to offer classes and advice to new immigrants to help them to adapt to their new surroundings. Thus, one goal of English language and citizenship classes was to make new immigrants aware of the social norms of the United States (typically those of white, native-born, Protestant middle-class people). The settlement houses also served to integrate newcomers into the community, introducing them to better-established immigrants from their own native countries. The underlying philosophy was that these efforts could reestablish social controls and connections, helping immigrants to keep the healthy behaviors they once had and counteract the anomie inherent in urban living.[4]

Today, immigration and urbanization, in the United States and other developed countries are much more complex than they were in the nineteenth century. For example, many immigrants come from urban situations in their home countries and may have already experienced the complexities of urban life or have been exposed to modernizing influences of contemporary developed societies.[5] In addition, globalization and increased media saturation have resulted in fewer differences between where many immigrants have come from and where they have arrived. In a world where U.S. retailers and fast-food providers have penetrated vast areas of the globe and where communication between countries is cheaper and easier, it may be that the dislocating effects of immigration are less severe than they once were. Not all immigrants share these advantages, of course. Some are refugees, fleeing war and bearing the psychological effects of civil strife. Still others are immigrants from rural areas without any prior experience with urban living or Western ways.

In the twenty-first century, the conceptual framework for how to understand the immigrant experience has changed to the idea of acculturation, the shifting of cultural values and social norms from those of the former country to that of the new. However, some oppose that terminology as being irrelevant to the general experience of immigrants.[6] In addition, we also know now that there is what is known as the healthy immigrant effect; people who immigrate tend

FIGURE 11.1   Latino Immigrants in the United States:
Key Health Indicators

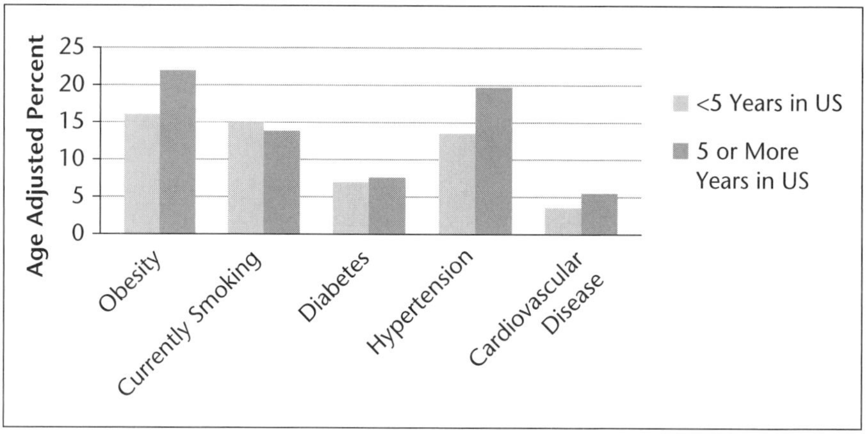

Source: CDC

to be healthier both physically and mentally than residents in their former country and those in their new country.[7] This gives some immigrants a resiliency that may protect them from some of the worst effects of urbanization and immigration. It may be that as immigrants assimilate and adapt to less healthy behaviors more prevalent in the United States, these protective effects wear off (see Figure 11.1). Their children are also less likely to have these health advantages.[8] It may also be that discrimination and racism eventually erode these protective immigrant effects.[9] Whatever the processes, however, services to immigrants are still important.

Biophilia

There have been concerns that city living itself is bad for mental health. The rise of the environmental movement in the last several decades of the twentieth century prompted new ideas about the effects of urban living that were different from anomie. The problem was now characterized to be not a surplus of contact with strangers, but a lack of contact with nature. The ubiquity of urban environments—concrete, asphalt, large buildings, and so on—meant that people had less or no access to green spaces, parks, and natural environments.[10] Extending the 1920s view of cities as overly developed and containing too many buildings and hard surfaces, with not enough land devoted to parks and other open spaces, it was now thought that too much day-to-day living with human-modified landscapes and not enough with natural landscapes might be bad for health.[11]

Beginning with the pioneering work of E. O. Wilson and others, it has been suggested that human beings have a natural need to be connected to nature. Called **biophilia**, this theory suggests that man-made environments are inherently deficient and unable to properly nurture human health and development.[12] This in turn can cause mental illness, poor school performance, and antisocial behaviors.

Perhaps, it has been suggested, a cause of the current problems of drug abuse, crime, and other poor behaviors is this lack of access to nature. A series of intriguing experiments provide support to this theory. One of the most influential was a study by Robert Ulrich, who explored the differences in experiences among patients who had gallbladder surgery in a Pennsylvania hospital.[13] He compared patients who had a view of nature from their hospital room windows with those whose windows looked out on a brick wall. He found that patients with nature views were more likely to recover quickly and less likely to need pain medication, particularly in the intermediate period several days after surgery but before the final days of hospitalization (the study was done at a time when gallbladder patients typically stayed in the hospital for two weeks—as compared to 2 to 3 days now). Ulrich and others built upon this research with a series of experiments in which they show individuals a variety of scenes—meadows, train stations, and so on—and then measure certain physiological responses, such as heartbeat rate. These studies suggest that looking at natural scenes is more conducive for recovery and health than looking at an urban scene. Blood pressure is reduced, skin conductance declines, and so on.[14] In a study of public housing residents in Chicago, it was found that those who had more access to landscaped areas reported better mental health outcomes than those who looked out over parking lots and other hard surfaces.[15]

In many of these experiments, it is important to consider that there were extreme differences in visual environments. It is not clear how these findings might be translated to more prevalent types of urban and suburban landscapes with their mixtures of land uses, or whether, for example, single-family homes and landscaped suburban lots provide better environments for mental health and healing than upper-income urban apartment dwellers' views of distant skylines. In other words, these findings are important but it is not clear how to translate them into urban design standards.

Richard Louv (2008) suggests that a syndrome he calls *nature deficit disorder* explains why people living in cities exhibit the antisocial behavior thought to cluster there. The lack of access to nature has been posited as a cause of attention deficit hyperactivity disorder, along with depression and other mental health and behavioral problems.[16] A cautionary note is that the existence of a nature deficit disorder has not been confirmed and is not a standard diagnostic classification. Furthermore, it does not explain the high rates of behavioral problems in rural environments. It is important that what may well be a very valid type of human desire, an innate love of nature and natural areas, not be so far extended that it is more reflective of an anti-urban bias on the part of researchers and policymakers.

What Is Healthier: Urban or Rural Living?

Biophilia and access to nature theory suggest that urban living is inherently unhealthy compared to rural environments and much of twentieth-century urban policy was predicated on the idea that cities were bad for health and that rural and suburban living was much better. In part, this reflects the reality of the nineteenth-century city, when death rates were substantially higher than in rural areas, a situation that persisted until well into the twentieth century.[17] The construct has been called the *rural health advantage*.[18] The theory is that access to clean air, sunlight, and natural environments, and reduced exposure to pollution, noise, and all the unpleasantness of city living, is better for human health.[19] This idea underpins much of current U.S. environmental thought and can be seen in well-meaning efforts to get inner-city kids out to rural camps in the summertime.

But are rural environments really healthier than urban environments? The evidence is not all that clear. Certainly some types of social distress, such as homelessness, drug abuse, and crime, appear to be more prevalent in cities. But partly this is a result of the concentration of poverty in cities and the visibility of social problems in urban areas.[20] For example, the crystal methamphetamine drug abuse problem surfaced in rural areas well before it spread to urban areas, but the very invisibility of social problems in rural areas helped to mask the issue. It is also easier to live in a city on a low income than it is to be poor in a rural area because of the greater prevalence of low-income housing, the plethora of social service agencies, and the ability to move around without a car, and thus many poor people move to cities. Economists would say the poor are making rational choices based upon the information and options provided to them. Thus, first of all, any analysis of the urban versus rural health has to control for poverty and income because it is well known that being poor is a risk factor for many poor behaviors and adverse outcomes. Another complication might be that all the other negative things that are often located in improvised areas such as hazardous waste facilities and trash transfer stations might be the factors are responsible for the lower mental health status or lower overall health status that is observed there. This would imply that it is not urban living itself that is the problem, but the clustering of unwanted land uses and problematic and disproportionate environmental burdens that are driving behaviors.

It is important to consider that urban living is not all bad. One of the greatest advantages of living in an urban area is that there is greater access to healthy food and medical services.[21] Even though, in far too many urban areas, there are many neighborhoods that don't have these types of services, they still remain more plentiful inside cities than in rural environments. There is also some evidence that social isolation, not being in close contact with other people, is bad for health. So this would also appear to be a benefit for people living in cities. In general, evidence suggests that though air pollution tends to be higher in cities, water pollution may be higher in rural areas. Rural areas have higher rates of motor vehicle accidents (people must drive more) and are less likely to have access to nutritious food and routine and emergency medical care. Urban residents walk more, rural residents less.[22] The debate continues.

FOCUS ON

Road Rage

Given the amount of time Americans spend commuting and the frustrations that can arise from accidents, traffic congestion, and transit delays, the potential for the stress of travel to build to the point that incidents between persons can happen is important. Not that this excuses any of the behavior on roads or on public transit.

One problem in assessing the incidence of road rage is that there is no clear consensus as to what it is. Generally, it is considered to be an acute episode of anger, sometimes accompanied by violence, threatening actions, or angry words, that occurs while driving, walking, taking public transportation, or otherwise traveling outside the home. Despite publicity, we don't really know how much road rage there is. Although the more extreme cases make the press, most incidents are probably not reported.

Solving the problem of road rage may be similarly difficult. One strategy would be to reduce the amount of impedance and other problems associated with commuting. But funding for infrastructure improvements is limited and, for the most part, further improvements to traffic flow are not likely. Helping people understand why and how they get angry may be effective, but again, there are most likely limits to this type of strategy.

Density and Health

The great failure of the family public housing program in the United States (see Chapter Five), along with perceived problems in congested tenement districts in the mid-twentieth century, prompted some researchers to study the effects of density on health. Interestingly, at first the studies seemed to suggest that there was an association between the two, but a reexamination of the evidence suggested no such association and the experience provides a cautionary lesson for those who wish to study the built environment or who plan to modify the built environment to promote health. Public health moves slowly when it comes to reaching conclusions about etiology and interventions.

The early evidence appeared to demonstrate that density was a problem. From the middle of the nineteenth century, if not earlier, medical and epidemiological studies suggested that the density in tenement districts was strongly associated with negative outcomes.[23] These high-density districts were the locations where disease and mortality were the highest, and so tenement reformers, zoning advocates, and housing specialists all sought to reduce the crowding in cities.

But it is very difficult, if not impossible, to conduct epidemiological research on housing and neighborhoods because it is too expensive and ethically wrong to randomly assign people to differing living environments. It is a basic human right to live where one wants to live and no funder or review board would allow such an assignment. To get around this problem, researchers in the 1950s and 1960s turned to studies of rats to see if animal experiments could provide evidence that would help increase understanding of human behavior. One of the most important of these studies, conducted by John Calhoun, looked at the effects of crowding on rats. The results were alarming. Overcrowded rats appeared to exhibit a range of antisocial behaviors including violence and inappropriate sexual behavior. He termed the location of the worst of these behaviors "behavioral sinks."[24] The lesson seemed to be clear for those who clustered in cities: living in an urban area promoted crime and deviancy. Later on, the results of these experiments were popularized among planners and architects by Edward Hall in his book *The Hidden Dimension*,[25] and for years, if not decades, it was thought that the link between density and health was firmly established. This assumption against density is one of the underpinnings of conventional U.S. zoning codes and many cities work to reduce densities in their jurisdictions. Overcrowding caused behavioral issues and because public housing was thought to be urban America's densest housing type, it provided a biological plausibility to the observed social problems concentrated there.

But a reexamination of the data and the experiments themselves found that the evidence was not so clear-cut. For one thing, simply overcrowding rats did not produce pathological behavior. So Calhoun began to withhold food. Again, pathological behavior did not develop. Next he limited the number of feeding stations, forcing rats to fight with each other to get access to scarce food. It was only when overcrowded rats were starved and provided limited feeding opportunities that the behavioral sinks developed. The problem was not density itself but density in the context of scarcity and problems with food access. The implications for humans living in cities were thus limited. Later, scientists challenged the appropriateness of rat models for human behavior altogether.[26]

Furthermore, examination of people in neighborhoods did not provide the corroborative evidence that was thought to exist in the real world. It was true that high-rise public housing did have serious crime issues and other social problems, but the densities of public housing were actually lower than the densities in other nearby urban neighborhoods that were safer.[27] Again, not density per se but perhaps the design of the buildings was causing the problem. It was also realized that the densities in poor urban communities in the United States are but a fraction of the densities found in many other countries where social pathologies did not seem to cluster. Therefore, any density-to-health pathway was socially mediated and not a biological imperative.[28] Overall, it was found that poverty was a much greater predictor of social problems than density or overcrowding and that once poverty and other social factors were controlled for, only a small association existed between overcrowded housing (persons per unit) and social problems. There was no association between overall population density (persons per square mile) and the social issues it was once thought to produce.[29] Over time, the role of density as a health problem has diminished in the health literature even though it may still be an unquestioned given among some urban theorists. It may also be one of the reasons why communities are so opposed to higher density. Thus, even though the evidence has been discredited and left aside by health professionals, its influence may persist.

High-Rises and Connections to the Street

Le Corbusier and his fellow Modernists thought high-rises and urban designs that set skyscrapers in parkland were an effective way to provide sunlight and ventilation to housing units and connect residents to nature. People living on upper floors could look out on the green space below and benefit from that view.[30] There may be some truth to this if the results of the view of nature and recovery from surgery study are valid. But by the mid-1960s, there was a growing dissatisfaction with the skyscraper-in-the-park urban design. Jane Jacobs strongly condemned this as being anti-urban and bad for cities. Jacobs, at least in her early writings, did not necessarily oppose high-rises, but she thought them to be not as desirable as walk-ups and thought they should never be built distant from the street.[31]

By the beginning of the twenty-first century, however, her ideas have often been interpreted to be strongly anti-high-rise. The biggest objection to living above the fifth floor of a building today is that it disconnects residents from the street.[32] The concern is that this is not only bad for maintaining the high degree of social observation of what is going on the street that helps make streets safer and prevent crime, but also that this disconnect is somehow bad for the mental health of residents. But although there is substantial evidence that living in high-rises is bad for low-income families with children, there is no evidence at this time to support the idea that living in a high-rise is bad for health overall.[33] One problem is that the very concept of a lack of connection to the street is difficult to define and its biological effects hard to operationalize. Another is that "a lack of connection" is difficult to measure and quantify. Furthermore, there are problems in assessing whether or not the lack of connection supposedly inherent in high-rise living is greater than other factors that promote disconnect from the street such as cell phones, single-family homes set apart by lawns, or cars. Though many urbanists continue to oppose high-rises because of this disconnect, in terms of health and scientifically validated issues, it may be better to be concerned about high-rise living for other reasons, such as wind and shadow effects.

Defensible Space

Some of the first modern health studies to explore the role of the built environment did not produce lasting results, but the extreme problems of urban living continued to encourage researchers to try to understand the role of the built environment in shaping behavior. These efforts continued throughout the mid-twentieth century and helped to increase our understanding of why public housing was so unsafe. For example, Oscar Newman, in a series of studies on New York City public housing, tried to determine if there were certain environments that fostered crime or promoted safety.[34] Eventually his work appeared to substantiate that certain types of architectural designs were better than others in terms of public and personal safety. Among the features that appeared to be safer were clear sightlines so that people could tell if any evildoers were lurking about and also that privatized space, regardless of who actually owned it, was safer than public space where no one felt responsible for its safety and upkeep. This concept is now called *defensible space* and it has a profound impact on multifamily housing architecture as well as urban design. For example, many public housing developments have been redeveloped so that a given entryway will only serve one or a few families and whenever possible, open spaces are given over to the private exclusive use of a single unit rather than shared by all the occupants of the development. Note that these alternatives also allow for more attractive landscaping than the alternatives: paved-over areas, high-intensity lighting, high fences, iron bars, and so on. Vegetation is selected so that it will not inhibit sightlines or lighting.

Defensible space was one of the concepts that underlay new urbanism and the federal program to renovate public housing known as HOPE VI.[35] The evidence supports the idea that small-scale, pedestrian-friendly environments are best for promoting health and socialization and they reduce crime and vandalism. In practice, defensible space involves giving individual people or families the responsibility for the use and maintenance of outdoor spaces whenever possible. The number of units per building entryway should be kept at a minimum and the yards outside the entrances should be deeded space. Parking, if provided, should be near units and within sight of them. It should be designed so that people feel safe as they travel from street to an entry to inside units. Many of these features are now prioritized in building codes as either being mandatory or strongly advised.[36]

The Role of Stressors and Allostatic Load

It has long been observed that life is full of stressors. Balancing job pressures and family responsibilities, coping with health issues, and trying to support families are all stressful. It is also understood that the poor face special stressors that are greater than those of the well-off. Not having a job can mean applying for public assistance, filling out long forms that threaten severe penalties for inaccurate information, waiting in line to speak to a staff person, and then worrying that there will not be enough money to buy food at the end of the month. Those who are working but have low incomes also face greater stresses. One of the greatest problems is the lack of control over one's working situation. Those in lower-paying jobs tend to have more rigid start times, less ability to refuse overtime work, and are less likely to have sick and vacation time, resulting in their having to work even when they are ill.[37]

In addition to individual stresses, low-income people can face a number of neighborhood problems including high crime, dependence on unreliable public transportation or being forced to pay for a car that they can hardly afford, abandoned buildings and vacant lots, and other stressors that can reinforce problems inside and outside of the home. People of color may face additional problems that lead to stress such as racism, discrimination, and the sense of isolation that can arise from being the only person of color in a given situation.[38]

People of both sexes can be subject to special stressors. Women may fear street crime, domestic violence, or harassment at work. Men may face stressors from competition with their peers. There are domestic stressors and stresses associated with being isolated. The range of stressors that may affect the homeless is even greater. The overall level of stress in a person's life has been termed *allostatic load*. The greater a person's level of stress exposure, the greater is their allostatic load.

This in turn suggests that their bodies are exposed to higher levels of psychosocial as well as social and external stresses.

The strong association between stress and health has been well documented; one of the reasons that almost all epidemiological studies control for race and income is that these factors can be proxies for all of the stressors in people's lives and represent the lack of resources they may have to meet the challenges posed by these stressors. In the past few years, the biological pathways responsible for this stress-to-health association have been identified. It is chronic stress, the constant and continuing stressors in people's lives, that may be most damaging to health, not the acute stress that might happen for a moment in time. Briefly, the biological pathway is that a stressful situation results in stimulation of the hypothalamus, which then signals the pituitary gland, which in turn causes the adrenal glands to secrete a hormone known as cortisol.[39] Even though it is essential to health, cortisol can cause a number of problems throughout the body, including high blood pressure, cardiac issues, renal problems, and other concerns. It may even be a factor in the development of Type II diabetes.[40]

Awareness of chronic stress as a problem has not necessarily led to adequate solutions. It is difficult, for example, to advise people to reduce the chronic stresses in their lives when they have very little control over the factors that led to that stress. There is a need to develop programs and policies to address the chronic stressors that affect so many and, so often disproportionately, the poor and persons of color. Of course, knowing that chronic stress has many potential health consequences may help frame research and interventions, and may add to our understanding of the concepts of cumulative risk in the problems of vulnerable populations.[41]

Rootshock and the Effects of Urban Renewal and Gentrification

The stresses associated with individual health outcomes could also be studied on the neighborhood level. Urban history in the United States is a constant story of neighborhood change as one racial/ethnic group is displaced by another. Often this displacement was voluntary, such as when the children and grandchildren of immigrants left old inner-city ethnic neighborhoods for new single-family homes in the suburbs. This type of change was seen as positive and health strengthening. But the United States has also seen episodes of forced neighborhood change which could be more rapid, have important economic consequences, and may have threatened the mental health status of residents and commuters.

Mid-twentieth century policies called urban renewal relied heavily on the massive demolition and displacement of entire communities, particularly those of African Americans. Urban renewal was used as a tool to eliminate or displace black neighborhoods; highways were often built through these communities because the land was cheap, the highway could be used as a barrier between blacks and whites, or, by building a highway in a certain location, a nonwhite community could be demolished. The noted community psychologist Mindy Fullilove described the psychological effects of these kinds of displacements as rootshock, meaning that when a community is displaced, it suffers from a collective stress that can lead to a feeling of grief and loss and a disconnect from its collective past as well as from larger society.[42] These effects were seen as early as the 1950s and were not exclusive to African American communities (as in the case of the displacement of an Italian and Jewish community in Boston's West End), but displacement disproportionately affected African American neighborhoods. It could well be that communities are still dealing with these kinds of issues even several generations after the neighborhoods were first destroyed. A lesson for those seeking to manipulate the built environment is that massive demolition and large-scale neighborhood change can have severe psychological impacts that can persist for decades, if not generations. Displacement is something that should be avoided.[43]

The era of large-scale publicly funded, intentional demolitions of neighborhoods is over. There is no longer the money to fund these types of programs nor the political will and ability to force the relocation of thousands of people by a single project. This does not mean that rapid and psychologically stressful displacement is not still occurring. Today the issue in many select urban neighborhoods is *gentrification*, the displacement of lower-income, often minority residents, by higher income, often white, newcomers.[44] Other areas can experience declines when local governments decide to deliberately withhold services.[45]

Many cities are actively promoting gentrification, seeing it as a way to improve their tax base and make their cities appear to be more economically viable. Upper-income families are seen as easier to service than lower-income families that tend to be larger, have children in public schools, require more police services, or pose other service provision issues.[46] In one sense there are two ways to raise the economic status of the community. One way, which is much more difficult, is to increase the earning power of current residents by bringing in jobs and increasing the skill set of existing residents. This can take time and enormous public investment that cities may not have. Many cities choose an alternative program of economic improvement by trying to encourage higher-income people to move into their communities. They may launch advertising campaigns to attract higher-income people, work to bring in developers who promise high-end shopping and other amenities, or give subsidies to developers or potential homeowners to locate in certain areas.[47] This later strategy can result in gentrification because as newcomers move in, housing prices can rise, forcing low-income renters to quickly have to seek new places to live and cause low-income homeowners to move as their property taxes rise. The psychological effect of these policies that result from gentrification have not been well studied at this time, but the fear is that they can lead to the same kinds of community psychological effects among the previous lower-income residents as did the older policies of urban renewal and highway construction.

Communities can pursue a number of strategies to protect residents from the effects of gentrification. Some cities have rent control, which can help make housing affordable even as potential higher-income renters want to move into a neighborhood. Other communities have adopted a robust policy of building subsidizing assisted housing so that even as the number of new higher-income units is increasing in the community, large numbers of lower-income residents can still be accommodated there. A third strategy is to have a community control land and own buildings.

Access to Open Space and Attention Deficit Hyperactivity Disorder

The past decade has seen research into the environmental influences on Attention Deficit Hyperactivity Disorder (ADHD). This is a syndrome of behaviors, often but not exclusively diagnosed in children, that may include an inability to concentrate, being easily distracted, having a hard time sitting still, and other similar symptoms. The percentage of children who may have ADHD may be as high as 4% of the population and as many as half of these children may go on to have ADHD as adults.

As noted above, though there are some who suggested ADHD is a form of nature deficit disorder and that it is the disconnect from nature that is responsible for the high rates we see of this disorder, there is little evidence to suggest that there is something in the built environment that causes ADHD at this time.[48] More study in this area is needed. However, there is some evidence that certain types of environments may assist in mitigating the impacts of the symptoms of ADHD. In particular, exposing ADHD children to natural environments may reduce the frequency and severity of symptoms and may make them more ready to learn in classroom situations.[49] Some have used nature walks and outdoor learning environments as a way to help ADHD children learn.

Noise Exposure and Health

Another pervasive feature of the modern urban environment is noise.[50] Motor vehicles, particularly trucks and buses, can be so loud as to make conversation

---

FOCUS ON

Healing Gardens

Given the influences of the built environment on mood and stress, there is a long history of designing and creating gardens to help those suffering from illnesses and their friends and loved ones. The idea of the healing garden extends back over a thousand years, reenergized by the research of Ulrich and others that access to nature can promote improved outcomes for surgery patients. As suggested by the University of Minnesota Sustainable Urban Landscape Information Series, a well-designed healing garden will be accessible for those with limited mobility and perception, be easy to maintain, environmentally sustainable, cost effective, and visually pleasing. (For more information, visit: http://www.sustland.umn.edu/design/healinggardens.html.)

Some healing gardens have been constructed adjacent to hospitals and clinics; others have been built out in the community in order to reach those who are not necessarily confronted by the challenges of acute illness. Others have been built in remote places, building on the long tradition of the healing garden in monasteries and religious institutions. Some gardens are aimed at special populations including nursing homes and schools. There have been gardens built on rooftops and in the courtyards of medical centers.

---

impossible. Noise from jets, airplanes, and helicopters may be so constant and so loud that living near an airport may be bad for health.[51] The concern is that noise exposures can lead to stress and cause the health issues outlined earlier, and that living near heavily traveled roads and airports can cause chronic noise exposures that lead to chronic stress, which is known to be so bad for health.[52] Communities have tried to address noise problems by banning takeoffs and landings at airports during certain hours, changing runways and operations, and by fighting the construction of airport expansions. Other neighborhoods have worked to address the noise from highways by having transportation authorities construct sound walls to keep the noise out of the neighborhoods.[53]

A similar issue in many suburban neighborhoods is the use of equipment for lawn and garden care because of concern for the serenity of neighbors. Though this noise tends to be acute rather than chronic and therefore have less of the chronic effects associated with highways, for example, neighbors can often be very annoyed by the sound of lawn mowers and leaf blowers. This has led some communities to consider bans on these types of equipment or restricting hours in which they can be used.

Health Facilities Design

The work by Ulrich and others has been extended into a new field of endeavor to increase the quality of the design of health care facilities. The architecture of hospitals has a long history that has paralleled the history of medicine itself. For example, during the time when tuberculosis was a major health threat, the design of tuberculosis sanitariums was a major focus that centered on how to get patients access to fresh air yet still keep them protected from the elements. As our understanding of disease has changed, and our understanding of how the environment of hospitals can influence health has changed, the importance of health facilities design has increased. Given the huge amount of data that are generated by the health care system, outcomes can be carefully measured against various environmental inputs. This has informed the state of the art of health care design.

A major problem in the health care system is that patients often acquire infectious diseases in a hospital or other health care setting when they are there for another reason. Collectively, these nosocomial infections result in millions of cases, cost billions of dollars, and kill thousands of people. Thus there is a major incentive to reduce hospital-acquired infections.[54] By studying how and where people become infected, there have been important changes in hospital design. For example, there has been a movement toward individual rooms as opposed to semiprivate rooms because such rooms isolate individuals and reduce their exposure to risk.[55] Changing ventilation and the circulation of air to reduce infections have also been demonstrated to be cost effective. In addition, providing facilities so that it is easier for doctors and nurses and others to wash their hands is also strongly effective against disease transmission. Collectively, these measures are dramatically changing how hospitals are designed.[56]

The advent of modern medicine with its heavy emphasis on medical equipment used to provide services and monitor patient status has resulted in a dramatic increase in the sound levels in many hospitals. Studies suggest that if decibel levels are too high, sleep is affected, patient comfort is diminished, and the risk of medical errors can increase. There is evidence that newborns, particularly those in neonatal intensive care units, are particularly sensitive to noise. In response, hospital designers have tried to modify the design of rooms and buildings so that sounds in one room do not affect those in another, along with increased soundproofing so that overall noise levels are reduced.[57]

Another major problem in the health care industry is occupational injuries. Musculoskeletal injuries associated with lifting, bending, and reaching are a particular issue for nurses and others who may have responsibility for lifting or transporting patients who may be very heavy. This has resulted in the design of a number of improvements to reduce the risks of these strains and to prevent injuries from happening.[58]

Evidence-Based Design

The revolution in changing how buildings are designed so that they are based upon experimental data has not been limited to hospitals. Traditionally, the fields of architecture and urban planning have not used standard epidemiological research methods to assess the efficiency of designs, buildings, or neighborhoods. Over the years they have tended to rely upon case studies and theoretical models for evaluating architectural practices rather than on the standard case-control and cohort studies that are at the center of medical research. The highly measured outcomes in the health care industry resulted in the use of those data to evaluate the built environment there first.[59] More recently, these techniques have expanded to other areas of design, where there are also large amounts of data that can be analyzed and the results of different environments compared.[60] These include educational environments and manufacturing facilities where outputs are heavily tested and measured. By carefully monitoring results along with controlling for key confounding factors, the built environment can be carefully evaluated. This allows for new changes in how schools are designed and how workplaces are set up. Test score results, productivity, and absences and injuries are among the outcomes studied.[61]

Summary

Concerns that the built environment may have an impact on mental health date back to a century ago when sociologists began to study how moving to the city affected rural migrants. Today, there are related concepts, including biophilia and nature deficit disorder. Current concerns include the concepts of defensible space and allostatic load. In addition, hospital design has begun to use epidemiologically derived data in what is known as evidence-based design to improve patient outcomes.

Key Terms

Anomie

Biophilia

Defensible space

Discussion Questions

1. Describe the ways that immigration might affect mental health.
2. What is biophilia?
3. Do you think there is such a thing as nature deficit disorder?
4. Are John Calhoun's rat studies a good model for predicting the behavior of people in U.S. cities?
5. Define defensible space.
6. What is allostatic load? How might it affect health?
7. What are some of the health problems associated with being a patient in a hospital?
8. Define evidence-based design.

For More Information

Design for Health. www.designforhealth.net.

Hall, E. T. *The hidden dimension*. (1969). New York: Anchor Books.

Hamilton, D. K., & Watkins, D. H. (2008). *Evidence-based design for multiple building types*. Hoboken, NJ: Wiley.

The Center for Health Design. www.healthdesign.org.

CHAPTER 12

SOCIAL CAPITAL

LEARNING OBJECTIVES

- Differentiate between environmental and biological determinism.
- Name key concepts in social capital theory.
- Describe how social capital is measured.
- Compare social capital bonding versus bridging.
- Identify the health effects of social capital.
- Define broken windows theory.
- Evaluate the role of neighborhood in the persistence of poverty.

Most of us exist in a web of connections with others. We have our family and friends, coworkers, and people we see on a daily basis and may not even know by name. Think about how these people affect your activities and preferences. Do they influence the music you listen to, the style of clothes you wear, or the place you would most like to live? Overall, consider their impact on your day-to-day practices that protect or cause problems with your health, such as reinforcing healthy eating habits or lending you cigarettes when you want to smoke. Look at others around you—do they appear to naturally collect into groups? Imagine if we could harness the power of these groups to promote health.

This chapter begins with the theory and historical beginnings of social capital, discusses environmental, biological, and social determinism theory, and explains key concepts related to social capital. It then describes how social capital can be measured and discusses potential negative impacts of social capital. Next comes an outline of the health benefits of social capital and an overview of some of the efforts to increase it. These are followed by sections on social norms and what is called broken windows theory. Then there is a consideration of how advertising can affect behavior. The final sections of the chapter discuss the concept of the culture of poverty, past efforts to break up poor communities, and an experiment to move poor families out of **concentrated poverty areas** known as the Moving to Opportunity Program.

Theory and Historical Beginnings

The study of human behavior has greatly benefited from the work of a wide variety of disciplines. One field that has had particular influence is that of economics. Both concerned with human behavior and based on an easy to quantify metric—money—economics developed a set of powerful tools that can be used to increase our understanding of human behavior and assist in studying the health effects of the built environment.

One important term that owes its derivation, in part, from economics is **social capital**, the strength and capacity of a network of human interactions and the associations in that network. Social capital can assist network members to either protect their health or make them more prone to risk behaviors. The concept of financial capital is straightforward. It is the amount of money or assets an individual, family, or society has that can be used to pay for goods and services, invest in new business enterprises or capital-intensive infrastructure, or save to meet future needs. Those with higher levels of financial capital, (also known as wealth), or increased access to financial capital, tend to have better health outcomes and are less likely to participate in risky health behaviors.[1]

Another important concept is *human capital*, the overall amount of skills and knowledge possessed by an individual or group. The investment in education is a prime example of human capital. Though the value of a college degree can be monetized in terms of increased lifetime earnings, it is difficult to quantify all the personal and social benefits of a college education; there is evidence that college educated persons are less likely to smoke, more physically active, report fewer sexual risk factors, and so on.[2] This quantifiable and qualitative set of skills a person or community possesses collectively makes up what can be characterized as a person's or society's stock of human capital.

Social scientists and public health workers have turned to the theoretical construct of social capital to describe how societies—ranging from international or countrywide networks, states or neighborhoods, or even small groups such as gangs or students in a single classroom—establish social norms, promote or inhibit risk behaviors, or influence health outcomes. The use of social capital has become a powerful tool for increasing our understanding of health and provides a useful basis for developing interventions.

Environmental Determinism Versus Biological Determinism

An important theme that has consistently been part of urban studies, sociology, and public health since their beginnings in the nineteenth century has been a search for what influences human behavior. In the health realm, individual behaviors, from physical activity to going to the doctor for preventive care, can have important effects on health. Therefore, researchers have asked questions such as why do some people act in their own best interest even when it may be uncomfortable, such as having blood drawn for cholesterol tests? Why do others do things that they know are bad for their health, such as start smoking? The idea that the built environment can shape human behavior arises from the theoretical construct known as *environmental determinism*. It is important to note that this term has never been meant to suggest that the environment is responsible for 100% or even a majority of the variance in human behavior. It only means that the environment contributes to the propensity for people to behave in certain ways.

Environmental determinism had its first great era of influence in the nineteenth and early twentieth centuries when urban reformers sought new laws to regulate the urban environment in order to address the appalling conditions in the tenement districts of large cities.[3] They aimed to improve housing in order to improve health. The middle and upper-middle classes also began to segregate themselves into enclaves that they believed promoted family life, moral correctness, and healthy living, a process that has continued for over a century.[4] Even misguided public policies such as Modernism and urban renewal had an underlying belief that the proper built environment could help make humanity better and create a healthier population.

The latter part of the twentieth century saw environmental determinism eclipsed by *biological determinism*; a large amount of research energy and resources have been spent on finding genes and biological structures and mechanisms that help influence violence, risk taking, and substance abuse. Some of these efforts have resulted in great advances in the understanding of the nature of health risks, increased ability to identify problems and plan interventions, and improved development of treatments. Researchers also use biomarkers and genetic testing to identify individuals who may be at greater risk for cocaine addiction or alcohol abuse. But again, there are limits to the influence of biology; it is not a 100% predictor of behavior or maladaption to social conditions.

The reestablishment of the built environment and health movement has given new life to theories derived from environmental determinism. In their current form, these ideas posit that both the built and the social environments can assist people to avoid risk behaviors or to promote healthy lifestyles.[5] They do not promise that everyone will meet physical activity guidelines in a new urbanist development; they only suggest that these behaviors become easier to adopt and maintain in some environments than in others.[6] One of the goals of built environment reformers in the twenty-first century has been to increase levels of social capital to help make people healthier.

Key Concepts

Social capital's influence on behavior and health is one aspect of social environmental determinism: an individual learns and adopts behavioral norms based on the actions and values of others around them as well as their interactions with their surrounding group of people.[7] Social capital theory also posits that connections with other people can help individuals adapt and maintain healthy behaviors. It also maintains that inappropriate behavior by others can prompt individuals to behave poorly themselves. If people see litter on the street, for example, they may be more likely to litter because they see that others believe that there is nothing wrong with it. They take clues as to what constitutes allowable, mainstream behavior from the environment around them. In another example, individuals may smoke because their close friends think smoking is okay or even desirable. Note that all these factors represent the interactions of an individual with people around them rather than anything internal to that individual such as genes or microbial action. One of the most important ideas in understanding social capital is that it is fundamentally a concept that has limited meaning when considered at the individual level. It is meant to describe the interactions and connections of individuals inside a larger, multi-individual network.[8] Though there are often efforts to measure the number and strength of connections an individual may have with others, social capital has no meaning when an individual is considered in isolation. It is a group-level variable. This does not mean that a value derived at the group level can't be assigned to individuals and used in epidemiological research, only that such assignment must be used and interpreted very cautiously.[9] Individuals can have varying degrees of social capital, but this is an indication of their relationships with others.

There are a number of subconstructs that make up social capital.[10] These are not discrete domains and in fact overlap each other. These subconstructs include trust, the degree to which individuals can predict the behavior of others in their group and to which the individual can rely on these behaviors for support.[11] There is **collective efficacy**, the belief that a group, when working together, can achieve goals and counteract internal and external threats (such as proposals to locate hazardous waste facilities in a community). This is a group-level corollary of **self-efficacy**, the belief on the part of an individual that he or she can achieve personal goals. Another important subconstruct is the richness and depth of the network, which is usually operationalized as the number of network connections. In general, as the number of connections between members of the group increases, so does the group's level of social capital. Another subconstruct is social support, the degree to which members of the group can be relied on when there are external threats or the degree to which individuals

FOCUS ON

Can Your Friends Make You Fat?

That's an intriguing finding from the results of a survey that used data from the famous Framingham Heart Study to study the influence of social ties on weight gain. The Framingham Study has been following residents of that Massachusetts town and their descendants for three generations. Participants receive periodic health assessments and have been surveyed repeatedly over time. In order to improve follow-up, participants are asked to name others who could provide contact information in case someone moves and doesn't provide a new address.

The study design used these contacts to construct a system of links and connections in the study population. They then looked to see if an increase in obesity among a study subject's friends was associated with an increased risk of weight gain for the subject. They found that having obese friends did indeed increase the risk of weight gain, even more than family or spouses did.

Some caveats should be kept in mind while interpreting the study. Although it controlled for individual characteristics, it did not control for neighborhood effects. It is possible that friends, even those who move across the country from each other, have similar tastes in neighborhood. There may also be issues with measuring the strength of associations between self-identified friends in the study population. Finally, this is only one study and it is important to remember that causality is rarely established by the results in one published article. Still, the results may be reflective of the power of social networks to influence health.

can depend upon other members of the network to assist them during times of emergencies. All of these may be related to health.

Measuring Social Capital

There are issues when it comes to measuring social capital because it is a group construct that can often only be measured by asking individuals about their beliefs, actions, and values.[12] In many studies, individual members are surveyed using a number of questions which are then grouped into scales, and these values are then averaged over the total numbers of the survey group.[13] Thus there may be a set of questions aimed to measure the extent to which individuals believe that their group can successfully meet external challenges; these responses are first tallied to form an individual scale and then grouped and averaged to give a single overall network value. The overall score of one group can be compared to that of another and thus the relative amount of social capital in one group can be compared to others. It should be cautioned that there are many different survey instruments that have been developed to measure social capital and that any single value derived from one scale cannot always be compared to a value derived from another scale.[14] One of the most widely used survey instruments is part of the General Social Survey, which has been asking questions that can be used for interpreting and measuring social capital for decades.[15]

The individual questions in these surveys vary in order to take into account the subconstruct that is being measured. For example, one common question is to ask if other members of the network (or community) can be trusted to obey the law. Another question often used is whether or not there are other members of the network from whom the individual could borrow money in an emergency. Regardless of which survey is used, compiling the answers to calculate overall social capital scores must be carefully considered. Often, a very serious issue is that of weighting, or whether or not each and every question should be weighted the same. This can become a problem when one subdomain has more questions than another and not weighting the questions results in giving greater or less weight to those questions in the domains with fewer or more questions.[16]

An alternative way to measure social capital is to ask how many organizations individuals belong to.[17] The thought is that each individual membership represents a social connection within the larger group, in this case usually referring to a neighborhood, city, metropolitan area, or state as proxies for all the other connections an individual may have. Social connections have been measured by asking individuals how many friends they have, how often they speak to relatives over the telephone, and how often they socialize with each other. Note how each of these questions aims to assess how the individual interacts with others in his network or group.[18]

Another method to measure social capital is to look at voter participation rates. A community that has a higher voter turnout may have higher levels of social capital, or potentially a higher degree of faith in the value of political processes that may reflect higher collective efficacy. An advantage of this method is that it relies on an external, publicly accessible data source rather than self-reported metrics. It does not need extensive surveying and the calculation of composite scores and scales. However, though there is most likely a correlation between voting percentage and other aspects of social capital, it is also potentially related to median income, citizenship status, and other factors that are not necessarily reflective of social capital. For example, an immigrant community may have low levels of voter participation because it has few adult citizens, but it may well have high levels of interactions within its group.

All of these measures have potential limitations. For example, the work of Robert Putnam—whose theories include the idea that the change in how people bowl (from the past when they participated in bowling leagues to the present where individuals simply get together with friends to bowl) reflects a decline in social capital (popularized in his book *Bowling Alone*)[19]—has been criticized because his observed changes in public participation and private groups may not reflect an underlying decline in social capital but may instead simply be related to the fact that women now have better employment opportunities, social norms have changed so that men now prefer to spend time with their families rather than with their peers in fraternal organizations, and that the changes in participation may simply reflect changes in leisure time tastes.[20] In another example, people in wealthier communities may report fewer people from whom they could borrow money because they have been less likely to ever have needed money, or because they have the ability to work with financial institutions or other means of accessing cash.

Is There Less Social Capital in One Type of Area Than Another?

Almost from the very beginning of modern U.S. suburbia after World War I, sociologists and urbanologists expressed concerns that the quantity and quality of the human interactions in suburbs was not as great as those found in cities.[21] There was also the feeling that small rural communities might have a greater amount of human interaction with people who are known and trusted than in other places. Many of these concerns predate the articulation of the concept of social capital but they are ultimately questions of whether or not certain types of places promote greater social capital and other types of places inhibit it. One of the ideas of Jane Jacobs was that a variety of uses on a street, along with the constant interaction between community members and people on the street, would promote strong social norms that would protect the community against crime and violence.[22] She believed that streets with only single uses such as housing would not have sufficient human activity to create the great richness of interconnections that was necessary for healthy neighborhoods. She did not explicitly use the term *social capital* but that was part of the underlying construct of her theories.

Despite these concerns, there is little evidence that suburban residents have lower levels of social capital than urban dwellers or that people who live in rural communities have more social interactions than those who live in other types of places.[23] In general, it may be easier to have day-to-day social interactions in places with higher population density, but once a certain minimum threshold is passed, there may be no additional social capital benefits to greater density.

It must be emphasized, however, that there is little research in this area. There is some evidence to suggest that rural residents have overall lower health status and are more likely to report having poor risk behaviors than residents of suburban and urban areas. This may be related to greater rates of poverty and reduced access to services. It also may represent the physical difficulty in meeting up with family and friends posed by long distances and a lack of transportation alternatives.

Social capital in inner-city, impoverished neighborhoods is also complex.[24] In general, poor communities tend to have lower measured social capital. But to what extent does this reflect the problems associated with poverty? Because poor people tend to have lower social capital, how much of this lower overall social capital rate be attributed to the community and how much to the individuals?[25] The complex decline of inner-city economies, institutions, social relations, and other dimensions of effects are greater than what can be attributed to changes in social capital.[26] It is important to keep in mind exactly what is meant by social capital and what the goals are in a project used to measure or increase it. A major research need continues to be the role of the built environment, and its many features, in improving social capital.

Negative Effects of Social Capital

It is important to understand that not all aspects of social capital may be positive.[27] For example, ethnic neighborhoods, which were once very prevalent in U.S. cities, had rich networks of formal and informal ties that helped strengthen the overall social capital in the communities. However, these neighborhoods have been criticized because of the resistance to racial integration and the degree to which outsiders were not welcomed.[28] Networks and groups can also reinforce negative behaviors, as when a gang promotes aggression or when intolerance can lead to violence, crime, or other destructive behaviors.[29] There also must be a balance between the social norms promoted by a group and individual freedom. If social capital is so strong and the ultimate impact on behavior so great that individuals feel they cannot do things that they may want to do even if such things might actually promote health or increase economic freedom, then the social norms, and the underlying social capital, can become destructive.[30]

Bridging versus bonding is one way that social capital has been considered.[31] Bonding represents linkages within a group, often defined by shared factors of ethnicity, socioeconomics, religion, age, and so forth. Bridging refers to linkages between people of different groups. [32] To a certain extent, bonding is easier to accomplish than bridging, but bridging might be better for a community and bonding may be more likely to enhance negative impacts of social capital.[33]

Health Effects

The great value of social capital theory for understanding communities and promoting social change has prompted many researchers to look at the health effects of social capital on both individual and neighborhood health. This is not always easy to accomplish. For one thing, it is important that the individualized measures of social capital be operationalized at a higher level (neighborhood, city, state, and so on) and that these group-level effects are analyzed in a manner that does not violate the standard rules of epidemiological inference and statistical analysis. For example, many statistical methods are based on the assumption that individuals are entirely independent from each other, but social capital is a construct that is only understandable as a group-level variable and thus individuals in the same group from which a group-level social capital score is constructed may not be independent. One way to account for these group level effects is to use *multilevel modeling*. In this method, some variables are operationalized as individual factors and some as group factors and the statistical analysis takes this into account, treating groups of individuals as clusters. An example of this are studies of students in classrooms and schools. Each of these represents a separate level.

It is also very important that individual-level factors that might be related to group-level factors be controlled for in the study. Thus people with lower incomes and low educational attainment might end up living in communities with low social capital. But then the challenge is to distinguish between the effects caused by those lower incomes and low educational attainment from those that are the responsibility of the community with low social capital. This is not always easy.[34]

In general, it has been found that individuals in communities with lower social capital tend to have lower overall health status, fewer protective health behaviors, more harmful health behaviors, higher morbidity, and higher mortality after controlling for potential confounding individual factors. Lower social capital has been associated with increased mortality, higher rates of communicable diseases, increased smoking, reduced diabetes control, and other adverse health outcomes.[35] The relative degree to which these higher-level factors affect health in comparison to the influence of individual-level factors has been debated; however, the presence of one as an influence of health does not negate the presence of the other. Ultimately both social factors and individual issues must be addressed if health is to be maximized. Again, it must be considered that there are other factors influencing health. For example, certain communities may have higher smoking rates, but is this attributable to a lack of social capital, social norms that see nothing wrong with smoking, or a clustering of tobacco advertising in the neighborhood? It is not easy to disentangle these effects.[36]

Improving Social Capital

Given the potential powerful effects of increased social capital on health, behavior, and life outcomes, a number of efforts have aimed to improve social capital for both individuals and groups. At the very small level, the widely-used team trust-building activities, popular in business and work environments, have underlying goals to improve trust among members of the group and improve their communication skills, thus strengthening individual connections, ultimately increasing group efficacy, and helping the organization's members believe that they have the ability to work together to accomplish common goals.

There has been a long-standing goal of urban planners and public health professionals to improve social capital by manipulating the built environment. One important way to do this is to use the built environment to create opportunities for people to meet and interact with each other.[37] The idea is that the more individuals in the community gather together, the more social connections can develop, leading to a greater degree of trust.[38] Thus planners promote open spaces, plazas, sidewalks lined with amenities, small playgrounds, farmers markets, and other similar uses so that individual interactions can increase.[39] Public health has used group interventions, peer education, and community events to promote social capital and support healthy behaviors such as healthy diets, physical activity, or reduced smoking.

Changing group expectations was part of Saul Alinsky's community organizing philosophy and one of his underlying ideas in his influential book, *Rules for Radicals*.[40] In general, community activists understand that the very act of organizing has benefits to the community because it strengthens social ties, helps build community efficacy, and establishes trust inside the group. These higher-level interventions can be important for promoting positive neighborhood change and both urban planning and public health greatly rely on community organizing to promote their goals. Urban planners often work to promote community development corporations, neighborhood associations, and business groups to improve the local environment and promote economic activity. Part of these efforts are focused on increasing the social capital of the group by developing trust between group members, promoting collective efficacy, and strengthening the number of connections between individuals in the neighborhood.[41] Similarly, public health advocates often rely on community organizing to meet the health challenges among a particular group or in a specific area. Thus, one way of addressing the HIV/AIDS epidemic is to create peer education groups or promote the use of teen organizers to connect individuals to larger networks and to change social norms.[42] Changing these social norms and using peer pressure to promote better health have also been part of the reasoning underlying public health campaigns such as encouraging people to choose designated drivers and banning smoking in workplaces and homes. By using the power of groups to reinforce positive behavioral norms, health can be improved.

FOCUS ON

Dudley Street Neighborhood Initiative

One organization that has dedicated itself to building up social capital in its home neighborhood is the Dudley Street Neighborhood Initiative (DSNI) in the Roxbury/Dorchester neighborhood of Boston.[43]

DSNI had its roots in the disinvestment that afflicted the neighborhood in the 1950s to 1980s. Like many other urban communities, it saw a loss of households to the suburbs, racial change, a declining housing stock, speculation, abandonment, and arson. There were a large number of social service organizations, but many of these were thought by residents to be run by outsiders or not attentive to the concerns of community members. A final catalyst for change was a combination of gentrification in nearby neighborhoods and a city-sponsored redevelopment plan that many feared would lead to displacement in this neighborhood.

Residents elect the board of DSNI, which has had a number of important initiatives aimed at improving the social, physical, and built environment of the community. Social goals are reflected in the priority that DSNI places on hiring local residents for positions in the organization, the emphasis on youth organizing, and its commitment to holding all meetings with simultaneous translations into English, Spanish, and Cape Verdean Creole, the three main languages in the community. Physical environment actions have included efforts to eliminate trash transfer stations in the neighborhood, establishing a coalition with other communities to stop an asphalt batching plant, and a concentrated effort with local, state, and federal agencies to address the problem of pollution from auto body shops in the community. Built environment actions ranged from working to build housing on vacant lots (DSNI was granted the power of eminent domain by the City of Boston), a strong commitment to community agriculture, and a focus on transportation advocacy. Although the neighborhood remains home to many poor families, it is also a national model of how a community can use self-organizing practices to improve the lives of its residents.

Multiple Levels of Effect, Multiple Levels of Action

The degree to which social capital affects health may indicate that interventions to promote health cannot rely solely on individual behavior change.[44] An important example of this is smoking. Addressing tobacco use was initially an individual-level activity with warnings on cigarette packages, antitobacco television and radio advertising, medical interventions to promote tobacco cessation, and other similar actions. Collectively, these resulted in a substantial drop in tobacco use in the United States, but ultimately these efforts stalled and left the country with a still too high level of tobacco consumption. So antitobacco activists turned to group-level interventions, addressing the wide range of social norms and policies that collectively also influenced the decision of whether or not those individuals would smoke. These higher-level interventions have included raising cigarette taxes, laws against smoking in workplaces, and educational campaigns to emphasize the role of secondhand tobacco smoke on health—all of which, again, collectively have helped push U.S. tobacco use rates down to one of the lowest in the developed world. The initial tendency was to focus on individuals but that tactic had limitations. It was only after higher-level interventions were planned and implemented that the full reduction of smoking rates was seen.[45]

Neighborhood Empowerment

A major goal of community organizing and public health has been to mobilize communities to identify and address the problems confronting them (see Figure 12.1). The United States has seen a long period of community activism

FIGURE 12.1 Neighborhood Disorder, Social Capital, and Adolescent Alcohol and Drug Use

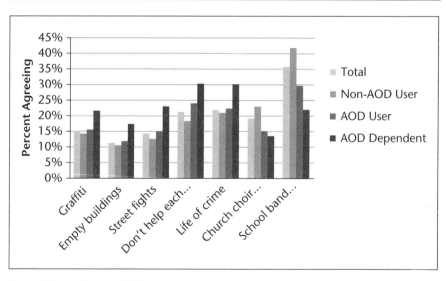

Source: Winstanely, et al., 2008

and community organizing in low-income communities ever since the codifi-cation of neighborhood organizing methods and strategies in Chicago in the mid-twentieth century. The overall objective of these strategies is almost always to increase neighborhood empowerment, assisting neighborhoods and their res-idents to acquire the power to implement their own solutions to problems by strengthening intraneighborhood ties (social capital) and convincing them that they have to power to protect themselves (collective efficacy).[46] These methods are also often used in social work and community development.[47]

The lack of attention to community empowerment often drives criticism of conventional public health research and interventions. In conventional public health activities, key decisions are often made by professionals, researchers, and funders, and the community has little say over the issues to be prioritized or how they should be addressed.[48] It is not that these other programs are not known to be necessary and effective, but they can often ignore major problems inside the community.[49] Thus a strategy to address diabetes in the neighborhood could contribute to increasing the overall health status of people in that neighborhood, but the community priority may be reducing the selling of drugs among its youth and that activity's associated addiction and violence problems. Given that resources are always scarce, who should decide whether the researchers or the community is right?

Even when programs match community priorities, they sometimes do not serve to ultimately empower neighborhoods and do not improve social capital. For example, if a program only hires people with master's degrees and does not engage local residents as more than research subjects, the long-term legacy of the program in terms of its influence on social capital may be minimal.[50] This is one reason that **community-based participatory research** advocates have suggested that whatever possible funding should flow to local community groups and that the program be structured so that the community can learn from the project and apply the tools in that project to other health challenges.[51]

Social Norms

One factor closely related to social capital is the idea of social norms influencing health behavior. In general, it is thought that these norms, the set of values and group ideas of what is acceptable behavior, have a very important role in protecting and promoting health.[52] For example, immigrants can maintain the health-promoting behaviors that they bring from their former country by settling in an immigrant community. Some of the former country's health-protective behaviors and values may persist, and others who share these values can support and reinforce behaviors through peer pressure.[53] Part of the assimilation process that often results in the acquisition of less healthy behaviors comes from the loss of such peer enforcement of social values and norms.[54] Thus public health interventions often look to support traditional social norms that reinforce positive behaviors.

Again, it should be noted, however, that social norms are not always a force for the good. For example, teenagers may want to drink alcohol because they see others in their peer group drinking. Similarly, group behavior can reinforce negative behaviors and create pressure on people who are trying to develop more positive lifestyles.

Broken Windows Theory

Individuals may decide appropriate behavior based on clues in the built environment around them. As mentioned, if an area is covered with litter, they may be more likely to litter. These neighborhood environmental influences on behavior are known as *broken windows theory*, a term based on the idea popularized by James Wilson that factors in communities—high levels of broken windows, abandoned buildings, graffiti, and other signs of disorder—promote antisocial behavior.[55] It is also often characterized as neighborhood disorder: the physical conditions in a community communicate social norms and influence the behavior and health outcomes of individuals.[56] One study found that neighborhoods with more disorder were associated with increased risk of gonorrhea, for example.[57]

These findings suggest that public health advocates should work with local governments on code enforcement and other actions that would maintain and restore abandoned buildings, reduce the amount of graffiti, and other similar actions.[58] These efforts can be taken too far, however. Broken windows theory has been used to justify actions against teenagers and minority group members who may not be breaking any law, but simply are perceived as a threat by other people inside or outside the community. Such action risks civil rights violations. In addition, the roots of crime and negative behavior are complex and may include factors in addition to disorder.[59] The presence of disorder may not be an indication of the social mores in that community. For example, many communities may have an ongoing problem with the illegal dumping of trash and construction debris, and although they may continually press city administrations to take action against these illegal actions, they may be unable to stop the dumping. The presence of disorder in this environment does not mean the community supports these behaviors; rather it may be indicative of how outsiders perceive the neighborhood or of other social, economic, justice, or political issues.[60]

Advertising and Behavior

A major concern in many communities is the proliferation of advertising that promotes unsafe behaviors such as smoking and alcohol consumption. In a sense, the built environment is dotted with reminders to partake of risky behaviors. Evidence suggests that African American neighborhoods and other poor communities are more likely to have outdoor liquor and tobacco advertising.[61] The concern is that these types of advertising reinforce risky behaviors and make it harder for those trying to control their alcohol consumption or quit smoking. These remind people of the existence of these products and communicate social norms that suggest certain types of behavior are socially acceptable. Some community activists have tried to work with billboard companies to reduce such advertising, and others have sought ordinances to mandate that these types of advertisements be prohibited near schools or in other areas.

Culture of Poverty Versus Poverty of Culture

The concern that some social norms can sometimes have negative influences has been incorporated into U.S. social policy for decades. Part of this reaches back to ideas on how culture influences poverty. In this context, culture does not mean symphony orchestras or other similar activities but instead refers to the overall complexity of human interactions, internal and external social norms for behavior, and the resulting behaviors. At one time, racist ideas permeated the study of non–Northern European societies and resulted in what is now considered to be a denigration of people who did not share Protestant white sensibilities. The thought was that many nonwhite peoples had a poverty of culture; in a sense they were somewhat less than totally human, and their lack of contemporary technologies was a reflection of their innate lower intelligence and lower levels of culture. These ideas are shocking to us today and were already under substantial challenge by the middle of the twentieth century.

Numerous groundbreaking anthropological studies—ranging from the work of Margaret Mead in the South Pacific to that of Oscar Louis in Mexico to that of Herbert Gans in the United States—demonstrated that low income people or people living in low technology environments had just as strong a sense of culture and just as great, if not greater, network of social interactions as did those living in contemporary high-income European communities.[62] Culture is a universal human experience and poor communities had a rich cultural experience that was equal to those of nonpoor communities.

The challenge became how to explain the persistence of poverty in a given location and across generations. Under the racist theories, poverty reflected the innate inability of people to better themselves. But mid-twentieth century progressives working in both community and government settings to address poverty rejected these ideas. Ultimately, it came to be believed that poverty existed and persisted because low-income people exhibit behaviors that ultimately result in their being unable to secure the life experiences and incomes that would lift them out of poverty. Eventually, the set of behaviors were termed a **culture of poverty** by Daniel Patrick Moynihan and others. A goal of much of U.S. social policy has been to engage the poor so that they could learn new behaviors mimicking those of more successful middle- and upper-income people.[63] Flowing from this theory are policies that seek to change the behavior of poor people, including boosting employment levels, reducing crime, and promoting health. These have ranged from time cutoffs after which people are no longer eligible for public assistance—it is thought that depending on welfare for too long a period fostered helplessness and poor personal habits—to programs that pay for students to get better grades, to other programs that seek to promote middle-class behaviors among the poor. It should be noted that the overall evidence underlying these policies has not been completely straightforward and that the whole process of adopting and implementing these programs has been highly politicized.[64] Their ability to change health by addressing this culture of poverty has been even less studied and is even more tenuously known.[65]

Dispersing Communities of Poor People

The idea of using public policies to address the problem of a culture of poverty has reached a climax of sorts in a long-term effort to reduce poverty by breaking up communities that have high levels of poverty. An underlying assumption is that if poor people live next door to nonpoor people, they will eventually learn how to act more like middle class people and thus adopt the behaviors of more successful households. Furthermore, the social norms of these nonpoor communities will serve to exert a social capital–like effect in which individuals will benefit from the greater social capital of their new communities.[66] These types of programs have been tried for generations. One of the goals of the federal urban renewal program the 1950s, for example, was to disperse poor people from their existing communities so that they would live among the nonpoor and thus could learn how to behave as nonpoor people behaved. The adults would benefit from both acquiring the behaviors of the nonpoor and from access to networks of jobs that were available in these other communities. In the 1990s, the HOPE VI program sought to change the economic mix of public housing developments by introducing nonpoor families into these developments, again with the idea that changing the concentration of poverty would be good for the poor.[67]

An additional reason for dispersing low-income communities was the finding that many people secure employment not from applying to help-wanted advertisements but via word of mouth from friends and family with jobs. But people living in poor communities have less access to already employed people and thus the network of potential employers they can access is smaller than if they lived in middle-class or wealthy communities. The fear was that simply living in a low-income community could limit one's employment opportunities and thus one's ability to earn an adequate income. Therefore the idea was that by dispersing poor people into middle-class communities, they could then have access to contacts of their employed neighbors.[68] Both higher incomes and more stable employment have been shown to be associated with improved health status.

As strong as this ideology is in the United States, it is not always applied in other countries. One alternative example is efforts to move slum dwellers in Mumbai en masse to new neighborhoods where basic city services can be delivered in the context of existing social ties which provide assistance to the poor. The community itself is maintained intact and without disruption.[69] Another policy is the microlending movement, which provides very small loans to individuals in groups in many less-developed countries. The microlenders depend on peer pressure from other low-income members of the group to help ensure that the loans are repaid. Again, this is a program that relies upon the connections between impoverished people to allow them to better themselves rather than calling for the severing of ties between low-income individuals so that they may acquire middle-class behavioral norms. These group-level interventions have been extended to the health realm as well, using peer support for health-promotion campaigns.

Moving to Opportunity Program

Though conducting experiments that involve assigning where people live is expensive and morally difficult, there was one major program in the United States that did assign people to various types of neighborhoods and then tracked certain outcomes among differing groups. This was the Moving to Opportunity Program (MTO). The program grew out of a lawsuit that accused the U.S. Department of Housing and Urban Development of fostering racial segregation by the way it allowed several local public housing authorities to operate. These local housing authorities were promoting racial segregation through illegal tenant assignment policies. As part of the settlement of the suit, HUD funded a program that involved three groups of low-income tenants. One group stayed in conventional public housing developments, while a second group was given a certificate that covered their rent, with most of these people going to similar low-income communities. A third group was given rent subsidy certificates but they were only allowed to secure housing in communities that did not have a high percentage of low-income households. MTO has provided some of the only evidence to see what happens to people when they move from a low-income community to one that is not low-income.[70]

In some respects, particularly the economic improvements that were the driving force behind implementing the program, MTO did not work. In general, the female heads of households in this study did not improve their employment status and did not increase their incomes. But physical and mental health measures in the study found that the physical and mental health status of the women in the study improved, and the school performance and health status of female children in the study also improved. There were not enough adult men to analyze in MOP and the effects on male children were not significant. These findings suggest that neighborhood can influence the mental health status of people and the way that it is thought to have been affected is by increasing participants' social capital.[71] These findings should be interpreted with caution, however, because it was a relatively small sample and has not been replicated. It is also not known if the benefits found came directly from a change in the built environment or from a change in the social capital of the participants' communities.

Summary

There have long been debates regarding social, environmental, and genetic determinants of health. One concept that has emerged is social capital, which aims to understand how a group and individuals in that group work together to protect health or maintain healthy behaviors. People who have higher rates of social capital tend to be healthier and have fewer poor health behaviors. Thus improving social capital has become a goal of both planners and health advocates.

Key Terms

Biological determinism	Environmental determinism
Collective efficacy	Multilevel modeling
Community-based participatory research	Self-efficacy
	Social capital
Concentrated poverty areas	Social norms
Culture of poverty	

Discussion Questions

1. What are the relative roles of social versus environmental versus genetic determinism in health outcomes?
2. Define social capital.
3. What are self-efficacy and collective efficacy? How might these protect health?
4. Describe the difference between bridging and bonding social capital.
5. Identify some of the ways social capital is measured. What are the relative strengths and weaknesses of these methods?
6. What are some of the ways that the built environment may promote social capital?
7. What is broken windows theory?
8. What is a "culture of poverty"? How might a culture of poverty affect health?

For More Information

de Souza Briggs, X., Popkin, S. J., & Goering, J. M. (2010). *Moving to opportunity: The story of an American experiment to fight ghetto poverty*. New York: Oxford University Press.

Gittell, R., & Vidal, A. (1998). *Community organizing: Building social capital as a development strategy*. Thousand Oaks, CA: Sage.

Lin, N., Cook, K. S., & Burt, R. S. (2009). *Social capital: Theory and research*. New Brunswick, NJ: Transaction.

Medoff, P., & Sklar, H. (1994). *Streets of hope*. Boston: South End Press.

Putnam, R. (2001). *Bowling alone: The collapse and revival of American community*. New York: Simon and Schuster.

CHAPTER 13

ENVIRONMENTAL JUSTICE

LEARNING OBJECTIVES

- Describe the beginnings of the environmental justice movement.
- Identify how the demographics of the environmental justice movement differed from that of the mainstream environmental movement.
- Describe the principles of the environmental justice movement.
- Assess the results of the 1994 Executive Order on environmental justice on at-risk communities.
- Discuss the problems in defining disproportionate burden.
- Compare the impacts of poverty versus income on environmental exposures.
- Assess whether low-income communities should accept hazardous waste.

Consider the many environmental problems in this country and elsewhere. Would you think they are randomly distributed, or do environmental risks seem to cluster in certain communities? Are there some neighborhoods that seem to be healthier and have more amenities such as parks? Why might this may be the case? Is it that some people want to live in more polluted places? Or are there social and economic forces that help create these inequities?

As we shall see, issues relating to environmental justice often arise from problems in the built environment: hazardous waste dumps, uranium mining, and bus depots, for example. In the effort to improve their local communities, environmental justice activists helped connect problems in the built environment to issues in the social and physical environment, providing an important contribution to all these fields.

This chapter begins with a history of the environmental justice movement, followed by a discussion of the 1991 environmental justice principles and the 1994 Executive Order that together helped produce a nationally consistent consensus on some of the overall themes of the environmental justice movement. Next is an overview of some of the key issues regarding current environmental justice

science: the problems of unequal access to amenities, disproportionate environmental burdens, issues with assessment, the debate between the importance of
race and income, and whether proximity is a good proxy for exposure. Then
we address issues of historical precedence: which came first, pollution or the
community? This is followed by a discussion of legal enforcement issues. Next is
a consideration of whether poor communities should accept hazardous waste as
an economic development strategy. The chapter concludes with an assessment
of the effectiveness of the environmental justice movement.

The Environmental Justice Movement

A recurring theme in this book is that certain groups, particularly low-income
individuals and people of color, are at increased risk of poor health and are more
likely to live in areas with poor environmental conditions (see Figure 13.1). The
term **environmental justice** refers to both the idea that all people have an equal
right to a clean and healthy environment and the unfortunate reality that some
groups bear a disproportionate burden of exposure to environmental problems.[1]
In general, environmental justice advocates are concerned that people of color
(Asians, blacks, Hispanics, and Native Americans) and low-income and working-
class people are more likely to live in communities and neighborhoods that have
higher levels of environmental problems (air and water pollution, more hazardous
waste sites, and so on), are less likely to have access to enforcement mechanisms

**FIGURE 13.1   Selected Characteristics of Neighborhoods with
Commercial Hazardous Waste Facilities**

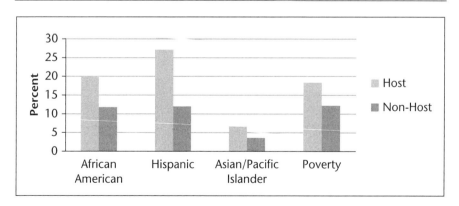

Source: United Church of Christ—Toxic Waste and Race

(administrative and legal relief), and less likely to have access to environmental amenities (parks, clean water, and the like).[2] Thus environmental injustices both result from and contribute to disparities in health and inequality in society as a whole. The goal of the environmental justice movement is to reduce these disparities so that everyone can benefit from a clean and healthy environment.[3]

The emergence of a strong environmental movement in inner cities, poor rural communities, and Native American tribal lands has greatly broadened and strengthened U.S. environmentalism.[4] Although it is important to remember that people of color have always had a strong commitment to the preservation of environmental quality, it was the development of the environmental justice movement that energized these communities and assisted the connection and extension of the activities of mainstream environmentalists back into cities and communities of color.[5]

A History of the Environmental Justice Movement

People of color have long been concerned about the environment. For example, the 1960s farm worker movement in California included exposure to toxic pesticides as part of its agenda.[6] But it wasn't until the mid-1980s that the environmental justice movement began to take form. It had its roots in a number of local problems in communities across the United States. Then these groups learned about other communities' struggles and they began to understand that there were similarities between their seemingly disparate problems.

Among the issues were problems with both legal and unregulated dumping of toxics and hazardous waste in African American communities in the rural South. Often, these were permitted by local, county, and state jurisdictions that had little or no representation of the poor rural areas that received these wastes.[7] For example, Warren County, North Carolina, was selected to be the site of a major landfill that was to receive hazardous wastes that included PCBs and other toxics that were being removed from hazardous waste sites in other areas of the country.[8] The dumping sparked large-scale actions in the local community that included demonstrations, letter-writing campaigns, and other types of protests. Local residents sought the assistance of allies in other states and civil rights activists rallied to the cause. Though these efforts were not successful, they sparked a rise of concern about the disposal of hazardous wastes in African American communities across the country. Similar actions occurred in Sumter County, Alabama, and other areas in the rural South, and communities began to realize that these campaigns were necessary because of the lack of political power to impact the siting decision-making processes.[9] These local concerns with built environment quality translated into an understanding that it was linked to social issues and physical environment problems.

At the same time, another effort to meet challenges posed by features of the built environment was taking form in the rural Southwest. For decades, uranium mining and other mineral extraction activities on Native American lands were despoiling formerly pristine areas with little benefit to local tribal groups.[10] Workers were poorly protected, environmental protections were limited, and the long-term health of communities was at risk. In response, new coalitions were formed to change how tribes considered mining proposals and efforts were renewed to protect environmentally sensitive areas. In many cases, the rights to mine the land and the royalties from these activities had been negotiated by the federal government with little input from tribes. Revenues often were placed in trusts that failed to distribute the funds to individuals living in the surrounding communities. When many of these operations were permitted, there were few environmental protections and even though there were new regulations that had been adopted over time, a great amount of environmental damage had been done and more continued. A new wave of action spread across the rural West.[11]

Environmental activism was not limited to rural parts of the United States but also gained traction in urban areas where problematic land uses and other built environment–related problems were a concern. One of the first communities to recognize that they had environmental injustices was in a heavily Latino area of Southern California. Residents of East Los Angeles began to realize that their neighborhood was being unfairly targeted for new highway construction and the building of new prisons and jail facilities. Already the site of heavy industry and trucking-related activities, the Mothers of East Los Angeles was organized in 1986 to fight the siting of a new state prison. But the organization quickly broadened its agenda to include the many other environmental problems in the community. This organization represented an important demographic shift from the traditional environmental groups that had tended to be mostly representative of the middle class and led by men. The East Los Angeles group was led by Latina women and it included both English- and non-English-speaking members, some born in the United States, some immigrants. The group understood that the environmental concerns of the community were related to the other social and economic threats in the area.[12]

Residents in this community connected the problems of the physical environment—factory pollution, hazardous waste sites, and so on—to social environment issues—poverty and racism—and the built environment—highways and prisons. This is an example of how the work of environmental justice activists would help to transform the broader environmental movement. In a sophisticated understanding of the problems that affected them, the women of East Los Angeles helped move concerns regarding social justice and the built environment into the traditional physical environment–related sphere of effort.

New York City's West Harlem community was another area where the built environment posed risks. Residents thought they had a high burden of asthma and they were aware that the area was a dumping ground for unwanted facilities that helped to keep a metropolitan area functioning: bus parking lots, sewage treatment plants, and the like. Separately, health care providers were aware of the asthma burden in the area, neighborhood leaders knew about the bus depots, and other people were working on lead paint issues. But despite concerns about the various environmental and health problems in the area, there was no systematic collection of data that confirmed the existence of these issues nor had the interrelationships of these problems been characterized. To meet these challenges, a group of concerned activists began to work together to try to understand what was special about the conditions in the neighborhood that was harming health.[13] This group was predominately African American and, again, most of its leaders were female. Once more, the demographics of an environmental justice group were different from those of a mainstream environmental organization's leadership.

As the West Harlem neighbors examined the data from various sources, they found that conditions were much worse than any one set of residents or health care providers in the community had known. For example, Harlem had the highest rate of asthma hospitalizations in New York City. These findings, along with other environmental concerns, led to the founding of West Harlem Environmental Action (WEACT) to organize residents, secure health services, manage research on the health and environmental problems of the community, and address the disproportionate burden of environmental problems in the neighborhood. As word spread of WEACT's activities, communities of color in urban areas across the country were inspired to similarly organize themselves. One of WEACT's major accomplishments was that it learned how to manage health researchers so that community residents were in charge of the research process and they were the ones who owned the results of studies. Rather than the traditional model in which researchers will study a community and then leave, providing no long-term lasting benefits to the neighborhood they had studied, WEACT's methods were to eventually help change how scientific research on environmental problems was conducted in the United States and elsewhere.[14] As a result of this paradigm shift, new research methods were developed and the scientific understanding of the problems posed by diesel exhaust, substandard housing, and other factors was substantially advanced.[15]

Though individual communities of color across the United States thought they were bearing a disproportionate burden of hazardous waste facilities, it was not until a report commissioned by the United Church of Christ titled *Toxic Waste and Race* was released in 1987 that activists across the country realized the full extent of the injustice in the siting of these legally authorized facilities.[16] The report, since updated, documented that Latino, African American, and Native American communities were more likely to be the sites of these types of facilities than white communities. The report demonstrated that the problems in any one area did not exist in isolation; instead there was a systematic national disproportionate burden on built and physical environments of communities of color. Activists across the country became concerned.

Along with this increased awareness of environmental problems, there was a growing dissatisfaction among newly energized activists of color with the current state of the environmental movement. The mainstream movement was perceived to have an anti-urban bias, or at least was heavily suburban oriented, had few employees who were members of minority groups, and had failed to protect low-income neighborhoods and communities of color from the burden of environmental problems.[17] Slowly, an independent movement began to form. Groups began to teach other communities about their issues and demonstrate to them what they could do to make their local environment better.

The 1991 Principles of the Environmental Justice Movement

One of the first major achievements of this multi-ethnic wave of activism was the 1991 First National People of Color Environmental Leadership Summit in Washington, D. C. It brought together a wide range of local activists who had begun to realize there were shared concerns for the environment and a similarity of underlying problems that linked their local issues. The gathering saw the adoption of a set of principles and when participants returned to their local communities, new groups were formed and existing organizations found new energy and inspiration. The environmental justice movement was born and soon began to change the U.S. environmental movement itself.[18]

During the three days of the 1991 summit, participants finalized and adopted a set of 17 principles that have helped frame environmental justice since that time. These principles are important not only because of this historical influence but also because they help increase the understanding of how the concept of the term "environment" is operationalized. Most important, the principles assert the right of all people to live in a healthy environment, free from environmental burdens, with access to clean air, safe drinking water, and amenities.[19] This was later shortened and elaborated to all people have the right to a clean and healthy place to live, work, play, and go to school. The principles also connect existing environmental inequities to historical processes, drawing connections between current problems and past injustices. They establish links between contemporary environmental problems and ongoing social, political, and economic problems. They draw parallels between the problems in the United States and global issues. While broadening the U.S. environmental movement, environmental justice advocates succeeded in making the environment an international movement as well. After the principles were adopted, they became a fundamental text of the environmental movement and the U.S. environmental movement was eventually transformed.[20]

1994 Executive Order

In the three years after these principles were adopted, the environmental justice movement spread to almost every major metropolitan area and state in the country. All over the United States, groups began to organize, informed by the strategies and successes of the original environmental justice organizations, and they began to investigate or call to be investigated the environmental issues in their communities. A wave of activism began to transform the urban environment and bring new energy to address long-standing problems. Local organizations quickly began to understand that the federal government had systematically failed to address the environmental concerns of communities of color and in urban areas. Because of rapidly increasing networks of organizations and communication between organizations, it was understood that this was not a problem that was local but was national in scope. There was a need for federal action to protect the health of communities of color.

In the winter of 1994, the National Institute of Environmental Health Sciences (NIEHS) convened a conference on how to conduct science to understand environmental justice issues and they made a special effort to include a number of representatives from local environmental justice organizations in the discussions. During the conference, some of these representatives were invited to the White House to witness President William Clinton signing an executive order calling for the consideration of environmental justice issues in certain decision-making instances. The order did not only cover the United States Environmental Protection Agency, but also called on other agencies to incorporate environmental justice concerns into their regulatory processes. The Executive Order, which is still in force, also sets up an appeal process and a legal process when groups feel that environmental injustice has occurred and where there is a need for appropriate federal involvement.[22]

FOCUS ON

The Principles of the Environmental Justice Network

Preamble

WE, THE PEOPLE OF COLOR, gathered together at this multinational People of Color Environmental Leadership Summit, to begin to build a national and international movement of all peoples of color to fight the destruction and taking of our lands and communities, do hereby re-establish our spiritual interdependence to the sacredness of our Mother Earth; to respect and celebrate each of our cultures, languages and beliefs about the natural world and our roles in healing ourselves; to ensure environmental justice; to promote economic alternatives which would contribute to the development of environmentally safe livelihoods; and, to secure our political, economic and cultural liberation that has been denied for over 500 years of colonization and oppression, resulting in the poisoning of our communities and land and the genocide of our peoples, do affirm and adopt these Principles of Environmental Justice:

1. **Environmental Justice** affirms the sacredness of Mother Earth, ecological unity and the interdependence of all species, and the right to be free from ecological destruction.

2. **Environmental Justice** demands that public policy be based on mutual respect and justice for all peoples, free from any form of discrimination or bias.

3. **Environmental Justice** mandates the right to ethical, balanced and responsible uses of land and renewable resources in the interest of a sustainable planet for humans and other living things.

4. **Environmental Justice** calls for universal protection from nuclear testing, extraction, production and disposal of toxic/hazardous wastes and poisons and nuclear testing that threaten the fundamental right to clean air, land, water, and food.

5. **Environmental Justice** affirms the fundamental right to political, economic, cultural and environmental self-determination of all peoples.

6. **Environmental Justice** demands the cessation of the production of all toxins, hazardous wastes, and radioactive materials, and that all past and current producers be held strictly accountable to the people for detoxification and the containment at the point of production.

7. **Environmental Justice** demands the right to participate as equal partners at every level of decision-making, including needs assessment, planning, implementation, enforcement and evaluation.

8. **Environmental Justice** affirms the right of all workers to a safe and healthy work environment without being forced to choose between an unsafe liveli-hood and unemployment. It also affirms the right of those who work at home to be free from environmental hazards.

9. **Environmental Justice** protects the right of victims of environmental injus-tice to receive full compensation and reparations for damages as well as quality health care.

10. **Environmental Justice** considers governmental acts of environmental injustice a violation of international law, the Universal Declaration on Human Rights, and the United Nations Convention on Genocide.

11. **Environmental Justice** must recognize a special legal and natural relation-ship of Native Peoples to the U.S. government through treaties, agreements, compacts, and covenants affirming sovereignty and self-determination.

12. **Environmental Justice** affirms the need for urban and rural ecological poli-cies to clean up and rebuild our cities and rural areas in balance with nature, honoring the cultural integrity of all our communities, and provided fair access for all to the full range of resources.

13. **Environmental Justice** calls for the strict enforcement of principles of informed consent, and a halt to the testing of experimental reproductive and medical procedures and vaccinations on people of color.

14. **Environmental Justice** opposes the destructive operations of multi-national corporations.

15. **Environmental Justice** opposes military occupation, repression and exploitation of lands, peoples and cultures, and other life forms.

16. **Environmental Justice** calls for the education of present and future gen-erations which emphasizes social and environmental issues, based on our experience and an appreciation of our diverse cultural perspectives.

17. **Environmental Justice** requires that we, as individuals, make personal and consumer choices to consume as little of Mother Earth's resources and to produce as little waste as possible; and make the conscious decision to challenge and reprioritize our lifestyles to ensure the health of the natural world for present and future generations.[21]

Unfortunately, the results of the executive order have been mixed.[23] On the positive side, the EPA and other agencies now routinely try to incorporate environmental justice concerns into their regulatory and decision-making process. There is no longer a need on the part of community groups to convince the EPA that there are environmental injustices in this country and a disproportionate burden of environmental problems experienced by certain groups. However, there has been little action to substantially reduce these injustices. What little evidence that exists suggests that there has been no change in the disproportionate impact of environmental problems and that there are few concrete regulatory practices that can be identified as having been modified because of environmental justice concerns. Because many of the responsibilities for health protection lie on the state or local level, conditions in many areas have not improved.[24] But the environmental justice movement remains strong and energized.[25]

Unequal Access to Amenities

The rise of the built environment and health movement has created the understanding that it is not just the presence of negative things in a community that are important but that there are certain amenities that can strengthen the health of neighborhood residents.[26] What has become clear is that there is not only a disproportionate burden on communities of color but also that these communities are more likely to lack basic amenities associated with the built environment, including parks, playgrounds, or even clean drinking water.[27] Other studies suggest that low-income and nonwhite communities are less likely to have hospitals, pharmacies that stock pain killers, supermarkets, and other features of modern life that support health.[28]

Part of this understanding came from the early work of the Bus Riders Union in Los Angeles, who successfully filed a suit against the Metropolitan Transportation Authority claiming that they were draining resources from the bus system, which served a primarily low-income and minority ridership, and were investing dollars in a suburban rail system that was serving higher-income white communities.[29] This and other injustices helped bring on a new awareness among activists that communities had the right not to be polluted but also had a right to basic city services. Again, the effort in one area inspired other groups across the country to work on similar issues.[30]

Disproportionate Burden

A key feature underlying the existence of environmental injustices is that communities of color bear a *disproportionate burden* of environmental problems in the United States.[31] But this has been fairly difficult to document. For example, there is no consistent definition of what is a disproportionate burden.[32] Though national data indicate that certain groups consistently are exposed to more toxins and environmental threats, often there is no cross-media (air, water, and so on) compilation that can demonstrate there is inequality in exposures overall. Part of the problem is that there is no scientifically validated way to add up these individual risks from different media. For example, there is the hazardous waste and race data first identified in 1988 and updated in 2008, which shows there is a disproportionate likelihood of hazardous waste facilities in communities of color. And there are air pollution data that suggest that people of color are more likely to live in places with higher air pollution burdens, but it has proved difficult to collect and quantify the extent of disproportionate burdens across environmental media.[33] How should hazardous waste exposures be considered alongside air pollution data, for example? There are different measures, different scales, different health effects, and so forth. This does not mean that these disproportionate burdens do not exist, only that we lack the statistical and scientific tools to properly identify these burdens at this time.[34] But the environmental justice movement has moved beyond trying to prove a disproportionate burden to urging local, state, and federal agencies to clean up or regulate the problems in communities of color. In one sense, proving national disparities is irrelevant. Communities simply want their local issues addressed.[35]

Assessing Health Effects of Multiple Exposures

A major problem when it comes to looking at how areas are affected by contamination, and one that is related to the issue of disproportionate burden, is how to measure and assess multiple threats in combination. Many communities do not face just one problem; they often have a multitude of issues potentially affecting health through multiple pathways involving large numbers of chemicals. Many chemicals have not been adequately studied and the full range of health effects of most chemicals, even those that we know are hazardous, are not always well characterized,[36] so the effect on a particular community or its residents is not clear. Another problem is that these chemicals are usually considered in isolation. It is rare that complex mixtures of chemicals are studied. But given that there are multiple threats in an area, how do we know that we are adequately protecting human health?[37] The answer is that the science does not exist to allow anybody to tell a community that their health is not at risk in these circumstances.[38]

Judging a health risk for a vulnerable population adds another dimension to the problem. Current risks are not the only problem; a lifetime of risks may be affecting the health of a community.[39] Most likely there are few, if any, studies that have worked on the health consequences of exposure to a specific chemical among vulnerable populations—and there may be many chemicals that might be safe if they were encountered at concentrations found in these neighborhoods in isolation, but little is known about what these effects may be in a population that is already suffering from a high burden of disease and also lacks the resources to adequately protect its own health. This is an issue that communities struggle with and something that regulators are trying to understand as well.

Race Versus Income

It should be noted that the underlying concepts of environmental justice science have not been without controversy. Perhaps the major criticism of the environmental justice movement has come from those who maintain that it is income rather than race that is responsible for the unequal burdens that some communities face. There is some evidence to support this claim. For example, income does appear to be an important factor when studies of the distribution of burdens are conducted, though race also is shown to be a predictive factor. In general, studies that use a more fine-grained definition of local community—such as census tract or block group—tend to find a greater predictive power for income than for race, while studies that use a larger geographic definition—such as zip code, groups of census tracts, or wider buffers—often find that race is more important than income. But most studies tend to find both have predictive power.[40]

The distinction between income and race is important because even though discrimination by income may not be desirable, it is not prohibited by law and the U.S. constitution. On the other hand, race is a protected class and discrimination based on race is actionable in court (though difficult to prevail). Income is not and thus individuals and communities would not be protected by federal and state law if they are discriminated against because they are poor.[41]

Environmental justice advocates counter that though race and income are separate constructs and not all poor people are members of minority groups and not all persons of color are poor, the two are highly correlated and thus the distinction is somewhat arbitrary. Another argument against the idea that environmental justice is only an income problem is that although the distinction may be important for certain narrow legal issues, as a moral and ethical issue it is not. Burdening people because they are poor is no more morally or ethically acceptable than burdening them because of their race. The outcome is the same and the advocacy would be nearly identical.[42] Furthermore, given the difficulty of pursuing environmental justice cases in the courts using race-based issues—almost no suits have succeeded—environmental justice advocates argue that the legal basis for the distinction is meaningless anyway. This debate is ongoing.

Is Proximity the Same as Unequal Exposure?

It is extremely difficult to prove causality using scientific and epidemiological methods; environmental justice issues, which are complex and often occur along with other pressing environmental and social problems, may be even more difficult to study.[43] The current types of statistical and research tools available to government agencies, research scientists, and local communities often lack the ability to identify with statistical precision that a specific facility or chemical is causing a specific problem in a specific community. In many cases, it is impossible even to establish or document that the community has a problem. Small numbers, the multitude of burdens, the high level of residential mobility, and the expense of health and environmental research often make small-scale studies difficult to design or may mean that they will not be able to confirm that any problem exists. The study sample size may simply be too small to give any possible power to identify associations between those potentially exposed to the chemical and the health outcome of interest. This does not mean there is not a problem or that the facility is not the cause of the health issue; it only says that we do not have the ability to study these problems at this time. Furthermore, as we have seen, the field of the built environment is fairly new and many chains of causality are yet to be established.

In response, communities and researchers often turn to using proximity as a proxy for unequal burden.[44] If a hazard is present in the community, it is assumed to also be a problem or contributing to the health and environmental problems in that community. These assumptions are usually based on accepted risk factors. For an example on the local scale, if a type of power plant is known to release particulates that (because of rodent and epidemiological studies conducted elsewhere), are known to exacerbate asthma, then it is assumed that an existing or proposed power plant in another community will also release particulates and these particulates will contribute to the burden of asthma in that community. A national example would be the documented problem that communities of color and/or low-income communities are more likely to be sites of hazardous waste facilities.[45] The very presence of these facilities is assumed to be a burden on surrounding neighborhoods.[46]

But these assumptions are often challenged, by both researchers and operators of facilities.[47] Local facility operators often claim that their particular facilities pose no burden on the surrounding communities and that the direct health impacts of their particular operations have not been scientifically documented. The very high levels of other pollutants in many of these communities are often used against these neighborhoods: they are already polluted, and so what is the burden of one more facility?

Such problems often push the solution to these issues into the realm of politics rather than science or, in other words, the way to protect a community may lie in administrative, legal, and political processes rather than in the power of epidemiological-based research. Clearly, many types of facilities are so highly regarded as detrimental that any community with sufficient economic and political power will fight them with every tool available: lawsuits, campaign contributions, media support, personal contacts, and so on. Communities that lack these resources are often the places that have higher rates of poor health and, environmental justice advocates have noted, it is impossible to disconnect unequal environmental burdens from broader social and economic disparities. Thus the solution to these problems may rest in addressing the other types of disparities by assisting at-risk communities to access the types of assistance that more affluent communities use to protect themselves. These might include pro bono legal and technical services, door knocking and community organizing, actions designed to publicize problems or secure media coverage, and the like. Though communities can use health studies as evidence for problems to assist them to persuade authorities to act, they might best not wait for or rely on these studies to demonstrate that a problem exists.[48]

Which Came First, Industry or People?

Another criticism of environmental justice science is temporal: hazardous waste facilities and polluting industries were in place before communities of color grew up around them. Thus neighbors moved into the community by choice after having considered the potential pollution in an area and weighing alternatives.[49] Part of the economic-based reasoning underlying this criticism is the assumption that the real estate market takes into consideration the pollution burden in a community and, as a result, housing prices are lowered. Persons considering moving into the polluted community make a judgment that the savings in housing costs adequately compensates them for potential problems resulting from the pollution. Therefore there is no inequity, as the increased health risks were considered to be balanced by the cheaper housing.

There are several assumptions underlying this argument. First, it assumes that the hazardous wastes (or other unwanted land uses) were indeed present before the low-income or minority community moved in. Certainly in the case of newer facilities, this is not true. And in the case of many older hazards, this may be somewhat true—the communities may not have been nonwhite but they were most likely poor.[50] But this ignores the lack of choice for many people. U.S. metropolitan areas remain substantially segregated and the inability to afford or access alternative housing has long been a problem. Thus, even if residents moved in after the facility was sited, there is no guarantee that it was a freely made choice.[51] This argument also doesn't include the possibility that health information evolves over time and what may have been considered a minor risk may now be recognized to be a much greater health threat.

There is also the assumption that residents know about the hazards in their neighborhood. There is no reason to support this. The full extent of the problems posed by a hazardous waste site, for example, is usually only understood after an extensive and expensive site evaluation conducted by a licensed professional. The evaluation may not have taken place or the results of it may not be known by the community. Existing operating facilities may report their emissions through a public database, but neighbors may not have access to this database, may not know about the existence of the database, or may not be able to understand and interpret the results.

At least in the case of Los Angeles, it appears that the issue of temporality is complex. In a sense, communities of color and industrial neighborhoods grew up together: as more industry moved into a neighborhood, the numbers of minority groups increased or, as a neighborhood became more heavily nonwhite, the numbers of facilities increased.[52] It is difficult to say definitively which came first in any one area. There was also some evidence that suggests industry moves into communities when they are most vulnerable, as when they are undergoing demographic shifts and the newcomers may therefore not be aware of the problems about to burden them.

Environmental Enforcement

Even if we know that certain chemicals cause problems, it is not clear that there is the ability to address these exposures. Most environmental laws were not meant to ban all chemicals outright, but instead the regulatory process is set up to allow the use of many chemicals if their releases do not exceed a certain threshold determined to be safe.[53] As a result, a particular problem in communities of color is that many of the most problematic users who are producing some of the worst pollution are legally operating and have received all necessary permits from local, state, and federal government. Yet the releases by any of the facilities in a community do not rise above the thresholds allowed by the federal and state permitting authorities.[54] The permitting process does not necessarily consider other pollution sources in the community or the underlying vulnerable health status of that community. Health issues are not always adequately considered nor is the total pollution burden in a community always known. Each facility is addressed independently, for the most part. Given that there is a documented clustering of facilities in certain communities, the risks and burden of releases most likely cluster in these communities as well. Accidental harmful releases probably overburden these areas, too.[55]

Prompting local governments to more vigorously regulate undesirable land uses can be difficult. Local governments permit factories and waste sites through zoning powers but once the facility is operational, it is often left to state or federal authorities to monitor emissions and environmental impacts. The role of local government after that point may be limited. Therefore, the time to influence local governments to protect against environmental burdens may also be limited in duration, that is, during the zoning and permit approval process. At the same time, federal authorities may not see their responsibilities to be more than monitoring and perhaps citing violators of the law.[56] The role of public health departments is even more limited. They may have not traditionally played a role in siting decisions and may not have the technical ability to monitor emissions. These issues are national in scope, though they play out on the local level and they have yet to be fully addressed.

FOCUS ON

The West End Revitalization Association

Some of the most problematic land use problems occur in areas where local communities have little influence over local political institutions. Such is the case of the West End community in Mebane, North Carolina. The neighborhood is 90% African American and is on the edge of town, technically beyond the city limits but, because of North Carolina law, it is subject to the zoning and development authority of the city. Thus the residents have no vote in city elections but are partly under its jurisdiction.

This historically black community has a number of environmental justice–related issues including the siting of problematic land uses and a lack of infrastructure such as clean water and sewer service. Worse, a highway was planned for the community that would have destroyed homes, a church, and a historic cemetery. The community resolved to organize itself.

The result is the West End Revitalization Association (WEBA), a community-based organization that has had some important victories since its founding in 1994, including bringing federal agencies into their fight for environmental justice and partnering with universities to access their research and organization abilities. The community has become a symbol of how neighborhoods can empower themselves.[57]

Additional Limitations of Environmental Justice Actions

Though much of the work of environmental justice activists is inspiring and deserves praise for how they have worked to make the environment better for all people, at this time there appear to be limits on the ability of the environmental justice framework to solve all the physical, built, and social environmental issues confronting many low-income neighborhoods and communities of color.[58] One of the problems is that the complexity of the issues has demonstrated that causality is very difficult to prove. Even though it may be known that a certain chemical causes a known health risk and it may be noted that the health risk is very prevalent in a community around a known source of that chemical, that is still far from proving that a particular emission is causing a health problem. Another limitation is that it is very difficult to protect vulnerable populations.[59] As was discussed earlier, often locally unwanted land uses have been permitted by the local government, or even worse, in some areas of the countries such as North Carolina, cities have the right to approve the siting of facilities in communities outside the corporate limits. This is a particular problem because these committees do not have a voice in the politics of the cities and thus have no voice in the decision-making process.[60]

Another problem is that environmental equities are often the result of social incquities and environment regulations were not designed to address these underlying problems. Environmental laws cannot replace the effort to work for the reduction of economic inequality, for example.[61] There is also a realization that certain communities are extremely vulnerable to pollution even if that pollution source is thousands of miles away. For example, native communities in Alaska that depend upon subsistence fishing for food are finding that they are being poisoned by dioxins and mercury that was emitted in distant parts of the globe. Finally, the experience of environmental justice activists has demonstrated the limits of regulatory/scientific processes such as risk assessment. These tools have not yet been refined so that they can always adequately assure communities that their health is not in danger.

Should Poorer Communities Willingly Accept Hazardous Waste?

There have been suggestions that poor neighborhoods and less-developed countries should accept hazardous waste from wealthier communities and more developed countries as a tool for economic advancement.[62] If they are paid to accept waste, countries can get needed foreign currency so they can afford to pay for more imports and increased investment in local infrastructure and development. Such proposals, which have included poor communities in the United States as well as the international transport of hazardous waste, are derived from the economic concepts of competitive advantage and economic efficiency. These concepts, explained in more detail in Chapter Sixteen, suggest that certain places are more efficient at certain processes, and thus no government efforts should be made to discourage these advantages. In the context of hazardous waste, these concepts suggest that poor countries (and neighborhoods) are the best places to accept hazardous waste because it is cheaper to dispose of materials and chemicals in these places than to create hazardous waste facilities in more affluent areas or to detoxify these wastes. There are monetary and perhaps efficiency savings to economies as a whole because this transport is thought to be more economically efficient.

The greatest objections to these arguments are on ethical grounds: it is immoral to subject communities to what may be generations of, or permanent, risks simply because they are poor. They often did not create these wastes, did not profit from their manufacture and sale, and did not benefit from using the products that produced these wastes; therefore there can be no adequate compensation for receiving these wastes.

There are other problems.[63] Accepting hazardous waste may permanently hurt local economies because they may bring long-term pollution problems or the area might become permanently blighted. It is not clear that a current generation has the moral authority to place future generations at a disadvantage because these future generations have no voice in the decision-making process and may not benefit from taking on the burden. Another problem relates to the impact of allowing these policies on society as a whole. Promoting easy disposal of toxic waste may facilitate the continued use of these hazardous chemicals rather than replacing them with more environmentally benign alternatives. If the cost of disposal is too low, then potential alternatives that are more benign but more expensive may not be commercially viable and so pollution may continue. In addition, if the cost of this disposal does not include in its price the externalities of that disposal, such methods can end up resulting in more pollution.

The economic arguments also assume that the compensation to local communities takes place in the context of free markets with perfect information. But many potential recipient countries have corrupt or undemocratic governments and the recipient communities may not know the full health and environmental risks they are accepting.[64] Thus the underpinning assumptions of free markets may be violated: there is not full knowledge about the negatives of the deal and there may not be free participation in the exchange. The proposal also dismisses the risks involved to third parties from accidents and spills during transport. The transport of wastes can be dangerous because of potential accidents and there is no guarantee that damages from spills and other incidents will be paid even if they can be quantified. In any case international treaties have generally reduced (but not eliminated) the transport of hazardous waste and fewer communities are willing to accept these wastes domestically.[65] The issue has not been resolved, but its magnitude has been reduced.

Lessons

After over twenty years of environmental justice activism, there are a number of lessons that can be drawn from this history. One very important issue is that communities can learn from each other. Even before the rise of the Internet, efforts in one part of the country were informing parallel efforts in others. For example, because of the work of the Bus Riders Union in Los Angeles, a group in Boston was able to address one of the most important problems affecting low-income users of buses in that city: they convinced the Massachusetts Bay Transportation Authority (MBTA) to allow for transfers between buses and between buses and subways, substantially reducing costs for a poorly transit-served neighborhood that was inhabited mostly by people of color and had a high percentage of low-income households.

Another important lesson is that all segments of the community can participate in the effort to understand what is going on in the local environment. Elders in the community can provide information on historical uses, even if the facility has been long vacant. Young people often know of current problems, and young people have demonstrated a strong ability to educate their peers and other people in their neighborhoods about environmental hazards. Adults can organize and turn out to a meeting, even if they can't necessarily all vote in elections because of citizenship status or other factors. Faith groups have a preexisting network and a long-standing history in many communities that can help organize against threats. Most important, the environmental justice movement demonstrated that no community is truly powerless and that every community has assets that can be used to improve and protect the health of its residents.

Summary

People of color have long had environmental concerns, but beginning in the 1980s a series of issues sparked the rise of the environmental justice movement. Many of these problems relate to the built environment, including the siting of hazardous waste facilities, highways, bus terminals, and other undesirable land uses. A number of concerns related to documenting that inequalities exist, for example, there have been problems with measuring environmental burdens, concerns that undesirable land uses were sited first, and legal enforcement problems. Overall, however, there have been important advances associated with the rise of this movement.

Key Terms

Environmental justice

Disproportionate burden

Discussion Questions

1. How did the demographics of environmental justice organizations differ from that of traditional environmental organizations?
2. How were the principles of environmental justice developed?
3. Is race or income a better explanation for the distribution of environmental inequities?
4. Describe some of the methodological problems involved in measuring unequal environmental burdens.
5. What are the advantages and disadvantages of using proximity as a proxy for exposure?
6. Identify some of the legal barriers to using environmental justice issues to improve the environment in communities of color.
7. Debate: should low-income countries accept toxic waste from wealthier countries?

For More Information

Bullard, R. (1996). *Confronting environmental racism: Voices from the grassroots*. Boston: South End Press.

Earth Island Institute. www.earthisland.org.

Environmental Justice Resource Center—Clark Atlanta University. www.ejrc.cau.edu.

Environmental Protection Agency—Environmental Justice. www.epa.gov/environmentaljustice.

Gottlieb, R. (1993). *Forcing the spring: The transformation of the American environmental movement*. Washington, DC: Island Press.

Policy Link. www.policylink.org.

TOOLS AND
APPLICATIONS

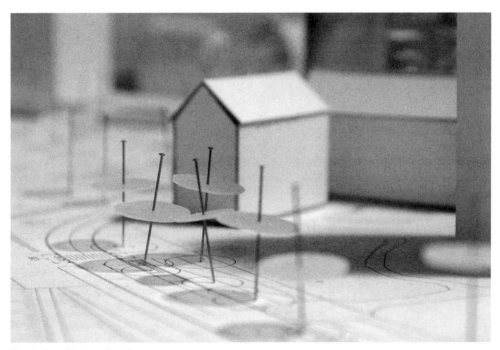

iStockphoto/© Leon Goedhart

CHAPTER 14

ASSESSMENT TOOLS AND DATA SOURCES

LEARNING OBJECTIVES

- List the steps of an environmental impact assessment.
- Evaluate the utility of environmental impact assessments for identifying built environment issues.
- Differentiate between environmental impact assessment and health impact assessment.
- Identify the steps of health impact assessment.
- Describe the steps of the Neighborhood Environmental Walkability Assessment.
- Discuss the advantages and disadvantages of cost-benefit analysis.
- Explain the strengths and weaknesses of different ways of measuring physical activity.
- Describe the strengths and limitations of national health surveys.

Let's reflect on how physically active you are and how you would measure your activity level as compared with that of others. Think about what you would want to know and how you might reduce biases and wrong answers. Consider how public health and urban planning professionals need to measure aspects of the built environment. What would be the features of a good measurement or policy tool? How might government and policy makers want to use this information in their work?

Communities, urban planners, and public health professionals have been asking for tools that they can use to evaluate the built environment, new development proposals, and programs and policies to manipulate the built environment to promote health. In response, there has been a reengineering of existing assessment tools and the development of new methods that can be used by policymakers and communities to gauge their current environment and the impacts of new proposals.[1] The tools described in this chapter are a very small fraction of those available, but they illustrate the range of methods that have been applied to the analysis of the built environment.

It must be stressed that these tools are not in themselves decision-making procedures. On the contrary, their goal is almost always limited to informing the decision-making process so that it can take into account the full range of what is known about current or potential impacts and conditions.[2] Also, these tools are only valuable to the extent that they are used to influence decisions.[3] Communities can be disappointed when an assessment reveals a potential problem but a project is approved anyway, but assessment tools only provide information about issues, they cannot prevent or remedy them. Similarly, each of these assessment tools has limitations on their scope and ability to adequately assess potential health and environmental problems.[4] There is no single assessment tool that can reliably identify all potential health and environmental problems and many health issues may be beyond the scope of many tools available today. Sometimes a community may rely on a tool that does not have the power or sensitivity to identify, describe, or assess a potential threat and so these tools must all be used with caution. They all have limitations and they are no substitute for thoughtful policy, project, and program assessment and development.

Tools to Inform Decision Making

Though all the assessment tools described in this chapter can be used to inform decision making, environmental impact assessment, health impact assessment, and other similar tools are usually commissioned directly in response to an individual development plan or policy that is being considered (see Table 14.1). The decision-making body needs information to help it reach a conclusion on how to act. Often, these tools do not generate new information on their own but rather collect information from other studies, apply findings from other places to the issue under consideration, or work to synthesize large amounts of information from diverse sources. They may ask for new studies, but they do not necessarily have to do so. For example, a city considering whether to approve a new shopping mall may apply standard equations for estimating traffic demand, use existing estimates of pollution produced per vehicle miles traveled, ask for the results of site evaluations for contaminants, and so forth.

Environmental Impact Assessment

The **environmental impact assessment** (EIA) process, established by the National Environmental Policy Act of 1969, has been adopted by many states through similar state legislation. Also called an environmental impact statement (EIS), this assessment tool has been used to evaluate specific development

Table 14.1   Characteristics of Health Impact Assessment and
Environmental Impact Assessment

	Health Impact Assessment	Environmental Impact Assessment
Mandatory in some jurisdictions		X
Usually voluntary	X	
Tied to existing environmental law		X
Flexible enough to include built environment research	X	
Goal is to inform decision making	X	X
High level of familiarity among policy makers		X
Strong emphasis on public involvement and information	X	

Source: National Center for Health Statistics

proposals to general plans for cities to the impact of major infrastructure improvements such as highways and dams. In general, a regulatory trigger, or minimum scale of potential impacts, must be met before an EIA is required. These thresholds generally relate to a project's size, projected air or water emissions, the extent of public funding for a project, and so on.

The EIA utilizes a very formal process that is often inflexible.[5] First, a project must be determined to have exceeded the minimum threshold requirements for an EIA. Only then must an EIA be developed. Next, there is a scoping phase where specific issues to be addressed are identified. In general, these must meet the regulatory authority of the Environmental Protection Agency (or whatever agency that will use the EIA in its decision-making process). This may mean there must be a preliminary determination of the project's potential impact in regards to the Clean Air Act, Clean Water Act, and the like, and there must be an identifiable connection to the statutory or regulatory power of an agency.

The scoping phase is critical since many mandated EIA processes insist that only issues identified in the scoping phase can be included in the EIA and once the scoping phase has been completed, it may be too late to consider additional issues. An EIA will include a statement of the purpose of the project, a description of the area around a project, a description of both the proposed project and a range of potential alternatives (sometimes including a no-build option), and an analysis of the potential environmental impacts of all these alternatives. Typically, a draft EIA is released for public comments before a final EIA is produced. If additional information is needed later, a supplemental EIA can be produced. Because most

EIAs are complex, they are usually produced by specialized consulting firms, but the agency with the regulatory authority over the project is responsible for its development. Again, these EIAs are meant merely to provide data to inform decision making and the EIA itself is not a decision-making tool. The EIA process has been criticized because of the lack of a mandated effective public participation process that can leave affected communities unaware of or dissatisfied with a final EIA report.[6] Another issue is that though they outwardly project scientific objectivity, EIAs often must incorporate subjective values and assessments.[7]

Using an EIA to analyze the built environment has had mixed success. EIAs can be useful for identifying certain types of impacts such as air pollution, storm water runoff, and the output of hazardous chemicals, and then, based on this information, projects can be approved, modified, or cancelled. But though they can be a powerful tool for analyzing potential environmental impacts that are within their legal jurisdiction, they are less useful in evaluating the very local impacts of development and designs of the built environment that are of highest importance in affecting local health, such as promoting access to nutritious food or addressing physical activity. Part of the limitations of federal-mandated and many state-mandated EIA reports has been that they are based upon the preexisting statutory authority of the federal and state governments, which may have focused on the great traditional environmental and health problems that were first identified in the 1960s and 1970s: clean water, clean air, and the effects on endangered species.[8] Thus the federal government can be involved in a development decision and require an EIA if there is a potential impact on air quality such that it meets the threshold requirements of the Clean Air Act. But there is no statutory justification for federal involvement in whether or not a development has sidewalks and thus promotes walkability or affects its potential for promoting obesity, for example. Nor can it generally consider the impacts on social capital or community efficacy, though these are often important public health concerns. Even though there is an overall government interest in promoting the general health of the population, many of the specific health impacts of the environment fall outside the strict limits of federal and state laws and thus are beyond the limits of the review in an EIA. The EIA process was not designed to consider these types of impacts. Therefore, health advocates have looked to other mechanisms beyond the EIA for evaluating new development proposals and the existing environment.

Health Impact Assessment

A new tool that is gaining popularity for assessing the built environment, and which is very different from environmental impact assessment despite its similar name, is a **Health Impact Assessment** (HIA).[9] HIA consists of procedures and guidelines which collectively can be used to evaluate new or existing projects' policies and programs. The objective of an HIA is to give communities and policymakers the information they need to understand what is happening, or may potentially happen, to the health of a population or community. The ultimate goal is to enable better development decision making and policy analysis. Health impact assessment is a voluntary tool, though some jurisdictions have been considering laws to make them mandatory for projects that meet certain minimum requirements. For the most part, it is up to a local jurisdiction or organization to decide whether to conduct an HIA or not, and unlike an EIA, there is no federal or state standard statutory threshold for their use at this time.[10]

HIA has been used in a number of different types of ways in the United States, including evaluations of housing affordability, mental health services, social capital impacts, access to schools, pedestrian injuries, and physical activity and obesity. Sometimes the focus of an HIA has been policy, as in an analysis of programs on low-income rental subsidies in Massachusetts. In other places, an HIA was commissioned to help analyze the impacts of a real estate proposal, as was an HIA developed to help the city of Oakland, California, analyze its proposed Oak to Ninth development.[11]

FOCUS ON

Oak to Ninth Health Impact Assessment

The U.C. Berkeley Health Impact Group prepared a Health Impact Assessment for the Oakland City Council in 2007. Led by Rajiv Bhatia, a group of students and associates prepared the HIA to help Oakland, California, understand a large project along the waterfront in that city. Consisting of 64 acres and originally planned to include two marinas, 3,100 housing units, 200,000 square feet of commercial space, and 30 acres of public open space, the project had the potential to have a substantial impact on its neighborhood.[12]

Among the findings of the HIA was that the project, on land owned by the Port of Oakland, had failed to comply with its previously approved Oakland Estuary Plan. The developers had failed to solicit community impacts and there were concerns about the financial feasibility of the final development program.

In order to address these findings, the HIA suggested that the plan for the development be reevaluated to meet the concerns raised in public hearings, a multistakeholder process be convened to resolve remaining issues, and that the public be better informed about the project as it went forward.

The steps for conducting a health impact assessment are screening, scoping, assessment, recommendations, reporting, and evaluation. In the screening step a decision is made as to whether an HIA is appropriate or practical. Important factors to be considered are whether there are sufficient resources to undertake an HIA and whether those with decision-making powers are willing to incorporate the HIA's findings into their approval process. A community may decide to undertake an HIA even if the relevant government authority is against one, but it may make data collection more difficult, the pace of the approval process may exceed that of the HIA (projects might come to a decision point before the HIA is completed), and it may be difficult to use the results to inform decision making.[13]

The HIA scoping step parallels the EIA scoping step, but with a very important difference. Rather than being constrained by the existing range of laws that provide legal justification for federal or state protection of the environment (Clean Air Act, Clean Water Act, and so on), an HIA can explore the full potential range of social, health, and environmental impacts that a community is concerned about regardless of whether there is a specific statute providing for government intervention. Therefore, many additional areas of potential impacts can be considered, such as noise, potential changes in quality of life and who lives in a community, and impacts on viewsheds, social equity, and environmental justice. Thus HIAs may be a superior tool for assessing a project's or program's impacts on obesity, physical activity, social capital, or the other factors associated with the built environment.

The assessment section is the portion of HIA where the actual impacts of a program, policy, or development are considered. This is very different from the formal risk assessment process that underlies many environmental decision-making laws and regulations, including those used by the EPA and other federal agencies. In general, the HIA assessment process is both broader and more comprehensive than formal risk assessment. The level of detail in HIA varies according to the needs of the community and the organization commissioning the HIA and the amount and quality of data available for the analysis. The data collected can be either quantitative, a series of measurements and models that provide hard numbers on potential impacts, or qualitative, describing the range, direction, and magnitude of potential outcomes.[14]

An HIA is meant to inform decision making and therefore it is very important that it lead to recommendations either for mitigation or regarding whether or not a particular initiative should be allowed to move forward. The HIA framework also recognizes that communities have a right to know and participate in decisions that potentially can affect their lives. Thus there is a strong emphasis on communicating the results and recommendations of an HIA back to the community and individuals who are going to be affected by the target process. The preparation of an HIA should therefore be an open process and all communications with the public affected by the issue being studied has to be understandable to the community and should address their concerns that they have outlined in the scoping step.[15]

Finally, there should be an evaluation of the HIA process and results. A goal of the evaluation is to enable future HIAs to better address the needs of communities. Among the questions that should be answered in the evaluation step are: Did the HIA provide the information that the community needed? Was the HIA completed a timely fashion? Did it contribute to better decision making?

Though useful, there are potential issues with HIAs. For example, they can take time to produce and thus developers and governments may oppose them or they may not produce evidence within a timetable that meets the limitations on how long a government has to approve or disapprove a project. They are also potentially expensive. Though some governments have allocated funds for an HIA, many may not have the resources to do so and developers may be reluctant to fund them out of their own budgets. The lack of a mandated process may make it more difficult to fund HIAs because there is no legal leverage to force one to be produced or to make an appropriate agency incorporate the findings of an HIA into its decision-making process. Again, the voluntary nature of HIAs may make the commissioning of one a political process and it may make it difficult for a government to agree to have one produced. The lack of knowledge of HIAs may contribute to this problem and if communities, government, and project proponents or opponents are not aware of HIAs or confuse them with EIAs, it may be difficult to develop a consensus to embark on an HIA process. Another problem is the lack of expertise in preparing an HIA. Though their use is growing, there were fewer than 100 HIAs completed in the United States in the year 2010. Finding personnel who have the expertise and knowledge to produce an HIA may be difficult in some areas. Despite these limitations, however, there is a likelihood that the use of HIAs will increase.

Information Tools

To a certain extent, the tools described in this section have been developed to assess or provide information on specific places or issues. Many times, they are used for evaluation, but they do not necessarily originate from the need by a public agency to come to a decision. They often result in the gathering of new information and data, and they may be undertaken by researchers, community groups, government agencies, foundations, or anybody who has a particular interest in an issue with the built environment. The results can be incorporated into EISs or HIAs, but they can also be stand-alone activities. For example, a local government may commission a study of a bike trail to assess how well a marketing strategy succeeded in bringing new users to the trail. Or a researcher interested in understanding the location of fast-food outlets in relation to high schools in order to study the impact of the local food environment on adolescent diets might use geographic information systems (GIS) to map locations of pizza, burger, and other restaurants. These are important data but not necessarily information that will be incorporated into the consideration of a new development or policy proposal.

Neighborhood Walkability Assessments

The preponderance of evidence that suggests that certain types of environments promote walking and physical activity while other types of environments inhibit healthy behaviors has resulted in the development of a series of tools to assess neighborhood walkability. One of the most widely used that is representative of the tools that have been developed for assessing the built environment is the Neighborhood Walkability Assessment Survey (NEWS) developed by Brian Saelens, James Sallis, and associates.[16] NEWS is based on the evidence for what influences individual walking behavior and the perceptions of pedestrians as they experience their environment. Originally developed to measure walkability for a general population, it has been adapted for special populations including the elderly and young people.[17] The survey is meant to be conducted while out in a community; it is not a tool that can be used inside a research office. The survey has sections on the types of residences; stores, facilities, and other land uses in a neighborhood; access to services; streets; places for walking and cycling; neighborhood surroundings; safety from traffic and crime; and neighborhood satisfaction. The total survey consists of over ninety questions. It has been tested for reliability, that is, its ability to identify conditions independent of the biases of any individual.

The first step in using NEWS is to adapt it for local conditions. Many of the features in NEWS are found in almost all neighborhoods, or their absence in a given neighborhood is of such importance that this absence should be noted. For example, the high utility of sidewalks for walking means that the sidewalk section of NEWS should be in virtually every survey. But other features may not be present in a local area, such as ravines and hillsides. Thus NEWS needs to be modified for most local uses. This might best be accomplished in consultation with members of the community to be surveyed and the scope of the final survey also will depend on the goals of the project.

The next, and most critical, step is the training of those who are going to administer NEWS to assess local conditions. Often it is conducted by local residents, but students and outside observers have administered it as well. It is highly important that each observer record a given type of local condition in the same way. The underlying epidemiological concept is called inter-observer validity or, in other words, the idea that two people will see the same feature and record it so as to give it as exact a score or result as possible. Training also reduces the amount of time it takes observers to survey communities. When resources permit, multiple observers should survey the same area so that results can be pooled or averaged, again with the goal of limiting observer biases and improving the overall validity of a survey. The results of NEWS and other similar surveys can be mapped using either computer technology or paper maps. Either way, the results can be used to identify particular places that have high or low walkability and whether opportunities exist for improvements. The results also have great utility in communicating issues to communities and policymakers.

Results from the NEWS surveys should be compiled and analyzed in a systematic manner. The NEWS Web site contains a suggested analytic framework. NEWS and similar tools end up producing lots of data, which lends them to computer analysis. The tool has been used to assess walking environments from Boston to San Diego and in Australia and Taiwan.[18]

Geographic Information Systems

The spread of personal computers with fast, powerful processors and access to the Internet has resulted in increasing use of **geographic information systems** (GIS) to identify, communicate, and analyze issues in the built environment.[19] There are a number of programs available for communities to use in this work that range from expensive and sophisticated programs to cheaper but perhaps less robust applications. In general, GIS involves collecting data, organizing it so that it reflects an underlying spatial order and is in a compatible electronic format, and then using the spatial relationships among different types of data to draw conclusions about the environment.[20] One fundamental concept of GIS is that there is a need for a geographical connection of data: data must be linked to an underlying geographic layer if it is to be spatially analyzed. Thus, a listing of traffic accidents without an identifying column of addresses or intersections cannot be used to analyze their geographic distribution, just as a map without health or physical environmental data is not valuable for health research or increasing understanding of community issues. It is only when there are both data layers and geographic layers that the power of GIS is possible.[21]

A particular advantage of GIS is that it allows for the combining of multiple layers of information.[22] For example, a database of traffic accidents that contains appropriate geographical information can be combined with demographic information obtained from the U.S. Census or similar data sources to develop population-specific accident rates or identify particular problematic intersections.[23] Simply considering the number of accidents by themselves may give misleading results because they do not produce any indication of the rate of accidents.

The range of uses for GIS is large. It has been used to map cases of a disease, abandoned housing, the location of liquor stores, and the extent of tree cover. It can help demonstrate that there are problems with access to supermarkets or hospitals or assist in understanding how multiple environmental health risks may simultaneously afflict an individual neighborhood, such as in the case of asthma and lead paint poisoning. However, there can be limitations to using GIS. The most useful GIS programs are expensive and can be difficult to master (though using them for basic mapping of census and other standard data can be fairly simple), data gathering can be time consuming, there may be problems with accuracy, and GIS poses its own set of statistical issues. Inaccuracies can also arise from the underlying geographic database or the data layers being added to the project.[24] For example, certain facilities may not appear in a database that is being used in the project.[25] The quality of the data used in GIS must be carefully assessed and potential limitations and biases identified. For example, census data may have problems with the undercounting of certain groups of people which may or may not affect results. In another example, a purchased list of businesses may be very useful for sales contracts, but it may not contain data on businesses owned by non-English-speaking people. The data collection process may have errors (addresses misreported, for example, or transcription errors). But even minor errors and inaccuracies can affect results.[26] There are a number of statistical issues that should be kept in mind when analyzing GIS results. These may be less of a factor when basic descriptive statistics are the goal of a project, but they may arise in both simple and complex projects.

One of the spatial statistical problems that can arise during GIS-related analysis is called the modifiable areal unit problem. This issue arises because local unit boundaries are inherently arbitrary and the question must be asked, if the boundaries were to be redrawn, would there still be differences between areas? Would the data change? This issue is hard to assess and account for.[27] Another set of problems arises from the statistical instability of small area samples.[28] They make differences hard to identify and interpret. These and other potential issues highlight the need for consultation with a GIS specialist or geospatial statistician when necessary.

Cost-Benefit Analysis

A tool that has been borrowed from the field of economics is that of **cost-benefit analysis**. The goal is to help decision makers understand whether or not all the potential benefits of a given program or policy, or set of options, exceed the costs.[29] For example, cost-benefit analysis has been used to assess the utility of programs to promote walking.[30] Actual cost-benefit analyses can be very sophisticated or fairly simple, and although simpler analyses may be faster and less expensive, they may also be more likely to be inaccurate. The two most important steps in a cost-benefit analysis are to identify potential costs and benefits and to quantify them. These steps can be very problematic because not only are potential costs or benefits often difficult to foresee, cost-benefit analysis typically has to assess the relative probability that these costs and benefits may occur. It is critical in any type of analysis to carefully and explicitly list costs and benefits and to justify how these were identified and assessed.[31] An opaque process may have a limited ability to influence policymakers or the public.[32]

A major challenge is that it may be difficult to transform a cost or benefit into a quantifiable dollar amount; that is, it can often be difficult to assign a dollar value to an item. The value of clean air, for example, is greater than the health costs of pollution or the damage that pollution may pose for wildlife, for example, and putting a dollar amount on these types of factors can be contentious. Furthermore, just because a factor cannot be easily quantified does not mean it does not exist or is not important. Social costs can be very difficult to quantify, but that does not mean they can be ignored. What is the value of a community? How can anyone put a value on the loss of neighborhood institutions or a lifetime of memories? Cost-benefit analysis cannot always address these types of concerns.[33] In addition, costs and benefits may occur very far into the future and will have to be translated into current dollars. In other words, the value of a $10,000 cost in Year 1 of a project is greater than a $10,000 cost in Year 10. The general way to address this is to use the net present value of distant events or to discount future costs and benefits by a standard percentage rate, but this might not reflect community values and priorities.[34] Discounting may also result in unacceptable burdens being placed on future generations.[35]

Another problem arises in the distribution of costs and benefits.[36] Who receives the benefits? Who pays the costs? These may not be the same individuals or communities. Cost-benefit analysis often does not take into account equity concerns and if it is used in ways that disproportionately harm a low-income community, it may even intensify inequities.[37] For example, the value of a home in a low-income community is almost always less than one in a high-income area, but is this fair to low-income residents? Using these values can result in a systematic burdening of low-income and minority communities. Despite these limitations, cost-benefit analysis is an important policy tool and provides essential information to those deciding between options and initiatives.

Physical Activity Assessment

Given the high degree of concern about physical activity's relationship to the built environment, there is a great need for instruments that measure physical activity in the general population, groups, and individuals. These assessments can take the form of surveys, observations, or measurement by instruments.[38]

The simplest way to measure physical activity is simply to ask people how active they have been.[39] Typically, the questions tend to be in the form of how many minutes was a subject moderately physically active, how many minutes were vigorously physically active, or how many minutes or miles did a subject walk in a given time. One widely used example of self-report is the International Physical Activity Questionnaire (IPAQ), available in multiple formats and multiple languages.[40] IPAQ contains questions on the duration, frequency, and intensity of physical activity. Many of these questionnaires use broad categories of physical activity such as light, moderate, or vigorous activity. Other surveys may ask provide subjects with a large number of specific activities such as walking, gardening, ballroom dancing, and so on, and then calculate physical activity based on subjects' responses.[41] Some surveys ask participants how they traveled during their normal school or work day.[42]

The concern with all self-reported survey questions is the accuracy of these self-reports. In particular, are people reporting more physical activity than they are actually performing and are these inaccuracies biasing or skewing the data so that inaccurate results are obtained from data analysis?[43] Subjects may overreport physical activity because they are trying to please interviewers, they may not accurately recall past activities, they may generally believe they are more physically active than they are in reality, or individuals may not have a good sense of the dimensions of their physical activity. One type of problem is known as recall bias; subjects may systematically be misremembering their past activities. Controlling for these inaccuracies may be difficult, but not doing so may reduce the validity of the study. However, self-report may be the easiest and cheapest way to collect this type of data, particularly for large numbers of subjects and in situations with limited funds and time.

A second way of measuring physical activity is through observation. This is most typically used for studies of playgrounds and parks or bikeways and trails. There are several methods that have been employed but they typically use a set of observers to periodically observe a facility at a predetermined set of dates and times, for example, data on a playground will be collected at 10 A.M. and 2 P.M. on Saturdays and Sundays, and at 3 P.M. and 5 P.M. on weekdays.

Sometimes these observations focus on the total number of users at a given time and place, or sometimes the observations are meant to determine how physically active people are at a given time and place. Small-scale studies can utilize observers measuring the physical activity of each subject in the study. Larger-scale studies, or studies of public places, often use a predetermined methodology for randomly selecting individuals among a group of people and that particular individual's rate of physical activity is assessed by a trained observer. The advantage of this type of measurement is that a well-trained observer may reduce the degree of bias in the study sample that may result from self-report and this methodology may be the only way that uses of public spaces can be assessed. The disadvantage is that it may be costly and is highly dependent on the quality of the training of observers of the study. Among the observational tools available is the widely used System for Observing Play and Recreation in Communities (SOPARC).[44] It was used in a study that compared physical activity levels at urban versus rural parks, for example.[45]

Another method to measure physical activity has been through the use of special equipment worn by study subjects. A relatively inexpensive methodology is the pedometer, which measures the number of steps a subject has made in a given time period. Many pedometers can be calibrated to reflect the length of a subject's stride and if the subject is shown how to properly wear the pedometer, the actual distance walked can be measured. For example, a study of the effectiveness of a cell phone–based intervention to promote walking used pedometers to assess the effectiveness of the program. The intervention used cell phone calls to encourage subjects to walk more and to follow-up with barriers to walking. The outcome of interest was the intensity and amount of walking. The evaluators had good data on the frequency and nature of the phone calls but then use the pedometers to measure the amount of physical activity among the subject population.[46] There may be difficulties in collecting the data from subjects, or ensuring that the subjects wear the pedometer. Another limitation may be that the pedometer may not adequately measure nonwalking physical activity or the vigorousness of walking or running.

More sophisticated are accelerometers, which are specialized instruments worn at the waist that measure almost all physical activity.[47] These can be extremely accurate and can provide very reliable evidence of minute-by-minute physical activity, including data on the intensity of the activity. One study that used accelerometry data to assess physical activity differences between black, white, and Hispanic girls found that there were important differences in barriers and correlates between these groups of adolescents.[48] Another used accelerometers to study the effects of friends on physical activity.[49] The drawbacks of accelerometers are that they are expensive, subjects must be trained on how to use them, subjects may forget to use them, and they also require special software to convert the data into usable forms.[50] However, these instruments may be the most accurate way to fully capture subjects' physical activity. It was by using accelerometers that researchers observed that self-reported physical activity was overreported.[51]

FOCUS ON

The Community Toolbox

The Work Group for Community Health and Development at the University of Kansas has created The Community Toolbox. Its aim is to empower communities, and those working with communities, to better shape community-based interventions.

The toolbox is organized as a series of sections with chapters on topics of interest. The sections include information on models for promoting community health, community assessment, promoting participation, strategic planning and organizational development, leadership training, community analysis, implementation, and many other issues.

The goal is to enable communities to improve themselves by communicating best practices and providing information that any community can use. For more information, see http://ctb.ku.edu/en/default.aspx.

Government Data Sources

The varying branches of government—federal, state, and local—collectively have large amounts of data on a wide range of topics that can be used to help assess issues associated with the built environment. Though the data can be difficult to identify and access, they often have the advantage of being cheaper than collecting new data. An important caution regarding all data sources is that the accuracy and potential problems with the data must be carefully considered when analyzing or communicating results derived from them to others.

The federal government collects large amounts of data. The agencies that collect this information include the U.S. Department of Transportation, the Bureau of the Census, the National Center for Health Statistics, and many others. Among the large national health surveys are the National Health and Nutrition Examination Survey,[52] the Behavioral Risk Factor Surveillance System,[53] and the National Health Interview Survey.[54] Other survey datasets include the Youth Behavioral Risk Factor Surveillance System[55] and the National Latino and Asian American Survey.[56] These are only a few examples of the types of data available, but they can provide important insights on the health effects of the built environment. A study using NHANES data, for example, found that people who lived in homes built after 1973 were less likely to walk. This study was interesting because it may be evidence that changes in the built environment after the early 1970s, which included greater use of dendritic street patterns, a higher degree of separation of land uses, increased urban sprawl, and other features of the built environment, may be associated with decreased physical activity.[57]

These data should be used with care. In general, there is a trade-off between finer geographic resolution and the availability and accuracy of data. National-level data tend to be easier to acquire (though there may be problems with using them to assess issues on the local level), and they may be fairly easy to work with; however, because they are survey data, they may need to be analyzed according to the guidelines accompanying the data. An advantage of these datasets is that they are publicly available, often the questions have been validated by other researchers, the findings can be compared to other research results, and assistance with data analysis is easily accessible. Similarly, data collected by the federal government but reported for states is often easy to acquire. Data from larger surveys such as the Behavioral Risk Factor Surveillance System (BRFSS) can even be used on the county level at times, for example, in the landmark 2003 study of urban sprawl and obesity.[58] Communities and researchers often need or want data on the very local level (block, neighborhood, or subneighborhood), but problems begin to increase rapidly when data on the sub-state-level are needed. National data sets such as the BRFSS may contain hundreds of thousands of subjects but may only have very few subjects in a local geographic area. They may not be able to release local data due to confidentiality concerns, or a local area may contain so few subjects as to be statistically unreliable.

States also collect data that may be of value for assessing the built environment or they may collect data from other sources that may be relevant to the built environment.[59] Agencies that may have useful data include state health departments, economic development agencies, school departments, and others. Depending on the location, states may be the best place to find data on hazardous waste sites, permitted facilities, natural resources, and other activities funded or regulated on the state level. Data provided by the State of California, along with other sources, was used to evaluate inequalities in environmental exposures in Southern California.[60] Again, there may be issues with privacy and accuracy regarding data on individuals. Some state governments have sophisticated programs and special agencies devoted to collecting, analyzing, and making data available. Others may not have these programs and agencies.

Local governments are also important data sources. They may have collected and analyzed data from a variety of sources that may be available upon request. In most places, local governments are the appropriate place to access data on land use patterns, street conditions, the location of parks, and so forth. They can be used to assess changes in a community's housing stock, for example.[61] The quality of these data may vary widely, however. In general, data may represent the best local information available, but there can be issues with accuracy, reliability, and consistency. The quality of this data is best assessed in collaboration with the government agency collecting the data and the community being assessed.

Summary

In order to better understand the impact of development and policy decisions, a number of tools have been developed to assist communities and policymakers to better understand potential impacts. These include environmental impact assessment, health impact assessment, and cost-benefit analysis. Other assessment tools aim to look at how the environment potentially affects physical activity and other health outcomes. Each of these tools has potential strengths and weaknesses. Also of assistance in planning and health assessment are a variety of federal, state, and local sources of data on health and the environment.

Key Terms

Cost-benefit analysis

Geographic Information Systems

Environmental Impact Assessment

Health Impact Assessment

Discussion Questions

1. List the steps of environmental impact assessment.
2. What are the differences between health impact assessment and environmental impact assessment?
3. What are the problems with using an environmental impact assessment to study the potential walkability of a development proposal?
4. Why do we need to train the people conducting a NEWS survey?
5. What are some of the issues in using cost-benefit analysis to study the built environment?

6. Why are there concerns with self-reported physical activity?
7. What are the problems of using national survey data to study small-area health problems?

For More Information

Active Living Research. www.activelivingresearch.org.

Center for Disease Control and Prevention. *Behavioral Risk Factor Surveillance System (BRFSS)*. www.cdc.gov/BRFSS/.

Health Impact Project. www.healthimpactproject.org.

International Association for Impact Assessment (IAIA). www.iaia.irg.

System for observing play and recreation in communities (SOPARC). www.activelivingresearch .org/files/JPAH_14_McKenzie.pdf.

The San Francisco Bay Area Health Impact Assessment Collaborative. www.hiacollaborative .org.

CHAPTER 15

HEALTH POLICY AND PROGRAMS

LEARNING OBJECTIVES

- Describe major types of health interventions.
- Name ways that public health education can promote increased understanding about health problems associated with the built environment.
- Explain how tobacco reduction efforts informed interventions to reduce the risk of obesity.
- Design a community-level intervention.
- Describe the range of school-based interventions.
- Identify issues related to using new laws to modify the built environment to promote health.

We have discussed a number of problems created by, and related to, the built environment in this book, some of which may seem overwhelming. But now let's talk about what we can do about making the built environment better. Think of the many ways communities can change. Most important, what would you do to create change in your neighborhood or among your friends and family?

We will begin this chapter with an overview of how public health develops and plans interventions. We will then discuss the Robert Wood Johnson Foundation's Active Living Research program because it has had a major impact on obesity research and because it was developed based on existing public health practice. Next is an overview on community, school-based, and individual interventions. The chapter concludes with a discussion of some of the legal issues that surround regulating the built environment and a new idea that calls for cities to incorporate health into their general plans.

Though public health had a long history of working on built environment issues, as the twentieth century progressed it became less involved with and finally became entirely disconnected from the field of urban planning after the mid-twentieth century.[1] Therefore, there is a special challenge involved in reconnecting public health to the built environment and urban planning.[2] A major obstacle has been the reluctance of public health departments and advocates to become involved in the day-to-day decision-making processes that shape the built environment.[3] Often, some may decline to contribute to development decisions or policy debates regarding zoning and building code changes because they believe they have no statutory power to intervene or no expertise to provide. But given the health implications of the built environment, public health professionals must work to educate the public, developers, and decision makers about the health consequences of their actions.[4] To facilitate this, it is very important that public health professionals understand their legal abilities and programmatic expertise regarding land use and built environment form. They must become motivated to use the basic tools of public health to help shape development and they should work to integrate public health concerns into urban planning.[5]

At the same time, urban planners need to understand that they have the power to improve or harm health. Even though many planners still see their actions as health neutral or irrelevant to environmental health issues, evidence suggests that development form does modify health risks and therefore planning decisions should incorporate what is known about the built environment and health. Guidelines that inhibit the ability to be physically active or overly separate land uses have the potential to harm health, whereas development that features mixed walkable communities can promote healthier living. Recall that the legal basis for zoning was, in part, the appropriateness of government restrictions to protect public health. Therefore, planners need to take into account what is now known to be health promoting and health limiting as they implement and develop new programs and policies. Of course this will be dependent on training urban planning professionals so that they understand the state of current science. Once urban planners are comfortable with their role in promoting healthy behaviors, they can help shape environments to actually become better for health.

The past decade has seen the growth and development of a number of programs, policies, and organizations that have specific and general goals of reuniting public health and urban planning to meet the health challenges of our time.[6] These have been situated in both the public and nonprofit sectors and these have included model projects that have a predetermined fixed life span and other programs that are meant to work with at-risk communities for an indeterminate future. These programs are also illustrative of how the vast range of public health and urban planning expertise and experience can be used to meet health threats.

Public Health Interventions

The field of public health has long used a variety of programs and interventions to protect and promote health. Many of these experiences can be used and brought to the field of health and the built environment. For example, one set of interventions aimed at promoting behavioral change is called the **health beliefs model**. In the case of the built environment and obesity, this may include the problem that if people do not believe that physical inactivity and obesity harm health, then they will be less likely to adopt behavioral changes that will address these issues.[7] Therefore, one role of public health should be to conduct research that identifies the various health impacts of the built environment and then get this information into the hands of the public so that they can incorporate that information into their daily living habits. In this way, they could become more likely to modify their behavior. For example, many people choose to move to distant suburbs because they believe that the negative consequences of a long commute are more than outweighed by the positive impacts of living in low-cost, low-density environments. This trade-off often results from individuals discounting or not knowing about the negative health impacts of a long commute (see Chapter Four). By communicating to the public that long commutes may create problems with participating in family activities, reduce the likelihood of having healthy nutrition and healthy meals, and severely cut down on the amount of time for physical activity, individuals can better assess whether or not they should move far away from employment opportunities. The thought is that once health beliefs about certain built environments change, behaviors and choices may change as well.

These effects cannot necessarily be universally applied. There are limits to using health beliefs models of change to reach young children, for example, because they may lack the ability to make rational choices. Furthermore, economic factors, such as falling costs for poorly nutritious foods, can be an incentive for children and others to buy nonnutritious snack foods.[8] These limitations suggest that there should be multiple programs to reduce the impact of complex health risk behaviors. Hence the simultaneous movements to keep high-calorie foods away from young people, place taxes on sodas, and reduce subsidies for corn, enact laws to mandate physical activity at schools, and so on.

Another way that public health often works to promote health is by changing *social norms*. For example, at one time special restraints for children in cars were rarely used and no one questioned parents if their children were not adequately placed in special child protection seats when they were being driven around. Today, child seats are the norm and any parent who did not use such seats for infants and small children would face social disapproval. Friends and relatives expect parents to act in certain ways, for example, to use car seats for their children. This change in norms helps reinforce healthy behavior. In addition, many states have passed legislation mandating that children be placed in car seats and the legislation itself both reflects changes in social norms and reinforces this healthy behavior.

Regarding the built environment, there is a great need to change public attitudes and conceptualizations of what constitutes a healthy living environment. Many, if not most, of the public believe that low-density, car-centric environments are much healthier than inner-city neighborhoods that have higher densities and feature public transportation.[9] This belief has been solidified into conventional zoning and building codes that currently reinforce the social norm to want to live in suburban environments.[10] One thing that public health can do is to work to change these social norms so that urban living is considered to be a desirable option for households and that those who can live in higher-density situations should do so. Changing these norms may result in individuals modifying their behaviors and may facilitate alternative codes and development decision making.[11]

Related to this is the development of new laws and regulations that promote health. Public health has long relied on laws to regulate behavior and address health risks. At the beginning of the twentieth century, public health advocacy focused on laws to protect workers, improve the safety of food, and mitigate many of the negative features of tenement living. Later on, public health advocacy included laws that aim to curb cigarette smoking, promote seatbelt use, and affect other issues. To address the health impacts of the built environment, public health may also need to be focused on changing the laws and regulations that shape building and neighborhoods.[12] This may include, for example, public health advocates working with mass transportation advocates to shift public funds away from highway construction towards transit.[13] Public health advocates should also be involved in reforms of building codes so that mixed-use and pedestrian-friendly development is easier to build. Public health advocates might also want to participate in discussions regarding new development proposals so that the health impacts of the built environment and the consequences of development decisions take into account what we know about the health effects of the built environment.[14] For example, they may want to be involved in programs that aim to ensure that sidewalks are safe and well maintained so that pedestrian use is maximized.[15]

Making the connection between different public agencies is not easy, but some have tried. The Massachusetts Department of Public Health (Mass DPH), for example, has implemented a number of activities to reconnect public health and urban planning. It has become a leader in facilitating meetings designed to bring together city and town zoning committees and public health boards. In Massachusetts, both planning and health are the responsibility of cities and towns, with no role for county government (except in the special case of a commission on Cape Cod). In practice, this means there are independent boards of health and zoning/planning commissions in each of the state's 351 cities and town, and in almost every case, the two organizations work in isolation from each other and without regard for the powers and priorities of the other. To bridge these gaps, Mass DPH has sponsored seminars that include outreach to both of these types of boards, encouraging them to jointly meet to identify common concerns, and has also worked to educate both groups about the influence of the built environment on health. This illustrates the power of outside conveners to bridge department isolation and create partnerships for change. In another example, Portland, Oregon, worked to create partnerships across city departments to address issues of the built environment and health.[16]

Robert Wood Johnson—Active Living Research

One of the most influential programs that has helped reconnect urban planning, public health, and other relevant disciplines to meet the challenge of physical inactivity and obesity has been the Robert Wood Johnson Foundation's Active Living Research Program at San Diego State University.[17] Active Living Research (ALR), along with several related programs, has played a major role in fostering research and action around using the built environment to improve health. The foundation's efforts in this area began out of its concern over the rising epidemic of obesity, particularly among children. Searching for an appropriate response, they looked at the tobacco-control movement for lessons on how to address obesity and physical inactivity. Their analysis showed that although there had been some gains made from emphasizing individual interventions (for example, focusing on individuals to assist them to stop smoking), there was a large potential for societal-level interventions. Initial efforts to reduce smoking included education to smokers regarding the health problems associated with tobacco use (warning labels on cigarette packs, television and radio commercials), and the development of individual interventions and drug therapies to assist people in quitting (tobacco counseling, nicotine patches). But though these interventions did succeed in reducing smoking rates, they left a substantial portion of the population smoking. A turn to other methods that worked to change behavioral norms and reduce the social acceptability of smoking included banning smoking in workplaces, making it no longer acceptable to smoke around children, and other types of actions that affected the community around smokers. These actions pushed U.S. smoking rates further down.

To replicate the successes of the antitobacco movement, the foundation sought to create models of interventions to address physical inactivity and obesity that affected the social structure in which people were situated. RWJF's effort to address obesity demonstrates that public health professionals can learn from the experiences addressing one issue and apply those lessons to other concerns.

ALR and its sister organizations have funded basic research, policy analysis, the identification of best practices, evaluation, and dissemination of results.[18] Basic research supported by ALR has included the development of baseline assessment tools and metrics for evaluating built environments. Its policy analysis projects have examined the role of recess policies, schoolyard renovations, and multiuse trails in increasing physical activity.[19] A set of grants sought to integrate health into other government agency agendas and change public policies.[20] In all of these projects, the ALR team worked to encourage grantees to evaluate results, to share information, and publicize findings.[21] An important result has been that the field of experts and the knowledge base of expertise have been dramatically expanded.[22] The foundation has not limited itself to research. It has funded programs to address childhood obesity among Latinos and blacks, promoted model types of infrastructure and design, and has sought to improve child nutrition.

Community Interventions

The built environment includes the neighborhood and community where people live. Though individuals may have certain abilities to change their behaviors—for example, they can try to eat better or exercise more—the broader environment provides the context for these behaviors and ultimately may provide important constraints on behavior. As we have seen, the built environment has a potentially important impact on diet and exercise. For example, as discussed in Chapter Nine, the goal of better nutrition and avoidance of high-calorie foods relies on the ability of an individual or family to purchase healthier alternatives.[23] If these are not present in the community, the diet of a household may suffer. Similarly, walking or physical activity may be highly influenced by the presence or absence of parks and playgrounds or the physical design of the community. Walking is much less likely if there are no sidewalks, no safe way to cross streets, and no destinations to walk to.[24]

Thus, programs and policies aimed to modify the communities in which people live are needed. Again, following the standard ways that public health has looked at interventions and behavioral change, these types of programs can include changing social norms to encourage physical activity and better nutrition, promoting government programs aimed to produce healthier built environments, supporting group actions to increase collective efficacy, providing model codes and ordinances to promote healthier eating and greater physical activity, and working with potential allies and others to produce a healthier environment. All of these methods have been applied to the built environment.[25]

Community coalitions working on food and fitness issues have been organized to address the constellation of health threats that exist in many low-income and inner-city communities. Many localities have an existing range of community institutions and partners that have programs and agendas that touch upon many aspects of the built environment or the health of people in that community.[26] There may be health clinics providing care to children and families, community development corporations building housing and promoting economic opportunities, job training organizations concerned that their graduates must leave the neighborhood to get to potential employment, afterschool providers who work with at-risk youth, and so on. Community coalitions to address health concerns, particularly issues that may be related to the built environment such as asthma, obesity, lead poisoning, and so forth, can work together to bring new attention to problems with the built environment or secure additional resources to meet the challenges confronting these communities.

School-Based Interventions

One area that has seen a great number of new policy initiatives to address the built environment and other correlates of obesity has been schools.[27] Most of these actions have included policies and programs to promote physical activity, provide healthier nutrition, or change how schools are constructed.[28] Given that children spend so much of their time in school and children's obesity rates have climbed so rapidly, schools are a very appropriate place in which to apply public health theory and practice.

As discussed in Chapter Nine, major efforts have focused on the types of food available for children at school, with the goals of providing more nutritious food, reducing the availability of less nutritious food, addressing the built environment surrounding schools, and assisting children to become more familiar with and to adopt healthy nutrition and physical activity behaviors.[29] In the past several decades, many schools had come to rely on the revenues from vending machines to supplement money raised from taxes and other sources. But often the food offered in these vending machines tended to be unhealthy sugared sodas, high-calorie and high-sodium content snacks, and heavily sugared and high-fat-content desserts. Advocacy to modify the food environment by changing vending machine offerings has focused on two goals. One is eliminating the machines altogether from schools or severely restricting access so that students can only get to the machines a few times a day. The goal is that the school environment will no longer include nonnutritious food. Sometimes, public health advocates have worked on this on a school-by-school basis, sometimes they have gone to the district level, and sometimes they have gone to state government to try to have laws passed to change all the schools in a state.

Another way in which vending machine issues have been addressed has been working with school administrations and the companies that supply vending machines to change the types of food and drink offered at schools. The goal of these programs has been to provide healthier alternatives for children.[30] They emphasize water and fruit drinks or healthier snacks such as yogurt and granola rather than the traditional offerings. There have been concerns that some of the alternative offerings are not as healthy or as environmentally friendly as they might seem. Many types of fruit drinks may have a higher sugar content and fewer vitamins than one might think would be the norm in natural alternatives to sugared sodas. There are controversies surrounding whether vending machines should offer bottled water, given that schools should be providing free and safe water for drinking. There have been concerns that students will not want these healthier alternatives and that the revenues from vending machines will be lost and school budgets suffer. But to date, it appears that children do like these healthier alternatives and schools can still rely on the revenues that come from their long-term contracts with vending machine companies. Most important, eating behaviors have improved.

A different type of common intervention focuses on increasing physical activity in schools.[31] In the wake of new laws to promote student achievement, many schools have dropped recess and reduced lunch periods so that more time is available to teach fundamental academic subjects.[32] Though well intentioned, the reduction in recess may result in children not meeting current guidelines for physical activity and could be contributing to the rise in childhood obesity. In response, public health advocates have turned toward promoting the beneficial impacts of recess and have worked to reestablish requirements for daily recess and physical education. Texas, for example, has strict laws mandating student activity that have helped to reestablish recess as a fundamental part of the elementary school day.[33] There is also a need to enforce existing regulations regarding physical activity and recess. Over the years, many schools have reduced or ignored their physical activity class requirements even though state and district rules may still be in effect. Therefore, public health departments may have to learn how to work with school personnel and parents to bring back physical education classes to make physical activity a part of each student's day.[34] In a sense, these are built environment interventions because they seek to reconnect students to sports, fields, playgrounds, gyms, and parks.

Some states have moved toward annual assessments of student height and weight, calculating Body Mass Index (BMI), and sending the results of these assessments home to parents.[35] These programs have been controversial because of concerns that students will feel stigmatized because of higher weight or that parents will be unable to adequately address or understand what their child's BMI report means. However, the state of Arkansas has found this assessment of student height and weight to be a central component of their successful effort to address that state's very high childhood obesity rate. Knowledge of the health risks of childhood obesity and an independent assessment of a child's health status may help parents meet the challenges of providing healthy food and greater physical activity.[36] They may also help promote the development of a public consensus that obesity is a priority public health issue and that an array of programs, including attention to the built environment, is important.

Another type of policy initiative has been to improve the physical state of schools, modifying the school built environment to promote healthy behaviors. Over the years, funding constraints have resulted in delayed maintenance for the outdoor portions of school campuses. Over time, this lack of maintenance has led to a severe deterioration of school outdoor environments. Children can no longer safely play outside because of broken or outdated equipment, decayed asphalt, playing fields that lack grass, or similar problems. When deterioration reaches a certain point, schools are reluctant to let children outside to play at all and the neighbors of these schools can no longer use them as a resource during nonschool hours. To address these problems, schools have turned to new ideas to restore the outside portions of their campuses. One innovative program has been the Boston Schoolyard Initiative (BSI). Many Boston schoolyards have suffered from decades of decay and, by the late 1990s, were often only used for parking.[37] Public and private institutions and individuals banded together to develop a program to restore these degraded play spaces. As a result, most of the schoolyards in this very diverse city have now been renovated and what were once dangerous places that contributed to the feeling that schools were partly causing blight in communities are now important resources to neighborhoods and heavily used by both children at schools and children in the surrounding community. There is also some evidence that the renovations have boosted school performance and the quality of life in the surrounding area.[38] Capital improvements and maintenance are expensive, but they are vital if children's health is to be protected.

One reason that walking to school has declined has been changes in school building policies. Over the past several decades, many states have mandated minimum square footage per student, resulting in a need for larger parcels of land to accommodate new schools. At the same time, policies encouraging larger schools (serving more students) have also led to an increase in school land requirements.[39] These trends have helped push schools to peripheral locations at the edges of communities or have resulted in fewer children being within walking distance of schools. In part because of concerns of rising childhood obesity rates, increasing transportation costs, and high levels of air pollution exposures associated with large-scale busing of children, there have been efforts to change the siting of schools.[40] These have included allowing for exceptions to minimum open space requirements or advocating for smaller schools.[41]

FOCUS ON

Soda and Beverage Taxes

Though strictly speaking not a built environment issue, some communities and states have proposed new taxes on foods that are thought to be unhealthy.[42] The public health rationale for these taxes stems from the success that raising taxes on tobacco products had on reducing cigarette smoking. As taxes on these products rises, consumption falls. Therefore, one way to reduce the consumption of sugary sodas and high-calorie snacks is to place a special tax on these products. But there are several issues to be considered before these levies can be put in place. One is the need to come up with a standard definition of these products so that the tax is targeted toward the unwanted foods and is not put on healthy staples. Another major problem is the political opposition from those who produce and sell these kinds of products and who have very legitimate concerns that their profits and economic livelihoods might be negatively affected. Though these special taxes have been proposed to a number of jurisdictions, they have yet to become popular.

Individual Level Interventions

Though much of the influence of the built environment takes place on the community level, there is still a place for individual interventions and actions to assist individuals in better adapting to their surrounding built environment in ways that promote their health. Again, many of these programs work to change health knowledge or behaviors. Others work to help individuals adopt and maintain healthy eating and physical activity behaviors. The range of these interventions extends well beyond efforts to modify the built environment.

A major challenge limiting the ability to increase public understanding of what constitutes a healthy built environment and the need to modify conventional building and zoning regulations to permit healthier development is the lack of funding to educate the public. Antitobacco advertising greatly benefited from cigarette taxes and other dedicated income streams to fund television and radio ads and billboards. There were also only a small number of tobacco companies, and so collecting taxes was easy and it was also fairly easy to target antitobacco warnings by placing them on cigarette packages. But these opportunities and revenue streams do not exist for those wishing to educate the public about the needs of the built environment. There is the long-established practice of using development impact fees to fund infrastructure and local government needs, but this source is highly variable, rising during times of economic upswings and falling when new development slows during recessions. There are also many competing uses for these funds and other constituencies may resent or resist efforts to use these revenues for public health–related programming.

Legal Basis for Built Environment Regulation

Changing the built environment can often result in compromises in the ability of owners to use their properties as they desire, resulting in court challenges or political opposition. Therefore the legal framework for implementing new regulations on the built environment must be carefully considered.[43] Communities, empowered by their states, have long had the ability to intervene in the built environment to promote health. Again, much of the history of the nineteenth and twentieth centuries is a series of efforts to implement new building and zoning laws. As a result of these efforts, there has been a slow increase in the ability of local governments to modify the built environment because of health. Throughout this time, there has been a general trend of the courts holding that promoting public health is a valid public purpose. However, this power must be carefully used and there is no guarantee that any new initiative will withstand legal scrutiny. Overregulation of land use can result in a severe political backlash and may well ultimately compromise the ability of local public health departments and local government to promote health. Therefore, it is wise to carefully consider the goals, language, and purposes of new laws and regulations.[44]

Often, there needs to be an explicit detailing of health problems and health-promotion goals that are the subject of the new law or regulation. By carefully demonstrating what is to be prevented, solved, or promoted, the legal justification for a new ordinance can be established. It is very critical that those working on a new proposed ordinance or law understand whether or not they have the legal or constitutional authority to regulate the issue they are trying to address. For example, the constitutional guarantees for freedom of speech may limit the ability of local governments to control advertisements for foods that they think are unhealthy. Sometimes the federal government preempts local government, as can state governments. Therefore, it is very important for public health advocates contemplating new legislation or ordinances to consult with those who have the legal knowledge to properly frame their new laws.

Inserting Health into City General Plans

Starting in California, there has been a recent movement to directly make public health a concern of cities' general plans. Since the 1970s, California has had strong statewide guidelines for its cities and counties regarding what must be in these plans that require not only land use but also housing, circulation, and other key features of the built environment.[45] Though not required, several cities have adopted health elements into their plans. For example, the City of Richmond, a community in the East Bay region of San Francisco Bay that has a substantial low-income and minority population, has begun to develop a health element for its general plan.[46] The element will include attention to both physical and mental health and will seek to identify ways in which the city can grow and adopt healthy built environment features such as bike paths, better nutrition, reduced chemical hazards, and reduced noise levels. Other communities are explicitly using health outcomes to modify code requirements to make streets more pedestrian friendly, for example.[47]

Summary

Efforts to modify the built environment, as well as to help people meet barriers posed by it, are shaped by public health theories of behavioral change. Many of these efforts have been informed by other public health campaigns such as anti-tobacco efforts. Some policies aim to shape community or school environments, whereas others seek to work with individuals to promote healthier behaviors.

Key Term

Health beliefs model

Discussion Questions

1. How might health beliefs affect a person's choice of neighborhood to live in?
2. What are the similarities between anti-tobacco and anti-obesity public heath efforts?
3. List community-based organizations that might be part of a neighborhood coalition to promote healthier built environments.
4. Name programs that aim to modify the school food and physical activity environments.
5. How might individuals improve their physical activity?
6. What is a health element of a general plan?

For More Information

American Public Health Association. www.apha.org.

Earle, S. (2007). *Theory and research in promoting public health.* Thousand Oaks: Sage.

Guttmacher, S., Kelly, P. J., & Ruiz-Janecko, Y. (2010). *Community-based health interventions: Principles and applications.* Hoboken, NJ: Wiley.

National Association of County and City Health Organizations (NACCHO). www.naccho.org.

Robert Wood Johnson Foundation. www.rwjf.org.

CHAPTER 16

SUSTAINABILITY

LEARNING OBJECTIVES

- Define sustainability.
- Explain the relationship between sustainability and equity.
- Describe the concept of an ecological footprint.
- Evaluate the role of the built environment in sustainability.
- Define green roofs.
- Explain how urban regreening programs could potentially contribute to sustainability.
- Describe the Leadership in Energy and Environmental Design program.
- List the potential health impacts of global climate change.

Have you ever worried about your impact on the environment? Consider all the efforts people make in their daily lives to reduce their contribution to pollution and the overuse of resources. Some people drive hybrid cars, others walk, bike, or take public transportation. Recycling bins are common and some cities post warnings about dumping chemicals into drains because they might pollute waterways. For the next 24 hours, keep a list of the many things people in your community are doing to reduce their environmental impact.

Sustainability, or the long-term ability to support the human population without seriously degrading the environment, is closely associated with the built environment. As we shall see, levels of sustainability are influenced by land use patterns, building codes, transportation infrastructure, and other aspects of the built environment. We will begin this chapter with a discussion of what sustainability is and how it relates to equity. Next we will explore measures of sustainability followed by an overview of different types of programs to increase it. We conclude with the issue of global climate change, its potential health effects, and how the built environment and individual efforts might help meet the challenges posed by this threat.

Defining Sustainability

What exactly is sustainability? Like so many other terms used in this book, it is a word that is used by different disciplines to mean different things. Among human service providers, for example, sustainability may have a fairly short time horizon and often refers to the ability to keep a program in operation once a pilot grant or a core service contract is completed.[1] Sustainability in the context of the built environment comes from the ecological science literature and refers to the long-term ability of an area to support its population without adverse effects on other people, species, or areas.[2]

Each of the parts of this definition is subject to interpretation. The time period over which sustainability is operationalized can vary by multiple orders of magnitude. One popular idea is that the effects of a policy, program, or development should be considered over the time period that would be lived by seven generations of humanity (an idea often attributed to the Iroquois Nations), or well over 200 years. Others use the term to refer to effects over a much shorter period of time, one that may be only twenty years or even less. There is no standard definition of the time frame in which sustainability is to be considered. Furthermore, it can be argued that it is impossible to forecast or predict very long-term problems and effects, and therefore the very distant future has too many unknowns to be considered. There is also the economic concept of discounting, the need to systematically reduce the value of future years' benefits and costs by a set annual percentage because the value of something in the future is less than the value of it today (see Chapter Fourteen). Some people in the sustainability movement find this discounting excessive or objectionable because discounting almost always assures that the effects of something in the very far future such as a century away have minimal value in today's dollars.[3] This potential misconsideration of future costs and benefits can result in poor policy and development decision making.[4] However these future costs are considered or how sustainability is thought of, it is important that these assumptions be made explicit during policy development and analysis.[5]

The ability of an area to support its population can also be subject to debate. For example, economists often speak about the relative efficiency of different areas. Some places, because of past investment, local climate, human capital, or other reasons, might be more efficient at producing a particular good or service than other areas. Though some environmentalists argue that every area should be self-sufficient, if one area can produce a good or service more efficiently than others, then it might make sense, from a global sustainability perspective, to produce that good or service in that more efficient locale and transport the goods or services to the less efficient area.[6] Overall, these issues are only slowly moving towards a consensus that would include those both in and outside of the sustainability movement.

Because the effects on other people or other points in time may not be known or well characterized, it can be difficult to gauge sustainability. That there is the potential for the long-term persistence of some chemicals and metals has been well described but the effects of many other materials, such as silver-based nanoparticles, are not known at this time.[7] Other effects are difficult to quantify. For example, the potential long-term impacts of carbon dioxide produced by the burning of oil can be identified, at least in general terms, but the effects of the depletion of energy resources on future generations is much less easy to characterize.[8] Yet these effects may be important. The ability to predict and measure effects on people over time and geography can be difficult. But this does not mean they do not exist.[9]

One of the most important ways to define sustainability arose out of the work of the United Nation's World Commission on Environment and Development, also known as the Brundtland Commission. It famously stated that sustainable development is that which meets the needs of the present without compromising the ability of future generations to meet their own needs. It goes on to declare that it is "Emphasizing the need for a new approach to economic growth, as an essential prerequisite for eradication of poverty and for enhancing the resource base on which present and future generations depend."[10] Note that this definition implies no time limit on effects, nor does it have limits on the types of effects or their geographic extent. It also includes important equity considerations.

Sustainability and Equity

Among the perhaps infinite number of ways a society could become sustainable, many would be undesirable. A major criticism of the sustainable environment movement, articulated by urban theorist Peter Marcuse and others, is that it could easily end up perpetuating existing social and economic inequities.[11] Simply continuing how certain segments of society are treated into perpetuity would be extremely unjust. Thus many in the sustainability movement have begun to incorporate measures of equity into their measures of progress toward sustainability and many statements of sustainability include strong commitments towards achieving social justice. However, not all statements on sustainability do so and when sustainability is translated down to the local policy level, equity issues can also fade in prominence.[12] Furthermore, as we will see next, sometimes the equity dimensions of sustainability become lost once measures of sustainability are created. One group of researchers who are concerned with both environmental justice and sustainability have developed the concept of "just sustainability" as an alternative that incorporates equity concerns into efforts to create models of long-term environmental action. This may help ensure that any effort to develop a sustainable future address current social, gender, racial, and other inequities.[13]

Measures of Sustainability

Quantifying sustainability impacts can be very difficult.[14] Though some processes are fairly well described, such as the impacts on polar environments of mercury emissions from lower latitudes, the causes and effects of other pollutants are not so clear-cut. Despite these problems, scientists and advocates for sustainability have tried to develop measures that allow for the quantification of impacts. In general, there is a trade-off between the simplicity of the measure and the need for incorporating into that measure all the varying factors that might go into a sustainable and just society. For example, it might be desirable to have a sustainability measure that consists solely of a single number. Think of a hypothetical example of a 100-point scale of sustainability where 100 was complete sustainability and zero was complete nonsustainbility. That might allow the public to quickly understand that from last year to this sustainability changed by so many units, for example, from 10 to 12. This would also allow easy comparison between areas. Metropolitan area X has sustainability of 7 whereas metropolitan area Y had a sustainability of 8. There is value in simplicity. The reality, however, is that sustainability is most likely a multidimensional concept and it might be that no single number could ever capture the complexity of what sustainability is. Thus, there is a trade-off between understandability and complexity, but this has not stopped the development of a number of measures of sustainability.[15]

Ecological Footprints

One growing effort to measure sustainability is the idea of *ecological footprint*, or the area of land that it takes to support an area's population, either for the area's total population (sometimes reported on a per capita basis) or for an individual's calculated support area.[16] The concept began out of the understanding that certain diets require fewer resources to support than others, for example, vegetarian versus meat-based diets. Based on what is known about human diets (most individuals don't vary greatly from the mean) and what is known about the ability of cropland to support agriculture and the amount of land it takes to support grazing animals or grow crops for grain-fed animals, the relative amounts of land needed to support various people in varied countries with varied diets can be fairly easily calculated, given the assumptions in these models. As would be expected, individuals who consume less food or who abstain from eating meat have a smaller ecological footprint than persons who eat more and who consume meat. By this measure, meat-eating countries would most likely have larger footprints than countries with a large percentage of vegetarians.[17]

But the impact of people on the environment is greater than just their diets, so beginning in the 1990s researchers began to expand the concept of **ecological footprint** to include the totality of humanity's impact on the environment. These broader measures of ecological footprints attempt to include transportation, consumer products, defense spending, and other similar impacts. The unit of reporting can be expressed in various ways, including land area, by measuring consumption in terms of how much energy is contained in the total amount of sunlight falling on a hectare (or acre) of land, the oil needed to support a given amount of activity, or the total amount of carbon dioxide that would be produced in order to support a person over the course of a year. The last measure has become particularly useful given the growing concern over global climate change.[18] The results can be startling: there are high disparities in consumption and impacts (see Figure 16.1). For example, by most measures, the ecological footprints of U.S. residents are much larger than those of other countries. It takes more land area, more barrels of oil, or more tons of carbon dioxide to support American lifestyles. But by other measures, however, we are not at the top of the footprint scale. For example, the amount of carbon dioxide produced per unit of

FIGURE 16.1   Selected National Carbon Footprints

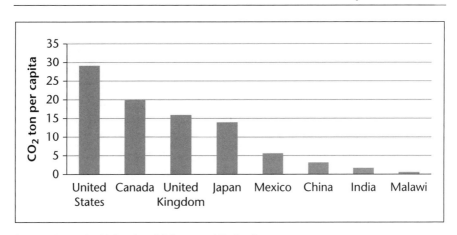

Source: Norwegian University of Science and Technology

Gross Domestic Product in the United States is lower than that of other countries due to certain efficiencies in the U.S. economy. However, because we have much higher incomes than other countries, our actual carbon dioxide use per capita is at the high end of the distribution. Some scientists have used the size of the United States' ecological footprint, as measured in hectares per person, to estimate what it would take in terms of land area to support the entire population of the world with the same degree of impacts of that of current U.S. society. The result predicts that the amount of land needed would be larger than size of the land area of the entire planet.[19] The implication is that the current U.S. ecological economy is not sustainable.[20]

A major issue is how to use the ecological footprint metrics. Individuals may find it difficult to change their carbon footprint (though a vegetarian diet would make an important difference), but many of the factors that lead to the size of a country's footprint are beyond the ability of any one individual to control, because they are highly related to income and population size.[21] For example, footprints are often the result of local, regional, state, and federal policies that collectively create land-use patterns or influence the built environment and they may incorporate the decisions of millions of individuals. Land use and the resulting transportation systems are heavy influences on the size of an ecological footprint, but individuals have a limited ability to change these by themselves. Another problem is that the footprint is an oversimplified measure and it cannot incorporate all the complexities of environmental impacts. For example, it does not incorporate into its value the extinction of endangered species.[22] Note that ecological footprint measures also fail to incorporate equity into the metric. The complexity of sustainability has been sacrificed in this effort to create a single understandable measure. The danger is that in this simplification process, equity may be forgotten.

On a national scale, lawmakers and policy developers have rarely used the ecological footprint framework to evaluate proposed developments or policies.[23] Either they are unaware of the policy tool or they do not see any political support to incorporate these tools into the decision-making process. Combined, these two problems suggest that there is a need for better education of the public and policymakers so that they understand the impacts of their lifestyles.

The last several years have seen the development of Web-based calculators that enable individuals to input key parameters of their lifestyles (where they live, total miles they drive, a description of their diet, and so forth) which will then produce an estimate of their ecological footprint. The scientific accuracy of these calculators has not been assessed, however. Nor have these been demonstrated to have the ability to influence individual human behavior. At this time, they may just be curiosities.

FOCUS ON

Impact on the Environment: Urban Versus Rural Residents

Sometimes it seems that some environmentalists are convinced that urban residents are worse for the environment than rural people. The thought is that the disconnect from the natural environments leads to less concern for the impacts of human activity on natural ecosystems. The argument is that urban residents consume more resources and create unnatural conditions. Is this true?

There is no reason to suspect that urban residents care less about the environment than rural residents. Voting for environmental measures and support for environmentally friendly candidates is stronger in urban areas than rural areas. Other competing concerns might sometimes obscure this support, but in general, environmentalism is strong in urban areas.

Do these concerns get translated into environmental action? On the one hand, urban residents tend to have lower recycling participation rates than suburban residents. Partly, this may be a reflection of a lack of space for recycling and the lower incomes of some inner-city communities. On the other hand, urban residents tend to drive less, take more public transportation, and use less energy to heat and cool their homes. The built environment in dense cities reduces their overall impact on the environment. Rural residents need to drive more and a single-family home uses more energy than an apartment or condominium. Thus the day-to-day impacts of urban dwellers may be less than those of rural residents.[24]

The Local Sustainability Movement

Rather than wait for a national set of policies that might promote sustainability, some communities have set out to develop programs and policies that would lead to greater sustainability on the local or regional level.[25] These local efforts received a major boost after the United Nations Summit on the Environment in Rio de Janeiro in 1992. An agreement that resulted from that meeting, adopted by over 150 countries including the United States, called on local communities to address sustainability in their own areas. The actual programs and policies that localities were to adopt were left to each community to plan and implement.[26]

Many local sustainability organizations in the United States have been non-profit, nongovernmental, voluntary organizations that consist of individuals and organizations interested in sustainability, social justice, and environmental issues. They tend to work on transportation, housing, open space, land use, and other topics related to the built environment. Their methods include public education, advocacy, model projects, and other similar activities. One of the earliest and most famous of these organizations is Sustainable Seattle, founded in 1991.[27] It works on sustainability issues in the Central Puget Sound area and its programs include indicator projects, outlining how the community is doing in terms of sustainability, the recognition of people and programs who are trying to increase the sustainability of the region, and connecting data with policy initiatives. It serves as a forum for those people and institutions in the region who are concerned about long-term climate change and who are working toward a more just and sustainable future.

Many cities and states have adopted policies with the explicit goal of promoting sustainability.[28] Sometimes these policies are an explicit and comprehensive statement of the goals of a sustainable future, sometime these policies tend to be focused on one or more main issues associated with sustainability, such as global climate change.[29] Some states, such as California, have adopted laws that will promote decreased greenhouse gas emissions with the goal of increasing that state's sustainability. Many local governments, including Chicago, have adopted a number of policies to modify their built environment with the goal of promoting sustainability as well. These include improving the energy efficiency of buildings, using fleets of alternative fuel vehicles, promoting green roofs (see below), changing zoning and building codes, planting trees, and so forth.

The Role of Environmental Design in Sustainability

Creating sustainability may mean changing the built environment or modifying the design of communities, but for many years standard development practices had little regard for their long-term environmental effects. Until well after World War II, many cities in the United States expanded without any consideration of their environmental impact on the land around them. Wetlands were drained or filled, forests cleared, and hillsides were graded without concern for the plant and animal populations displaced or the ecosystems destroyed. For example, coastal cities routinely filled in near-shore areas, producing new lands from Seattle's waterfront to the entire city of Miami Beach. In most of the United States, cities allowed new subdivisions to spread across the landscape and new streets were often added without accommodation to topography or local conditions.

This indifference to local environments began to change in the 1950s with the work of Ian McHarg and others. McHarg and his associates put forth the theory that humanity was part of local ecosystems, not outside of them. Therefore, how humanity built and designed its cities could be improved if they acknowledged the interrelationship of people and their natural environments. With the 1969 publication of McHarg's landmark book, *Design with Nature*, the concept of environmental design moved into the mainstream of landscape architecture and urban planning.[30]

Today, though there are many conflicts between developers who want to maximize the return on their investment in property and environmentalists and communities who value the special environmental attributes of a given parcel of land, the idea that there are certain types of landscapes that should be preserved has become widely accepted.[31] In most communities, this can mean that wetlands are preserved, streets are aligned to reflect local topography, and special environments are targeted for preservation in advance of development. These measures do not always work. Sometimes it is difficult to get developers and property owners to agree not to develop an area, or a local government may lack the resources to pay to preserve a piece of land. In general, current standard subdivision guidelines now incorporate many of the principles of environmental design and call for developers to set aside critical habitats and minimize the need for grading hillsides, cutting down trees, and other intensive modifications of the natural environment. Though these are often overridden by the appeal or regulatory process, at least these laws are in place.[32] It has become more difficult to legally destroy wetlands today, because, for example, federal and state wetland protection laws now help shape development.[33] In addition, as was discussed in Chapter Eight, public water suppliers often attempt to buy land for the development rights around critical water resources so that they are not contaminated. As we will see in the programs described below, there are number of ways in which sensitive areas are now protected.

Today, we have a deeper understanding of what may be the totality of what constitutes environmentally sensitive design. It is more complex than many realize.[34] It includes preserving sensitive areas, enhancing biodiversity, designing neighborhoods with a variety of housing types, promoting sustainable development, and much more. [35]

Greenbelts and Land Preservation

As was discussed in Chapter Three, a major goal of antisprawl advocates has been to promote more compact metropolitan area forms. But the preservation of farmland and sensitive environmental areas is more than just a matter of protecting the health of people in metropolitan areas; there is a sustainability impact as well.[36] The goal is to modify the built environment at the metropolitan level to reduce its environmental impacts. As neighborhoods spread out across the landscape, sensitive environmental areas are threatened and the need for car-based transportation systems increases. Some communities have looked at ways of curbing this expansion and trying to direct development into central areas or those with access to transit.[37] One of the most common programs is to simply purchase land that is threatened by a particular development. Some cities have gone a step further and have developed comprehensive programs to either purchase land, acquire development rights, or otherwise limit development on a broad area around a city so that further suburbanization is stopped.[38] As previously noted, Portland, Oregon, is famous for its very strict urban boundary beyond which no development is permitted.[39] San Jose, California, purchased land or development rights in the hillsides and bayside surrounding its urban core.[40] Both cities have seemed to be successful in slowing or reversing the amount of sprawl.

As we discussed in Chapter Three, these efforts have not been without controversy. Critics suggest that these efforts hurt the poor because they limit the availability of housing and thus cause housing prices to increase.[41] The amenities provided by open space are mostly on the edge of the metropolitan area and tend to accrue to those wealthy enough to afford these communities, whereas those in the inner city are potentially confronted by increased traffic and pollution. The effects of greenbelts on housing prices has been studied extensively with some studies suggesting that housing prices do increase and others suggesting that they do not.

These programs can be hard to implement because they require extensive financing and the political will to implement.[42] Often, land preservation is financed through property or parcel taxes which many find objectionable. But without financial incentives, it can be difficult to persuade landowners not to develop their properties. Other potential problems are that large-scale land purchases can be expensive and government may lack the ability to protect the land that has been purchased. Despite these issues, many of the other programs and policies that have been used to promote healthier neighborhood environments can also be used to shape urban form for sustainability, including housing moratoriums, density bonuses, mixed-use development, transit-oriented development, and smart growth. This demonstrates that there are potentially multiple benefits rising from these types of programs.[43]

Green Roofs

The effort to improve sustainability does not have to take place on the global or regional scale; it can also take place on a building-by-building basis. A major problem that has been identified in the past several decades is the **urban heat island** effect.[44] In general, urban areas are warmer than the surrounding countryside because their large amounts of paved surfaces and big blocks of buildings absorb and retain heat. Modern roofing technologies, particularly the use of asphalt and black rubber roofs, are a particular problem because they absorb a large amount of sunlight, slowly releasing it as heat, and thus are a major contributor to higher urban ambient temperatures.[45] Another problem is the storm runoff from roofs. Impervious roofs increase the volume of storm water and add to the problems associated with heavy rain events.

A solution to these problems is the **green roof**. These are roofs that are planted with vegetation, the most famous of which is the rooftop garden on Chicago's City Hall. Green roofs can take many forms: they can be planted with native vegetation adapted to maximize local climate conditions, or they can be almost the equivalent of public parks, containing grass, trees, and heavily manicured landscapes. The design and construction of green roofs is more than a matter of simply hauling dirt up on the roof and planting trees. They must be carefully designed so as to avoid structural or maintenance problems. A roof must be assessed to determine if it can support the weight of soil, and the drainage of the roof and the selection of plantings must be carefully considered.

The limitations of green roofs are both sociopolitical and technological. Many jurisdictions do not require green roofs, so property owners do not think to install them. Other building owners may fear there might be safety issues or may be concerned that they could face special legal liabilities if rooftops become heavily used or leak. Addressing these types of concerns may mean promoting and publicizing model projects, adopting zoning changes or the modification of building liability laws, or new programs that provide public funds for projects that aim to retrofit existing roofs.[46]

Other problems can be technologically related. Many existing buildings have been built with high pitched roofs that have little ability to support vegetation. Others lack the structural ability to withstand the weight of soil, plantings, and water that a green roof would require unless they are substantially rebuilt. Roofs in arid parts of the United States may not be good candidates for green roofs if these new plantings would require irrigation to support vegetation or would present a fire hazard during dry spells.[47]

A simpler, but not as thorough alternative to green roofs, has been to require that developers and property owners use light colors for their roofs.[48] This can mean painting a rubber roof or using a cover that will reflect, rather than absorb sunlight. The goal is to prevent sunlight from being absorbed and converted into heat. These programs often rely on simple changes in local building codes and mostly apply to new construction or new roofs rather than requiring property owners to retrofit existing roofs.

Urban Greening

Another built environment program that some communities have used to promote sustainability has been urban regreening efforts. Recognizing that cities are a landscape that offers both hard and soft surfaces, cities are looking at their public and private spaces to find policies that can reduce their impacts on the environment. Extensive street tree programs in the first half of the twentieth century produced lush plantings along major thoroughfares and in many residential areas. But a series of pest invasions and disease outbreaks, including Dutch elm disease and the wooly algid that attacks hemlocks, along with declining municipal budgets that have vastly curtailed city tree-planting programs, resulted in many cities having lost a substantial part of their tree canopy by the beginning of the twenty-first century. This tree loss can result in reduced pedestrian activity, warmer temperatures, increased air pollution, and a reduced capacity to absorb carbon dioxide. Trees can also reduce the volume of rain water runoff, so deforested neighborhoods can lead to increased risks of flooding. Residential property values may decline as well and there is some concern that the loss of trees has been greater in poor neighborhoods and communities of color.[49]

In response, many cities have announced programs to replant street trees and other open areas. New York City has a goal of one million new trees and Los Angeles has set a similar target.[50] Programs of this scale require a substantial commitment of time and money, in part because it will take many years for these plantings to be completed and decades for them to reach their full scale of impact. They require the cooperation of residents and businesses to maintain and support plantings, the adoption of new programs that will help nurture trees, and the long-term financing of tree planting and maintenance operations. Of New York City's one million trees, for example, approximately 220,000 will be street trees, another 320,000 will be planted on public property, and 400,000 will be on private property.

These programs differ from earlier tree-planting efforts in several important ways. The toll of past epidemics, which was particularly noticeable on streets that had been planted with a single species of tree, has prompted a rethinking of how to select trees, with a new priority given to the planting of a variety of trees so that all will not die if a new disease or pest strikes. Local species adapted to local conditions are now prioritized over imported species that can become pests or prove to be less adapted to local climate conditions. For example, cities once planted Norway maples, but these have been found to create problems because they are invasive and can aggressively crowd out other trees.[51] Similarly, cities in warmer climates once planted eucalyptus trees, but these have fallen out of favor because they can be major consumers of water or pose a fire danger during times of drought. Local arborists, who have experience with such issues, have become essential members of coalitions to support regreening.

There are still some unknowns regarding how to best manage a citywide tree-planting program.[52] For example, is it better to use resident labor to plant trees because neighbors will then be more likely to protect and maintain the trees? Or does all the time and money it would take to train volunteers, distribute trees, and monitor planting techniques render city contractor plantings more likely to thrive? It is hoped that these new programs will help suggest some answers to these questions.

Cities have also come to realize that these programs are long-term efforts.[53] It takes many years before the amount of carbon dioxide used in the growing, transport, and planting of a tree is matched by the amount of carbon sequestered in a tree's overall biomass. Thus tree plantings today may not result in an overall net reduction in carbon dioxide for decades.[54] This should not deter these efforts, however. Given the long-term benefit of tree planting, the benefits most likely far exceed the cost.

Green Building Design

In the effort to promote sustainability, architects and designers have turned to what is known as green building design to reduce the impacts of development on the environment. The goal is to make a building contribute to sustainability while still ensuring that occupants are satisfied with the building.[55] In general, there are several ways in which a building can have an impact on long-term sustainability, and architects try to reduce the environmental impacts at each stage in the development, construction, maintenance, and demolition of a building.[56]

Green building design must begin during the development stage, when a building site is selected, the intensity and range of uses outlined, and the buildings are sited on a parcel. Many green buildings have been criticized because even though they may maximize energy efficiency and minimize local environmental impacts, their locations are so far from existing city services or so distant from potential users that their regional or global environmental impacts far exceed their local environmental benefits. If everyone must drive several miles or more to a green building, is it really green?

It is very important to consider the environment impacts of the development even before the building is occupied. During the building development phase, materials to be used are specified and the procedures to be followed during the construction process are detailed, all with the goal of reducing the effects of later phases. Designers often require that recycled building products or locally produced materials be used in the construction. These plans often specify low-impact processes and materials such as solvent-free adhesives. They have the goal of reducing impacts on the environment during and after construction. They may also call for more efficient heating and cooling systems, thicker insulation, and higher efficiency lighting to reduce energy costs and use in the completed building.[57]

To ensure long-term sustainability, green building designers work to reduce the burden of maintenance. Often, it is a reduction of operating and maintenance costs that offsets higher development and construction expenses which makes green building economically feasible. Designers may include more windows, which can allow for natural sunlight and ventilation, reducing energy costs. They may seek to incorporate designs that reduce the requirement for problematic maintenance procedures or reduce the need for solvents during maintenance and cleaning. It may be necessary to train building maintenance staffs in how to operate and maintain these unfamiliar processes and operations. Specialists in building design and construction may be necessary as well.[58]

Finally, designers have looked at end-stage costs of demolishing a building if and when it reaches the end of its useful life.[59] These end-of-life costs are more difficult to quantify. First of all, it is not clear what the useful life span of a building is. Most buildings can be used for decades, if not indefinitely, if they are well maintained and a regular schedule of capital improvements is adhered to. Some housing in older cities is now centuries old with no sign of being in need of demolition, for example. The other issue is how to discount for costs that will take place far into the future. The value of a dollar saved decades from now is less than the cost of a dollar spent today. Inflation will erode the value of a dollar over time and it can be hard to quantify the loss of current purchasing power for future savings. Still, designers have sought to make it so that buildings can be more easily demolished if they need to be by reducing the amount of hazardous materials or using materials that can be easily recycled.

Leadership in Energy and Environmental Design. Overall efforts to promote green building and promote more sustainable built environments received a substantial boost when the United States Green Building Council, a nonprofit organization of builders and developers, established **Leadership in Energy and Environmental Design (LEED)**, a voluntary program of certification for buildings that achieved certain standards, agreed upon in advance, regarding design, construction, and energy efficiency. Its aim is to encourage the establishment of best practices and the development of energy efficient and environmentally friendly buildings and communities.

The original LEED certification was for the new construction of office buildings, but it has since been extended to cover a wide variety of building types, such as residences, schools, and so on, and even for entire neighborhoods.[60] The initial guidelines have been evaluated over time and the guidelines for any one category are subject to periodic revision. There are varying levels of LEED certification: silver, gold, and platinum, depending on the degree of efficiency the project incorporates. Architects and planners can become certified in LEED operations.

A given LEED set of guidelines is a list of items that the developer of an individual building can select from with each item having points attached to it. To achieve LEED certification, a project must reach a minimum number of points.[61] These point systems are voluntary, but they must be certified by a professional trained in how to monitor and assess compliance with LEED building practices. The guidelines give points for the use of natural lighting, higher levels of insulation, and more efficient heating and air conditioning, for example. This allows builders to select which features they want to incorporate into their development based on local conditions and costs. But these choices have been criticized because in certain cases they may have allowed some builders to be certified even though some of the LEED-approved features used are fairly minimal. However the guidelines are evolving to take these concerns into account.

The LEED–Neighborhood certification was developed in part because the initial LEED building guidelines ignored the context in which a building was sited, allowing for the granting of LEED certification of a building that might have high internal energy efficiency, but one whose occupants had to rely on private automobiles for driving long distances to get to it. Although this may still be an issue for individual buildings, the LEED neighborhood guidelines are an attempt to address these concerns. LEED neighborhood guidelines address street connectivity, access to public transit, storm water impact mitigation, and other items that reflect a wide variety of sustainability and environmental issues. Other items address social justice concerns, including, for example, points for providing affordable housing.

LEED was developed to be a voluntary program, a certification process that was to operate outside of government programs. But in the last decade, a number of jurisdictions have decided to adopt LEED standards as part of their local building codes, in a sense requiring new buildings to qualify for LEED standards, even if they do not formally apply. Other jurisdictions have decided to give bonuses in the form of allowing higher densities or reduced impact fees for buildings that meet LEED certification.

A concern with LEED is that there is no requirement that the long-term upkeep of the features that qualified for LEED certification be maintained. A building could be constructed with high-efficiency lights, for example, but no one goes back to determine if the lighting has been maintained so that the promised energy savings have been delivered.[62] Again, LEED is an evolving proccss.[63]

Xeriscaping

As discussed in Chapter Eight, outdoor water use can represent a significant portion of residential water consumption, particularly in warmer areas with large lots for single-family homes. Thus, modifying the built environment can reduce water use. As aquifers are depleted and other sources of drinking water are overstressed, some communities are adopting ordinances requiring that the use of water for the irrigation of yards be reduced.[64] Sometimes, these ordinances require reductions in the amount of land used for lawns. Other communities require that native plants or other types of vegetation adapted to need less water be used for landscaping. The use of these types of vegetation is known as xeriscaping.[65]

It can be quite jarring for those communities used to lush, green lawns to see front yards planted with native grasses that may turn brown during the summer months, or with cacti and succulents. Therefore, these ordinances should be accompanied by extensive public education.[66] Even voluntary attempts to adopt xeriscaping can sometimes lead to conflicts. Some localities have ordinances prohibiting xeriscaping and requiring lawns, some homeowner associations and condominium associations have regulations mandating lawns; thus, persuading individuals, homeowner associations, and local governments to change their landscaping can be difficult. It is best to consult with local experts to determine what types of vegetation will thrive under local conditions. In general, plants native to an area, or that are native to areas with similar climates, work best.[67]

Global Climate Change and Greenhouse Gases

Given the evidence that the buildup of carbon dioxide in the atmosphere produced by human activity is leading to increasing temperatures around the globe, there is a grave need to address the problems associated with global warming. The association between the built environment and energy use, in building systems and in transportation, has led to a reexamination of the sustainability impacts of communities and individual buildings. The resulting actions are of two types: programs and policies to reduce greenhouse gas emissions, and efforts to mitigate the impacts posed by global climate change.[68]

There are number of ways that global climate change may affect health. Increasing temperatures may result in a greater number of heat-related deaths, increased vulnerability to other extreme weather events, new risks of vector-borne diseases in places that had previously not seen them, amplified vulnerabilities in global food supplies, and higher rates of cancer caused by higher temperatures and greater volatilization of solvents and other chemicals.[69] All these issues point to why those concerned with public health should include global climate change as part of their agenda and why urban planners who are concerned about health should be working to mitigate the impacts of development decisions.[70]

FOCUS ON

Hybrid and Electric Cars

Given what we know about the health effects of cars powered by gasoline, it is no surprise that many people are proposing that we use hybrids and electric cars as alternatives to internal combustion engines. An important issue is whether these cars would, in fact, provide environmental improvements and promote health.

Hybrid cars, those that use electric energy and recapture energy during deceleration and braking, are much more energy efficient than conventional cars. Despite the issues associated with their batteries, they most likely do have a reduced impact on the environment. All-electric vehicles, assuming that they will be powered by electricity generated by power plants, have an impact that is dependent on the source of that electricity. Wind- and solar-generated electricity, to the extent it powers the grid in the area where the car was charged, is certainly more benign. Natural gas and renewable energy produces much of the country's electric power. Even coal-fired plants might be easier to make more environmentally friendly as it is technically easier to clean up a single large source (a power plant) than a multitude of small ones (cars).

But consider that the health impacts of cars are greater than their air pollution contributions. Switching to electric cars would not change land use patterns, contribute to an increase in physical activity, reduce accidents, or help slow the growth of sprawl. Many of the issues outlined in this book would not be affected by changing the power sources of private automobile.

Limiting Greenhouse Gas Emissions

As global temperatures increase, the need to develop programs and policies to reduce the emissions of carbon dioxide, methane, and other greenhouse gases increases as well. Again, sustainability advocates have looked to the built environment for solutions. This has proved to be a challenge. There needs to be action at the international, national, state, and local levels as well as changes by individuals. But each of these has problems. For example, the main vehicle by which international agreements are reached is the treaty. The most famous greenhouse gas treaty was the Kyoto Protocol which the United States never signed. Furthermore, many signatories did not meet their obligations under the protocol. Negotiations for a new treaty have been slow and it is not clear that the United States and other countries will be willing to sign a treaty that will significantly reduce their greenhouse gases at this time.[71]

On the national level, there are limits to what the federal government can do.[72] One of its greatest tools is its ability to set fuel efficiency standards for cars. Given the large contribution of transportation to global warming, this is very important: The U.S. EPA set higher fuel efficiency standards for cars in 2009. But the relationship between fuel efficiency and total emissions is complex and greater fuel efficiency can also lower the cost of driving per mile, potentially increasing overall vehicle miles traveled and blunting the impacts on the environment. The federal government could enact carbon taxes or some sort of charge on oil and coal use, but it is not clear that the United States has the political will for this at this time. It could create a cap-and-trade system similar to that for sulfur emissions from power plants. This system sets up an overall amount of greenhouse gas emissions, allocates these emissions across industries and companies, and allows for the creation of a market through which the permits for these emissions can be traded. The goal is to create an economic incentive for reductions in emissions.[73] But efforts to implement a cap-and-trade system for carbon dioxide have stalled.

One of the greatest drivers of greenhouse gas emissions in the United States results from local land use policies and other factors of the built environment that created the need for automobiles and promoted single-family houses.[74] Together these lead to increased fossil fuel consumption for transportation, heating, and air conditioning. But the federal government has no role in local land-use policies beyond its funding of highways that have made suburban sprawl possible. Traditionally, local land use is the responsibility of states that have delegated this power to county and city governments.[75] Changing land use may well require concerted actions on the part of each of the 50 states in this country that would then have to translate down to changes in land use by thousands of local jurisdictions.

Planning for Global Climate Change

Rising temperatures pose a number of potential problems for the built environment, such as an increase in extreme weather events (floods, hurricanes, and heat waves), and rising sea levels that could potentially overwhelm coastal cities and development.[76] Planning for the infrastructure that can withstand floods and hurricanes is a costly and time-consuming endeavor (see Chapter Six). Creating the political climate to address the impacts of global warming by modifying local infrastructure is going to be difficult as well.[77] Planning for heat waves involves identifying those individuals who are at risk during these events and planning for action in advance of an emergency (see Chapter Six).[78]

Protecting communities from rising sea levels is going to require complex engineering and planning. Many major cities, including New York, Boston, Miami, and of course, New Orleans, are especially vulnerable. Protecting these cities will require expensive and large-scale infrastructure improvements as well as finding the money to pay for these features.[79] Many seaside resort communities are in similar vulnerable positions and the cost of protecting people and property in these areas will be even more difficult to meet.

Individual Efforts

Most of the efforts outlined above are actions that government or coalitions of individuals can take to reduce the environmental impacts of contemporary life. But there are also a number of additional actions that individuals can do to reduce their impacts on the environment.[80] From changing diets, to recycling, to changing where households decide to live, individual decisions can have an important impact on how people affect the environment and consume resources. Providing a social framework that supports such individual efforts may be a role for the built environment. Those actions that promote walking and alternatives to cars, that create and nurture local sources of agriculture, that result in greater energy efficiency for housing and residential construction might make it easier for individuals to reduce their impact on the environment and perhaps contribute to a more sustainable and just future.[81]

Summary

Sustainability, which can have different meanings depending on the context in which it is used, is often defined as the ability of a community to meet the needs of its residents over the long term without harming the environment or other communities. One important consideration in sustainability is equity, or how all people might fare in a sustainable community. There are a number of measures of sustainability, including what is known as an ecological footprint. Many of the features, programs, and policies designed to promote healthier built environments have also been used to promote sustainability. These efforts have been highlighted because of concerns with global climate change.

Key Terms

Ecological footprint

Green roof

Leadership in Energy and Environmental Design (LEED)

Urban heat island

Discussion Questions

1. How would you define sustainability?
2. In what ways might sustainability promote equity? How might it make equity less likely?
3. Define an ecological footprint.
4. Name some of the ways in which local communities might make themselves more sustainable.
5. List some of the benefits of, and problems with, green roofs.
6. What is LEED?
7. Why should public health advocates be concerned about global climate change?

For More Information

Agyeman, J., Bullard, R., Evans, B. (2003). *Just sustainabilities: Development in an unequal world.* Cambridge, MA: MIT Press.

U.S. Green Building Council. www.usgbc.org.

National Research Council. *Adapting to the impacts of climate change.* (2011). Panel on Adapting to the Impacts of Climate Change. Washington, DC: National Academies Press.

Cantor, S. L. (2008). *Green roofs in sustainable landscape design.* New York: Norton.

McMichael. A. J. (2003). *Climate change and human health: Risks and responses.* Geneva: World Health Organization.

Accessibility. In transportation planning, the ability to reach desired destinations including employment, schools, grocery stores, parks, family, and friends, and other reasonable places a person may go as part of day-to-day life.

Anomie. An idea that refers to the psychological disconnect and distress that happens to people who live in cities, particularly those moved there from rural settings. It arises from a combination of the loss of longtime social connections and the need to adjust behavior to meet the challenges posed by interactions with strangers.

Aquifer. The water that is stored in an underground feature as well as the feature itself.

Biological determinism. The idea that underlying biological factors such as genetics, cellular processes, and organ systems are responsible for disease, health, and behaviors.

Biophilia. The theory that human beings have an innate need to be in contact with nature.

Brownfields. Older, often abandoned, buildings and parcels where contamination from past successes or the fear of such contamination may inhibit development.

Built environment. All the human-made features on the planet, generally referring to stationary or fixed items. Also, the total sum of these features.

Collective efficacy. The belief that by working together as a group, people can achieve their aims or protect themselves from threats.

Combined sewer overflow. A situation where sanitary and storm sewers together discharge waste and storm water during periods of heavy rainfall.

Complete streets. The theory that a street should be designed so that it accommodates the needs of all transportation mode users including pedestrians, bicyclists, and public transportation riders as well as people in cars.

Community-based participatory research. A type of research that works to involve communities in research programs, including study design, data analysis, interpretation, and communication of results. This research should be for communities, not simply about them.

Community-supported agriculture. Programs that link consumers to local farmers so that the farmers have a guaranteed income stream and consumers have a guaranteed source of fresh produce.

Concentrated poverty. An area that has high rates of poverty. It also refers to the potential problem that people in these neighborhoods have little contact with those who are not poor.

Congestion charges. A program implemented in London and other cities that charges tolls on cars entering certain zone at certain times in order to reduce traffic or raise funds for transportation improvements.

Conventional development. The predominant pattern of development in the United States after World War II that prioritizes transportation by automobiles, emphasizes single-family homes, prefers large lot zoning, widely separates different land uses, and often features dendritic street designs.

Cost-benefit analysis. A policy tool that seeks to determine whether the overall costs associated with a policy or program are greater than the overall benefits.

Criteria air pollutants. Certain problematic pollutants in outdoor air for which the EPA has established standards of concentration. Criteria air pollutants include carbon monoxide, oxides of nitrogen, sulfur dioxide, ozone, particulates, volatile organic compounds, and lead.

Culture of poverty. The theory that there is an established culture among people who are poor and that poverty is transmitted across generations because of ingrained behaviors that keep impoverished people from improving their economic status.

Cumulative risk. All the environmental and social risks in a community or experienced by individual that collectively create threats to health.

Defensible space. Outdoor and interior areas that are given over to the control of individual persons or units so that they feel responsible for their care and upkeep. The goal is to reduce crime and vandalism.

Demand management. Transportation tools that aim to reduce the number of cars on the road, particularly during times of heavy traffic.

Disproportionate burden. The environmental doctrine that certain people and communities have more than their fair share of environmental problems and fewer amenities.

Ecological footprint. A way of measuring an individual's or community's level of environmental impacts that quantifies all the various impacts using a standard metric, such as barrels of oil or hectares of land.

Environmental determinism. The idea that forces outside the individual, including factors in the social and built environment, influence health and behavior.

Environmental Impact Assessment (EIA). A process, often legally mandated, that sets forth a procedure for collecting and assessing the environmental results of a policy or development decision. Usually these results are restricted to closely parallel existing environmental law.

Environmental justice. This term refers to both the idea that everyone has the right to a healthy environment and the fact that environmental burdens and amenities are more likely to be in some types of communities rather than others, often because of the racial or economic makeup of those at a disadvantage.

Equity. A concept that refers to the equal right of all people to live healthy, fulfilled lives.

Food desert. Refers to the fact that certain places, particularly those in low income urban and rural areas, do not have any way for the residents in these communities to put together a healthy meal. They may lack supermarkets and other sources of produce and nutritious food.

Food insecurity. The situation in which households cannot always afford to buy food for all the members in the household. The problem may be long-term, periodic, or occasional.

Food miles. A metric designed to identify how far food travels from source to consumer.

Form-based codes. Building codes that aim to shape development by emphasizing desired results rather than by prescribing detailed parameters for each type of development.

Garden cities. First proposed by Ebenezer Howard and associates, these were planned suburban developments that focused on providing healthy housing, jobs, and access to other parts of the metropolitan area.

Gentrification. A process by which higher-income and often nonminority households displace residents who are more likely to have low incomes and/or be of a minority race or ethnicity.

Geographic information systems (GIS). A computer-based type of software program that combines data with geographic information and allows for the simultaneous connection, display, and analysis of these two types of data.

Graywater. Water that is the result of recycled or reused processes.

Green roof. A building feature that usually includes plantings or other environmentally benign attributes designed to reduce runoff or absorption and re-radiation of solar heat.

Greenbelts. Areas around a neighborhood, city, or metropolitan area that are purposely left undeveloped or used only as parks, open space, agriculture, and similar types of non-built-up activities. They aim to create a boundary around a city and reduce sprawl.

Health. More than just the absence of disease, health refers to the ability of an individual to live as well as he or she can across his or her life span.

Health beliefs. The ideas that an individual or community may hold about health or what causes good or poor health (for example, the belief that smoking will cause cancer).

Health impact assessment (HIA). A usually voluntary process that allows for a community or policymakers to systematically collect information on and assess the potential health, social, and other impacts of a project, program, or policy.

Integrated pest management (IPM). An alternative to heavily using pesticides, IPM seeks to involve residents and building managers in preventing pest infestations, using pesticides as only a last resort, and using safer pesticide application processes if necessary.

Intermodal Surface Transportation Efficiency Act (ISTEA). Passed in 1991, this federal law changed transportation planning and funding so that alternatives to cars, including bike trails, pedestrian infrastructure, and other features, were allowed and encouraged.

Leadership in Energy and Environmental Design (LEED). A program of the Green Building Council, LEED aims to produce more environmentally friendly building and neighborhood designs by promoting voluntary compliance by developers and others.

Liquefaction. The problem that occurs during earthquakes when certain soils become saturated by ground movement and lose their ability to support infrastructure and buildings above them.

Locavorism. The idea that food is best produced and consumed locally.

Miasma theory. The belief that bad smells and noxious odors cause disease.

Mobility. The transportation concept that stresses the need for travel itself rather than the goals that produced that trip.

Model tenement movement. A nineteenth-century progressive movement that thought that by creating special apartment buildings, it could demonstrate that developers could make a profit on providing quality housing for the poor and that the poor could have their health improved by living in these units.

Modernism. A twentieth-century design and architecture movement that sought to connect health and social goals to building and product design. Its architectural style emphasized access to sunlight and ventilation and strongly discouraged ornamentation.

Multilevel modeling. A set of statistical methods that recognizes that because standard analysis relies on subjects being independent from each other, other means of analyzing groups of subjects are necessary. The classic example would be a study of education policy that considers students grouped in classrooms, grouped in schools.

New urbanism. A late-twentieth-century architecture and planning movement that sought to reject conventional development and emphasize traditional small-town and urban neighborhood idioms. It often features small streets, prioritizes pedestrian movement, and encourages mixed uses.

Nonpoint pollution sources. Small-scale pollution sources that include septic systems, individual households, or other hard-to-identify and individually potentially benign sources of pollution that collectively can have important effects on water or air quality.

Ozonation. A water treatment process that involves introducing ozone into water to kill microorganisms.

Physical environment. The traditional chemical and biological agents that affect health, including water and air pollutants, radiation hazards, and other similar factors and features.

Planned unit development. A type of development that allows for a project to be considered as a whole rather than having each component of the project subject to the code as if it were independently built. This can lead to clustering of open space, semidetached homes, or other features that conventional zoning does not allow.

Race. An often-changing social construct that identifies an individual as a member of a particular group.

Rural health advantage. The idea, reflective of health conditions for much of the nineteenth century, that people in rural areas living longer and were less likely to suffer from diseases. This advantage disappeared in most developed countries by the mid-twentieth century.

Self-efficacy. The belief an individual has that he or she can protect or maintain his or her health or reach identified personal goals.

Shrinking city movement. An international phenomena that recognizes that the decline of certain urban areas is inevitable and that planning should be undertaken to meet the physical, social, and built environmental consequences of population loss and economic decline.

Sick building syndrome. A collection of illnesses that may affect the inhabitants and users of a building in varying degrees that may include respiratory, immune, or other symptoms. The illnesses are thought to be caused by contaminants in indoor air.

Smart growth. A set of planning goals that emphasize inner-city development, brownfields' reuse, transit, increasing density rather than peripheral, conventional development.

Social capital. The degree to which members of a group know, trust, and can rely on each other.

Social environment. Factors such as income, race, gender roles, customs, and so forth that provide the context in which human beings live.

Social norms. Formal and informal ways of acting that provide guidance for behavior.

Spatial mismatch. The problem that although much of the job growth in the past fifty years in the United States has been in peripheral areas far from the inner city, low-income areas in the city have the highest unemployment.

Storm surge. The degree to which a hurricane creates a bulge of high water that can inundate low-lying coastal areas or tributaries.

Sustainability. The ability of an area or society to support itself without compromising current or future environments.

Traffic calming. A set of design features that are intended to force or encourage cars to slow down and recognize the rights and needs of pedestrians and bicyclists.

Transit-oriented development. Development that tries to encourage higher intensity of uses around transit facilities by promoting walking, permitting higher densities, and so on.

Urban heat island. The situation that develops from buildings and paved areas being more likely to absorb heat than undeveloped land or open water. This results in higher temperatures in urban cores.

Urban sprawl. An overall metropolitan or neighborhood form that is dispersed, car centered, low density, and often highly focused on peripheries.

Weathering. The health concept that certain people, because of their past experience, diseases, or health risks, age and become more vulnerable to illness sooner than others.

Xeriscaping. Landscaping that uses native vegetation or other plantings that require less water or are adapted to arid climates.

Zoning. A legal process that assigns properties specific classifications, each with its own set of allowable land uses, permissible densities, required setbacks, parking requirements, and so forth.

REFERENCES

Preface

1. Botchwey, N., Hobson, S., Dannenberg, A., et al. (2009). A Model Curriculum for a Course on the Built Environment and Public Health: Training for an Interdisciplinary Workforce. *American Journal of Preventive Medicine*, *36*, pp. S63–S71.

Chapter One

1. Levinson, D., & Gillen, D. (1998). The full cost of intercity highway transportation. *Transportation Research Part D: Transport and Environment*, *3*, pp. 207–223.
2. Fox, D. M., Jackson. R. J., & Barondess, J. A. (2003). Health and the built environment. *Journal of Urban Health*, *80*, pp. 534–535.
3. Dannenberg, A., Jackson, R., Frumkin, H., et al. (2003). The impact of community design and land-use choices on public health: A scientific research agenda. *American Journal of Public Health*, *93*, pp. 1500–1508.
   Frumkin, H. (2002). Urban sprawl and public health. *Public Health Reports*, *117*, pp. 201–217.
4. Folkman, J., Hahnfeldt, P., & Hlatky, L. (2000). Cancer: Looking outside the genome. *Nature Reviews Molecular Cell Biology*, *1*, pp. 76–79.
5. Welman, B., & Wortley, S. (1990). Different strokes from different folks: Community ties and social support. *American Journal of Sociology*, *96*, pp. 558–588.
6. Lipfert, F. (1994). *Air pollution and community health: A critical review and data sourcebook*. New York: Van Nostrand Reinhold.
   Downey, L., & Van Willigen, M. (2005). Environmental stressors: The mental health impacts of living near industrial activity. *Journal of Health and Social Behavior*, *46*, pp. 289–305.
7. Smedley, A. (2005). Race as biology is fiction, racism as a social problem is real. *American Psychologist*, *60*, pp. 16–26.
   Ford, C. L., & Harawa, N. T. (2010). A new conceptualization of ethnicity for social epidemiologic and health equity research. *Social Science and Medicine*, *71*, pp. 251–258.
8. Alexander, G. R., Wingate, M. S., Bader, D., & Kogan, M., D. (2008). The increasing racial disparity in infant mortality rates: Composition and contributors to recent U.S. trends. *American Journal of Obstetrics & Gynecology*, *198*, pp. e1–e9.
   Williams, H., & Powell, I. J. (2009). Epidemiology, pathology, and genetics of prostate cancer among African Americans compared with other ethnicities. *Methods in Molecular Biology*, *472*, pp. 439–453.

9. Carlson, S. A., Brooks, J. D., Brown, D. R., & Buchner, D. M. (2010). Racial/ethnic differences in perceived access, environmental barriers to use, and use of community parks. *Prevention of Chronic Disease*, *7*, p. A49.

10. Massey, D. (2004). Segregation and stratification: A biosocial perspective. *Du Bois Review*, *1*, pp. 1–19.

11. Massey, D. Segregation and stratification.
Massey, D., & Denton, N. (1993). *American apartheid: Segregation and the making of the underclass*. Cambridge, MA: Harvard University Press.

12. Li, F., Harmer, P., Cardinal, B. J., Bosworth, M., & Johnson-Shelton, D. (2009). Obesity and the built environment: Does the density of neighborhood fast-food outlets matter? *American Journal of Health Promotion*, *23*, pp. 203–209.
Lee, I. M., Ewing, R., & Sesso, H. D. (2009). The built environment and physical activity levels: The Harvard Alumni Health Study. *American Journal of Preventive Medicine*, *37*, pp. 293–298.
Booth, K. M., Pinkston, M. M., & Poston, W. S. (2005). Obesity and the built environment. *Journal of the American Dietetic Association*, *105*, pp. S110–S117.

13. Lannero, E., Wickman, M., van Hage, M., Bergstrom, A., Pershagen, G., & Nordvall, L. (2008). Exposure to environmental tobacco smoke and sensitisation in children. *Thorax*, *63*, pp. 172–176.

14. Aquilina, N. J., Delgado-Saborit, J. M., Gauci, A. P., Baker, S., Meddings, C., & Harrison, R. M. (2010). Comparative modeling approaches for personal exposure to particle-associated PAH. *Environmental Science and Technology*, *44*, pp. 9370–9376.

15. Bhata, C. R., & Guo, J. Y. (2007). Modeling residential sorting effects to understand the impact of the built environment on commute mode choice. *Transportation Research Part B: Methodological*, *41*, pp. 506–526.
X Cao, S. H. (2006). The influences of the built environment and residential self-selection on pedestrian behavior: Evidence from Austin, TX. *Transportation*, *33*, pp. 1–20.

16. Cohen, D., Spear, S., Scribner, R., Kissinger, P., Mason, K., & Wildgen, J. (2000). "Broken windows" and the risk of gonorrhea. *American Journal of Public Health*, *90*, pp. 230–236.

17. Vitruvius, P. (1999). *Ten books on architecture*. New York: Cambridge University Press.

18. Corburn, J. (2004). Confronting the challenges in reconnecting urban planning and public health. *American Journal of Public Health*, *94*, pp. 541–546.

19. O'Toole, R. (2002). Special interests run with faulty obesity data. *Cascade Commentary*, *2002, 9*, p. 1.
Frumkin, H. (2003). Healthy places: Exploring the evidence. *American Journal of Public Health*, *93*, pp. 1451–1456.

20. Vlahov, D., Gibble, E., Freudenberg, N., & Galea, S. (2004). Cities and health: History, approaches, and key questions. *Academic Medicine*, *79*, pp. 1133–1138.

21. Vlahov, D., Galea, S., & Freudenberg, N. (2005). The urban health "advantage." *Journal of Urban Health*, *82*, pp. 1–4.

22. Corburn, J. (2004). Confronting the challenges in reconnecting urban planning and public health. *American Journal of Public Health*, *94*, pp. 541–546.

23. Leibold, M. A., Holyoak, M., Mouquet, N., et al. (2004). The metacommunity concept: A framework for multi-scale community ecology. *Ecological Letters*, *7*, pp. 601–613.

24. McHarg, I. (1969). *Design with nature*. Hoboken, NJ: Wiley.

25. Wright, F. L. (1938). Broadacre City: A new community plan. *The Architectural Record*, pp. 243–255.

26. Kawachi, I., Kennedy, B. P., & Glass, R. (1999). Social capital and self-rated health: A contextual analysis. *American Journal of Public Health*, *89*, pp. 1187–1193.

27. WHO. (1946). *Preamble to the Constitution of the World Health Organization*. Official Records of the World Health Organization, no. *2*, p. 100. Geneva: World Health Organization.

28. Kunstler, J. H., & Salngaros, N. (2007). The end of tall buildings. In A. Chavan, C. Peralta, C. Steins (Eds.), *Planetizen's contemporary debates in urban planning*. Washington D.C.: Island Press.

29. Agyeman, J., & Evans, T. (2003). Toward just sustainability in urban communities: Building equity rights with sustainable solutions. *Annals of the American Academy of Political and Social Science, 590*, pp. 35–53.
   Bassett, M. T. (2000). The pursuit of equity in health: Reflections on race and public health data in Southern Africa. *American Journal of Public Health, 90*, pp. 1690–1693.
   Zimmerman, R. (1993). Social equity and environmental risk. *Risk Analysis, 13*, pp. 649–666.

30. Verbruggen, A. (2008). Renewable and nuclear power: A common future? *Energy Policy, 36*, pp. 4036–4047.

31. Marcuse, P. (1998). Sustainability is not enough. *Environment and Urbanization, 10*, pp. 103–112.

32. Lefebvre, H. (1974). *The production of space*. Oxford: Editions Anthropos.

33. Botchwey, N. D., Hobson, S. E., Dannenberg, A. L., et al. (2009). A model curriculum for a course on the built environment and public health: Training for an interdisciplinary workforce. *American Journal of Preventive Medicine, 36*, pp. S63–S71.

Chapter Two

1. Vitruvius, P. (1999). *Ten books on architecture*. New York: Cambridge University Press.

2. Mumford, L. (1961). *The city in history: Its origins, its transformations, and its prospects* New York: Harcourt, Brace & World.

3. Melosi, M. (2008). *The sanitary city: Environmental services in urban America from colonial times to the present*. Pittsburgh, PA: University of Pittsburgh Press.

4. Melosi, M. (2005). *Garbage in the city*. Pittsburgh, PA: University of Pittsburgh Press.

5. Rosen, G. (1993). *A history of public health*. Baltimore, MD: Johns Hopkins University Press.

6. Rasmussen, S. E. (1951). *Towns and buildings*. Cambridge, MA: MIT Press.

7. Hayden, D. (2003). *Building suburbia: Green fields and urban growth, 1820–2000*. New York: Vintage Books.

8. Stanislawski, D. (1946). The origin and spread of the grid-pattern town. *Geographical Review, 36*, pp. 105–120.

9. Hebbert, M. (1999). A city in good shape: Town planning and public health. *The Town Planning Review, 70*, p. 450.

10. Hall, P. (1988). *Cities of tomorrow: An intellectual history of urban planning and design in the twentieth century*. Malden MA: Blackwell.

11. Tarr, J. (1985). Industrial wastes and public health: Some historical notes, Part 1, 1876–1912. *American Journal of Public Health, 75*, pp. 1059–1067.
   Tarr, J. (1996). *The search for the ultimate sink: Urban pollution in historical perspective*. Akron, OH: University of Akron Press.

12. Rosen, G. (1993). *A history of public health*.

13. Mumford, L. (1961). *The city in history*.

14. Tarr, J. (1996). *The search for the ultimate sink*.

15. Boyer, M. C. (1986). *Dreaming the rational city: The myth of American city planning*. Cambridge, MA: MIT Press.

16. Mumford, L. (1961). *The city in history*.

17. Rasmussen, S., E. (1951). *Towns and buildings*.
    Tarr, J. (1996). *The search for the ultimate sink*.

18. Marx, K. (2004). *Wage labour and capital*. London: Kessinger.

19. Szreter, S. (1988). The importance of social intervention in Britain's mortality decline 1850–1914: A reinterpretation of the role of public health. *Social History of Medicine 1*, pp. 1–38.
    Szreter S. (1997). Economic growth, disruption, disease, and death: On the importance of the politics of public health for development. *Population and Development Review, 23*, pp. 693–728.

20. Goldin, C. (1993). The political economy of immigration restriction in the United States, 1890 to 1921. *National Bureau of Economic Research, Report No.: W4345*.

21. Ibid.

22. Gomez, J. E., Johnson, B. A., Selva, M., & Sallis, J. F. (2004). Violent crime and outdoor physical activity among inner-city youth. *Preventive Medicine, 39*, pp. 876–881.

23. Melosi, M. (2001). *Effluent America: Cities, industry, energy, and the environment*. Pittsburgh, PA: University of Pittsburgh Press.

24. Barnes, D. (2006). *The great stink of Paris and the nineteenth-century struggle against filth and germs*. Baltimore, MD: The Johns Hopkins University Press.

25. Mearns, A. (1866). *The bitter cry of outcast London*. Boston: Cupplers, Upham.

26. Rosenberg, C. (1959). The cholera epidemic of 1832 in New York City. *Bulletin of the History of Medicine, 33*, pp. 37–49.

27. Rosenburg, C. (1987). *The cholera years: The United States in 1832, 1849, and 1866*. Chicago: University of Chicago Press.

28. Dubos, R., & Dubos, J. (1952). *The white plague: Tuberculosis, man and society*. New Brunswick, NJ: Rutgers University Press.

29. Ibid.

30. McKeown, T., & Record, R. (1962). Reasons for the decline of mortality in England and Wales during the nineteenth century. *Population Studies, 16*, pp. 94–122.

31. Szreter, S. (1988). The importance of social intervention in Britain's mortality decline 1850–1914.
    Szreter, S., & Mooney, G. (1998). *Urbanization, mortality, and the standard of living debate: New estimates of the expectation of life at birth in nineteenth century British cities*. Economic History Review, *51*, pp. 84–92.

32. Tesh, S. (1995). Miasma and "social factors" in disease causality: Lessons from the nineteenth century. *Journal of Health Politics, Policy, and Law, 20*, pp. 1001–1024.

33. Chadwick, E., & Flinn, M. W. (1965). *Report on the sanitary condition of the labouring population of Great Britain*. Edinburgh: Edinburgh University Press.

34. Southwood Smith, T. (1830). *A treatise on fever*. London: Longman, Rees, Orme, Brown, Green.

35. Shattuck, L. (1850). *Report of the Sanitary Commission of Massachusetts*. Boston: Dutton and Wentworth, State Printers.

36. Riis, J. (1890). *How the other half lives*. New York: Scribner.

37. Carmona, M. (2002). *Haussmann: His life and times, and the making of modern Paris*. Chicago: Ivan R. Dee.

38. Fisher, I., D. (1986). *Frederick Law Olmsted and the city planning movement in the United States*. Ann Arbor: University of Michigan Press.

    Olmsted, F. L. (1970). *Public parks and the enlargement of towns*. New York: Arno Press.

39. Tarr, J. (1984). *The evolution of urban infrastructure in the nineteenth and twentieth centuries*. In R. Hanson (Ed.), *Perspectives on urban infrastructure*. Washington, D.C.: National Academies Press.

40. Ibid.

    Tarr, J. (1989). Infrastructure and city-building in the nineteenth and twentieth century. In S. Hayes (Ed.), *City at the point: Essays in the social history of Pittsburgh*. Pittsburgh, PA: University of Pittsburgh Press.

41. Hall, *Cities of tomorrow*.

    Boyer, *Dreaming the rational city*.

42. Szreter, Economic growth, disruption, disease, and death.

43. Lubove, R. (1961). *Lawrence Veiller and the New York State Tenement House Commission of 1900*. *The Mississippi Valley Historical Review, 47*, pp. 659–677.

44. Howard, E. (1965). Garden cities of to-morrow. Cambridge, MA: MIT Press.

45. Fishman, R. (1982). *Urban utopias in the twentieth century: Ebenezer Howard, Frank Lloyd Wright, Le Corbusier*. Cambridge, MA: MIT Press.

46. Unwin, R. (1920). *Town planning in practice: An introduction to the art of designing cities and suburbs*. Princeton: Princeton University Press.

47. Perry, C. (1929). City planning for neighborhood life. *Social Forces, 8*, pp. 98–100.

48. Lubove, R. (1962). *The progressives and the slums: Tenement house reform in New York City, 1890–1917*. Westport, CT: Greenwood Press.

49. Blackmar, E. (1995). Accountability for public health: Regulating the housing market in nineteenth-century New York City. In D. Rosner (Ed.), *Hives of sickness*. New Brunswick, NJ: Rutgers University Press.

50. Day, J. (1999). *Urban castles: Tenement housing and landlord activism in New York City, 1890–1943*. New York: Columbia University Press.

51. Veiller, L. (1910). *Housing reform: A hand-book for practical use in American cities*. New York: Russell Sage Foundation Charities Publication Committee.

    Veiller, L. (1914). *A model housing law*. New York: Russell Sage Foundation.

52. Dubos, R., & Dubos, J. (1952). *The white plague:*

53. New York Times. (1922 June 25). The zoning law and its benefits. *New York Times, Sect. RE1*.

54. Bassett, E. (1936). *Zoning*. New York: Russell Sage Foundation.

    Schilling, J., & Linton, L. (2005). The public health roots of zoning: In search of active living's legal genealogy. *American Journal of Preventive Medicine, 28*, 96–104.

55. Silver, C. (1997). The racial origins of zoning in American cities. In J. Manning-Thomas and M. Ritzdorf (Eds.), *Urban planning and the African American community in the shadows*. Thousand Oaks, CA: Sage.

56. Wolf, M. A. (2008). *The zoning of America: Euclid, V. Ambler*. Lawrence: University Press of Kansas.

57. DuBois, W. E., B. (1899). *The Philadelphia negro*. Philadelphia: University of Pennsylvania Press.

58. Boyer, M., C. (1986). *Dreaming the rational city*.

59. Massey, D., & Denton, N. (1993). *American apartheid: Segregation and the making of the underclass*. Cambridge, MA: Harvard University Press.

60. Polednak, A. (1996). Segregation, discrimination and mortality in U.S. blacks. *Ethnicity and Disease, 6*, pp. 99–107.
    Polednak, A. (1997). *Segregation, poverty, and mortality in urban African Americans*. New York: Oxford University Press.
61. Huxtable, A. L. (2004). *Frank Lloyd Wright*. New York: Viking Penguin.
62. Scully, V. (1960). *Frank Lloyd Wright*. New York: Braziller.
63. Wright, F. L. 1938. *Broadacre City: A new community plan*. The Architectural Record, 243–255.
64. Doremus, T. (1992). *Frank Lloyd Wright and Le Corbusier*. New York: Van Nostrand Reinhold.
65. Wilk, C. (2006). The healthy body culture. In C. Wilk (Ed.), *Modernism: Designing a new world 1914–1919*. London: V&A.
66. Hitchcock, H.-R., & Johnson, P. (1935). *The international style*. New York: Norton.
67. Benton, T. (2006). Building utopia. In C. Wilk (Ed.), *Modernism: Designing a new world 1914–1919*. London: V&A.
68. Hall, P. (1988). *Cities of tomorrow*.
69. LeCorbusier. (1929). *The city of to-morrow*. Cambridge. MA: MIT Press.
70. Venturi, R. (1966). *Complexity and contradiction in architecture*. New York: Museum of Modern Art Press.
71. Le Corbusier. (1923). *Towards a new architecture*. New York: Dover.
    Le Corbusier. (1929). *The city of to-morrow*. Cambridge, MA: MIT Press.
72. Fishman, R. (1982). *Urban utopias in the twentieth century:*
73. Corburn, J. (2004). Confronting the challenges in reconnecting urban planning and public health. *American Journal of Public Health, 94*, pp. 541–6.
74. Wood, E. E. (1919). *The housing of the unskilled wage earner*. New York: Macmillan.
75. Bauer, C. (1934). *Modern housing*. Boston: Houghton Mifflin.
76. Bristol, K. (1991). The Pruitt-Igoe myth. *The Journal of Architectural Education, 44*, pp. 163–71.
77. Neuman, M. (2010). City planning and infrastructure: Once and future partners. *Journal of Urban History, 9*, pp. 42.
78. Goodman, R. (1972). *After the planners*. New York: Simon & Schuster.
79. APHA. (1938). Committee on the Hygiene of Housing. *American Journal of Public Health, 28*, pp. 351–372.
    Senn, C. (1951). Hygiene of housing: Contribution of the American Public Housing Association to housing evaluation. *American Journal of Public Health, 41*, pp. 511–515
    Winslow, C.-E. (1947). Health goals for housing. *American Journal of Public Health, 37*, pp. 653–662.
80. Kaplan, H. (1966). Urban renewal in Newark. In J. Q. Wilson (Ed.), *Urban renewal: The record and the controversy*. Cambridge, MA: MIT Press.
81. Lopez, R. (2009). Public health, the APHA, and urban renewal. *American Journal of Public Health, 99*, pp. 1603–1611.
82. Baum-Snow, N. (2007). Did highways cause suburbanization? *Quarterly Journal of Economics, 122*, pp. 775–807.
83. Zipp, S. (2010). *Manhattan projects: The rise and fall of urban renewal in cold war New York*. New York: Oxford University Press.
84. Jacobs, J. (1961). *The death and life of great american cities*. New York: Vintage Books.
    Manshel, A. (2010 June 29). Enough with Jane Jacobs already. *The Wall Street Journal*, Sect. D8.

Chapter Three

1. McDonald, J. (2008). *Urban America: Growth, crisis, and rebirth*. Armonk, NY: M. E. Sharpe.

2. Danziger, S. (2008). *Working and poor: How economic and policy changes are affecting low-wage workers*. New York: Russell Sage Foundation.

3. Grant-Meyer, S. (2000). *As long as they don't move next door. Segregation and racial conflict in American neighborhoods*. Lanham, MD: Rowman & Littlefield.

4. Massey, D. (2010). *New faces in new places: The changing geography of American immigration*. New York: Russell Sage Foundation.

5. Frey, W. H., Liaw, K.-L., Wright, R., & White, M. J. (2005). Migration within the United States: Role of race-ethnicity. *Brookings-Wharton Papers on Urban Affairs*, pp. 207–262.

6. Smith, N. (1996). *The new urban frontier: Gentrification and the revanchist city*. New York: Routledge.

7. Chevan, A., & Stokes, R. (2000). Growth in family income inequality, 1970–1990: Industrial restructuring and demographic change. *Demography*, *37*, pp. 365–380.
   Denton, N. (1999). Half empty or half full: Segregation and segregated neighborhoods 30 years after the Fair Housing Act. *Cityscape*, *4*, pp. 107–122.

8. Sugrue, T. (1996). *The origins of the urban crisis: Race and inequality in postwar Detroit*. Princeton, NJ: Princeton University Press.

9. Wallace, R. (1988). A synergism of plagues: Planned shrinkage, contagious housing destruction and AIDS in the Bronx. *Environmental Research*, *47*, pp. 1–33.

10. Smith, *The New Urban Frontier*.

11. Dalbey, M. (2008). Implementing smart growth strategies in rural America: Development patterns that support public health goals. *Journal of Public Health Management and Practice*, *14*, pp. 238–243.

12. Bruegmann, R. (2005). *Sprawl: A compact history*. Chicago: University of Chicago Press.

13. Hayden, D. *Building suburbia: Green fields and urban growth, 1820–2000*. New York: Vintage Books. (2003).

14. Jackson, K. (1985). *Crabgrass frontier: The suburbanization of the United States*. New York: Oxford University Press.

15. Frumkin, H. (2003). Healthy places: Exploring the evidence. *American Journal of Public Health*, *93*, pp. 1451–1456.

16. Kunstler, J. (1993). *The geography of nowhere: The rise and decline of America's man-made landscape*. New York: Simon & Schuster.

17. Kay, J. H. (1998). *Asphalt nation: How the automobile took over America, and how we can take it back*. Berkeley: University of California Press.

18. Duany, A., Plater-Zyberk, E., & Speck, J. (2000). *Suburban nation*. New York: North Point Press.

19. Dannenberg, A. L., Jackson, R. J., Frumkin, H., et al. (2003). The impact of community design and land-use choices on public health: A scientific research agenda. *American Journal of Public Health*, *93*, pp. 1500–1508.

20. Loukaitou-Sideris, A. (1997). Inner-city commercial strips: Evolution, decay, retrofit? *The Town Planning Review*, *48*, pp. 1–29.

21. Gordon, P., Richardson, H. (2001). The sprawl debate: Let markets decide. *Publius*, *31*, pp. 131–149.

22. Bruegmann, *Sprawl*.

23. Dannenberg, A., Jackson, R., Frumkin, H., et al. (2003). The impact of community design and land-use choices on public health: A scientific research agenda. *American Journal of Public Health, 93*, pp. 1500–1508.

24. Frumkin, H., Frank, L., & Jackson, R. (2004). *Urban sprawl and public health: Designing, planning and building for healthy communities*. Washington, D.C.: Island Press.

25. Sugrue, T. *The origins of the urban crisis.*

26. Duany, et al. *Suburban nation.*

27. Gutfreund, O. (2004). *20th-Century sprawl: Highways and the reshaping of the American landscape.* New York: Oxford University Press.

28. Kay, *Asphalt nation.*

29. Ellis, C. (2002). Interstate highways, regional planning and the reshaping of metropolitan America. *Planning Practice and Research, 16*, pp. 247–269.

30. Hott, L., & Lewis, T. (1997). *Divided highways: The interstates and the transformation of American life.* A Hott Production of Florentine Films by Lawrence R. Hott and Tom Lewis. Edited by Diane Garey. A Coproduction of WETA-TV, Washington, D.C.

31. Jackson, *Crabgrass frontier.*

32. Hayden, *Building suburbia.*

33. Frumkin, *Healthy places.*

34. Frank, L., Sallis, J., Conway, T., Chapman, J., Saelens, B., & Bachman, W. (2006). Many pathways from land use to health. *Journal of the American Planning Association, 72*, pp. 75–87.

35. Hayden, *Building suburbia.*

36. McHarg, I. (1969). *Design with nature.* Hoboken, NJ: Wiley.

37. Hayden, *Building suburbia.*

38. Jordon, S., Ross, J., Usowski, K. (1998). U.S. suburbanization in the 1980s. *Regional Science and Urban Economics, 28*, pp. 611–627.

39. Jackson, *Crabgrass frontier.*

40. Sugrue, *The origins of the urban crisis.*

41. Heim, C. (2001). Leapfrogging, urban sprawl, and growth management. Phoenix, 1950–2000. *American Journal of Economics and Sociology, 60*, pp. 245–283.

42. Wheeler, S. (2008). The evolution of built landscapes in metropolitan regions. *Journal of Planning Education and Research, 27*, pp. 400–416.

43. Vlahov, D., Galea, S., & Freudenberg, N. (2005). The urban health "advantage." *Journal of Urban Health, 82*, pp. 1 4.

44. De Ville, K. A., & Sparrow, S. E. (2008). Zoning, urban planning, and the public health practitioner. *Journal of Public Health Management and Practice, 14*, pp. 313–316.

45. Duany et al., *Suburban nation.*

46. Frank, L., Engelke, P., & Schmid, T. (2003). *Health and community design: The impact of the built environment on physical activity.* Washington, D.C.: Island Press.

47. Kay, *Asphalt nation.*

48. Glazer, N. History's angel. (2007). In T. Mennel, J. Steffens, C. Klemek (Eds.), *Block by block: Jane Jacobs and the future of New York.* Princeton: Princeton Architectural Press.

49. Schwartz, J. (1993). *The New York approach: Robert Moses, urban liberals and the redevelopment of the inner city.* Columbus: Ohio State University Press.

50. Jacobs, J. (1961). *The death and life of great American cities.* New York: Vintage Books.

51. Flint, A. (2009). *Wrestling with Moses: How Jane Jacobs took on New York's master builder and transformed the American city.* New York: Random House.

52. Gopnik, A. (2007). Gothamitis. In T. Mennel, J. Steffens, C. Klemek (Eds.), *Block by Block: Jane Jacobs and the future of New York*. Princeton: Princeton Architectural Press.
    Manshel, A. (2010 June 29). Enough with Jane Jacobs already. *The Wall Street Journal*, Sect. D8.

53. Jacobs, *The death and life of great American cities*.

54. Kramer, J. (1962 December 20). All the ranks and rungs of Mrs. Jacobs' ladder. *The Village Voice*, Sect. 3, 34.
    Mumford, L. (1962 December 1). Mother Jacobs' home remedies. *The New Yorker*, pp. 148–79.

55. Hubbard, T. K., & Hubbard, H. V. (1929). *Our cities to-day and to-morrow: A survey of planning and zoning progress in the United States*. Cambridge, MA: Harvard University Press.

56. Bassett, E. (1936). *Zoning*. New York: Russell Sage Foundation.

57. Jacobs, *The death and life of great American cities*.

58. Weaver, C., & Babcock, R. (1979). *City zoning, the once and future frontier*. Chicago: Planners Press.

59. Katz, P. (1994). *The new urbanism: Toward an architecture of community*. New York: McGraw-Hill.

60. Duany, et al., *Suburban nation*.

61. Frank, L., & Engelke, P. (2001). The built environment and human activity patterns: Exploring the impacts of urban form on public health. *Journal of Planning Literature*, *16*, pp. 202–218.

62. Krasnowiecki, J. (1965). Planned unit development: A challenge to established theory and practice of land use control. *University of Pennsylvania Law Review*, *114*, pp. 47–97.

63. Cullingworth, J., & Caves, R. (2008). *Planning in the U.S.A: Policies, issues, and processes*. New York: Routledge.

64. Peise, R. (1989). Density and urban sprawl. *Land Economics*, *65*, pp. 193–204.

65. Duany, et al., *Suburban nation*.

66. Katz, *The new urbanism*.

67. Talen, E. (2005). *New urbanism and American planning: The conflict of cultures*. New York: Routledge.

68. Moule, E., & Polyzoides, S. (1994). The streets, the block and the building. In P. Katz (Ed.), *The new urbanism: Toward an architecture of community*. New York: McGraw-Hill.

69. Mumford, E. (2000). *The CIAM discourse on urbanism, 1928–1960*. Cambridge, MA: MIT Press.

70. CNU. (1996). *Charter of the new urbanism*. http://www.cnu.org/charter.

71. Duany, A., Sorlien, S., & Wright, W. (2008). *SmartCode v9.0*.

72. Rupasingha, A., Goetz, S., & Freshwater, D. (2006). The production of social capital in U.S. counties. *Journal of Socio-Economics*, *35*, pp. 83–101.

73. Cox, W. (2001). *American dream boundaries: Urban containment and its consequences*. Atlanta: Georgia Public Policy Foundation.

74. O'Toole, *The folly of smart-growth*.

75. Ellis, C. (2002). The new urbanism: Critiques and rebuttals. *Journal of Urban Design*, *7*, pp. 261–291.

76. Scully, V. (1994). The architecture of community. In P. Katz (Ed.), *The new urbanism: Toward an architecture of community*. New York: McGraw-Hill.

77. Parolek, D. G., Parolek, K., & Crawford, P., C. (2008). *Form-based codes: A guide for planners, urban designers, municipalities, and developers*. Hoboken, NJ: Wiley.

78. Burdette, J. (2004). *Form-based codes: A cure for the cancer called Euclidean Zoning?* Burlington: University of Vermont.

79. Flegal, K., Carroll, M., Kuczmarski, R., & Johnson, C. (1998). Overweight and obesity in the United States: Prevalence and trends, 1960–1994. *International Journal of Obesity and Related Metabolic Disorders, 22*, pp. 39–47.

80. Ewing, R., Pendall, R., & Chen, D. (2002). *Measuring sprawl and its impact*. Washington, D.C.: Smart Growth America.

81. Lopez, R., & Hynes, H. P. (2003). Sprawl in the 1990s: Measurement, distribution and trends. Urban Affairs Review, *38*, pp. 325–355.

82. Hox, J. (2002). *Multilevel analysis: Techniques and applications*. Mahwah, NJ: Erlbaum.

83. *BRFSS — Frequently asked questions*. (2003). Accessed March 20, 2003, at http://cdc.gov/brfss/faqs.htm#3.

84. *Calculated variables of the 2001 Behavioral Risk Factor Surveillance System Data File*. 2001. Accessed November 2003, 2003, at http://www.cdc.gov/brfss/technical_infodata/surveydata/2001/riskfactor_01.rtf.

85. O'Toole, R. (2002). Special interests run with faulty obesity data. *Cascade Commentary, 2002*, p. 1.

86. Ewing, R., Schmid, T., Killingsworth, R., Zlot, A., & Raudenbush, S. (2003). Relationship between urban sprawl and physical activity, obesity, and morbidity. *American Journal of Health Promotion, 18*, pp. 47–57.
Lopez, R. (2004). Urban sprawl and risk for being overweight or obese. *American Journal of Public Health, 94*, pp. 1574–1579.
Trowbridge, M. J., Gurka, M. J., & O'Connor, R. E. (2009). Urban sprawl and delayed ambulance arrival in the U.S. *American Journal of Preventive Medicine, 37*, pp. 428–432.

87. Lopez, *Urban sprawl and risk for being overweight or obese*.

88. Ewing, R., Brownson, R. C., & Berrigan, D. (2006). Relationship between urban sprawl and weight of United States youth. *American Journal of Preventive Medicine, 31*, pp. 464–474.

89. Kelly-Schwartz, A., Stockard, J., Doyle, S., & Schlossberg, M. (2004). Is sprawl unhealthy? A multi-level analysis of the relationship of metropolitan sprawl to the health of individuals. *Journal of Planning Education and Research*. Forthcoming.
Vandegrift, D., & Yoked, T. (2004). Obesity rates, income, and suburban sprawl: An analysis of U.S. states. *Health and Place, 10*, pp. 221–229.
Booth, K. M., Pinkston, M. M., & Poston, W. S. (2005). Obesity and the built environment. *Journal of the American Dietetic Association, 105*, pp. S110–S117.

90. Trowbridge, et al., *Urban sprawl and delayed ambulance arrival*.

91. Li, F., Harmer, P., Cardinal, B. J., Bosworth, M., & Johnson-Shelton, D. (2009). Obesity and the built environment: Does the density of neighborhood fast-food outlets matter? *American Journal of Health Promotion, 23*, pp. 203–209.
Clougherty, J. E., Wright, R. J., Baxter, L. K., & Levy, J. I. (2008). Land use regression modeling of intra-urban residential variability in multiple traffic-related air pollutants. *Environmental Health, 7*, pp. 17.
Lopez, R. P. (2007). Neighborhood risk factors for obesity. *Obesity* (Silver Spring, MD) *15*, pp. 2111–2119.

92. Parsons Brinckerhoff Quade and Douglas.(1996). Transit and urban form. Volume 1. *Transit, urban form, and the built environment: A summary of knowledge*. Washington, D.C.: National Academies Press.

Gordon-Larsen, P., Nelson, M. C., & Beam, K. (2005). Associations among active transportation, physical activity, and weight status in young adults. *Obesity Research*, *13*, pp. 868–875.

93. Morland, K. B., & Evenson, K. R. (2009). Obesity prevalence and the local food environment. *Health Place*, *15*, pp. 491–495.

    Frank, L., Kerr, J., Saelens, B., Sallis, J., Glanz, K., & Chapman, J. (2009). Food outlet visits, physical activity and body weight: Variations by gender and race-ethnicity. *British Journal of Sports Medicine*, *43*, pp. 124–131.

94. Leyden, K. M. (2003). Social capital and the built environment: The importance of walkable neighborhoods. *American Journal of Public Health*, *93*, pp. 1546–1551.

95. Floyd, M. F., Taylor, W. C., & Whitt-Glover, M. (2009). Measurement of park and recreation environments that support physical activity in low-income communities of color: Highlights of challenges and recommendations. *American Journal of Preventive Medicine*, *36*, pp. S156–60.

    Ries, A. V., Gittelsohn, J., Voorhees, C. C., Roche, K. M., Clifton, K. J., & Astone, N. M. (2008). The environment and urban adolescents' use of recreational facilities for physical activity: A qualitative study. *American Journal of Health Promotion*, *23*, pp. 43–50.

    Floriani, V., & Kennedy, C. (2008). Promotion of physical activity in children. *Current Opinion in Pediatrics*, *20*, pp. 90–95.

    Atkinson, J. L., Sallis, J. F., Saelens, B. E., Cain, K. L., & Black, J. B. (2005). The association of neighborhood design and recreational environments with physical activity. *American Journal of Health Promotion*, *19*, pp. 304–309.

96. Frank, L., Schmid, T., Sallis, J., Chapman, J., & Saelens, B. (2005). Linking objectively measured physical activity with objectively measured urban form: Findings from SMAR-TRAQ. *American Journal of Preventive Medicine*, *28*, pp. 117–125.

    Owen, N., Humpel, N., Leslie, E., Bauman, A., & Sallis, J. (2004). Understanding environmental influences on walking: Review and research agenda. *American Journal of Preventive Medicine*, *27*, pp. 67–76.

97. Mathews, A. E., Colabianchi, N., Hutto, B., Pluto, D. M., & Hooker, S. P. (2009). Pedestrian activity among California adults. *Journal of Physical Activity & Health*, *6*, pp. 15–23.

    Budd, G. M., & Hayman, L. L. (2008). Addressing the childhood obesity crisis: A call to action. *MCN The American Journal of Maternal and Child Nursing*, *33*, pp. 111–118, quiz 9–20.

    Schmalz, D. L., Deane, G. D., Birch, L. L., & Davison, K. K. (2007). A longitudinal assessment of the links between physical activity and self-esteem in early adolescent non-Hispanic females. *Journal of Adolescent Health*, *41*, pp. 559–565.

    Sallis, J., & Glanz, K. (2006). The role of built environments in physical activity, eating, and obesity in childhood. *The Future of Children*, *16*, pp. 89–108.

98. Galvez, M. P., Pearl, M., & Yen, IH. (2010). Childhood obesity and the built environment. *Current Opinion in Pediatrics*, *22*, pp. 202–207.

    Sallis, J. F., Bowles, H. R., Bauman, A., et al. (2009). Neighborhood environments and physical activity among adults in 11 countries. *American Journal of Preventive Medicine*, *36*, pp. 484–490.

    Jago, R., Baranowski, T., & Baranowski, J., C. (2006). Observed, GIS, and self-reported environmental features and adolescent physical activity. *American Journal of Health Promotion*, *20*, pp. 422–428.

99. Rodriguez, D. A., Aytur, S., Forsyth, A., Oakes, J. M., & Clifton, K., J. (2008). Relation of modifiable neighborhood attributes to walking. *Preventive Medicine*, *47*, pp. 260–264.

100. Ries et al., *The environment and urban adolescents' use of recreational facilities*.
Pate, R. R., Colabianchi, N., Porter, D., Almeida, M. J., Lobelo, F., & Dowda, M. (2008). Physical activity and neighborhood resources in high school girls. *American Journal of Preventive Medicine*, *34*, pp. 413–419.

101. Humpel, N., Owen, N., Iverson, D., Leslie, E., & Bauman, A. (2004). Perceived environment attributes, residential location, and walking for particular purposes. *American Journal of Preventive Medicine*, *26*, pp. 119–125.
Velasquez, K. S., Holahan, C. K., & You, X. (2009). Relationship of perceived environmental characteristics to leisure-time physical activity and meeting recommendations for physical activity in Texas. *Prevention of Chronic Disease*, *6*, pp. A24.

102. Handy, S. L., Boarnet, M. G., Ewing, R., & Killingsworth, R. E. (2002). How the built environment affects physical activity: Views from urban planning. *American Journal of Preventive Medicine*, *23*, pp. 64–73.

103. Grow, H. M., Saelens, B. E., Kerr, J., Durant, N. H., Norman, G. J., & Sallis, J. F. (2008). Where are youth active? Roles of proximity, active transport, and built environment. *Medicine and Science in Sports and Exercise*, *40*, pp. 2071–2079.
Gomez, J. E., Johnson, B. A., Selva, M., Sallis, J. F. (2004). Violent crime and outdoor physical activity among inner-city youth. *Preventive Medicine*, *39*, pp. 876–881.
Harries, K., D. (1980). *Crime and the environment*. New York: Charles, C. Thomas.
Casagrande, S. S., Whitt-Glover, M. C., Lancaster, K. J., Odoms-Young, A. M., & Gary, T. L. (2009). Built environment and health behaviors among African Americans: A systematic review. *American Journal of Preventive Medicine*, *36*, pp. 174–181.

104. Schilling, J., & Linton, L. (2005). The public health roots of zoning: In search of active living's legal genealogy. *American Journal of Preventive Medicine*, *28*, 96–104.
Talen, E. (2009). Design by the rules: The historical underpinnings of form-based codes. *Journal of the American Planning Association*, *75*, pp. 144–160.

105. Geller, A. (2003). Smart growth: A prescription for livable cities. *American Journal of Public Health*, *93*, pp. 1410–1415.
Tregoning, H., Agyeman, J., & Slenot, C. (2002). Sprawl, smart growth and sustainability. *Local Environment*, *7*, pp. 341–347.
Foster-Bey, J. (2002). *Sprawl, smart growth and economic opportunity*. Washington D.C.: The Urban Institute.

106. Phillips, J., & Goodstein, E. (2000). Growth management and housing prices: The case of Portland Oregon. *Contemporary Economic Policy*, *18*, pp. 334–344.

107. Feiock, R., Tavares, A., & Lubell, M. (2008). Policy instrument choices for growth management and land use regulation. *Policy Studies Journal*, *36*, pp. 461–480.

108. Denning, C., McDonald, R., & Christensen, J. (2010). Did land protection in Silicon Valley reduce the housing stock? *Biological Conservation*, *143*, pp. 1087–1093.

109. Aytur, S. A., Rodriguez, D A., Evenson, K. R., & Catellier, D., J. (2008). Urban containment policies and physical activity. A time-series analysis of metropolitan areas, 1990–2002. *American Journal of Preventive Medicine*, *34*, pp. 320–332.

110. Schuetz, J., Meltzer, R., & Been, V. (2004). 31 flavors of inclusionary zoning: Comparing policies from San Francisco, Washington, D.C., and Suburban Boston. *Journal of the American Planning Association*, *75*, pp. 441–456.

111. Paul, E. (2008). *Property rights and eminent domain*. New Brunswick, NJ: Transaction.

112. Cohen, C. (2006). Eminent domain after Kelo v. City of New London: An argument for banning economic development takings. *Harvard Journal of Law and Public Policy*, *29*, pp. 41.

113. Bengston, D., Fletcher, J., & Nelson, K. (2004). Public policies for managing urban growth and protecting open space: Policy instruments and lessons learned in the United States. *Landscape and Urban Planning*, *69*, pp. 271–286.

114. O'Toole, *The folly of smart-growth*.

115. Arrington, G., & Cervero, R. (2009). *Effects of TOD on housing, parking, and travel*. Transportation Research Board.

116. Dunham-Jones, E., & Williamson, J. (2008). *Retrofitting suburbia: Urban design solutions for redesigning suburbs*. Hoboken, NJ: Wiley.

117. Intense Transit Oriented Development for the Suburbs. (2009). Accessed July 19, 2010, at http://www.apa-tpd.org/Beststudent/2010/first_prize_paper.pdf.

118. Frumkin, et al., *Urban sprawl and public health*.

Chapter Four

1. U.S. Department of Transportation. (2009). *The "carbon footprint" of daily travel*. National Household Transportation Survey Brief. http://nhts.ornl.gov/briefs/Carbon%20Footprint%20of%20Travel.pdf. Washington, D.C.: U.S. Department of Transportation.

2. U.S. Bureau of the Census. (2007). *American factfinder*. Washington, D.C.: U.S. Bureau of the Census.

3. Texas Transportation Institute. (2007). Urban Mobility Study. http://mobility.tamu.edu/ums/.

4. Banister, D. (2008). The sustainable mobility paradigm. *Transport Policy*, *15*, pp. 73–80.

5. Gärling, T., & Schuitema, G. (2007). Travel demand management targeting reduced private car use: Effectiveness, public acceptability and political feasibility. *Journal of Social Issues*, *63*, pp. 139–153.

6. Hensher, D., & Puckett, S. (2007). Congestion and variable user charging as an effective travel demand management instrument. *Transportation Research Part A: Policy and Practice*, *41* pp. 615–626.

7. Litman, T. (2008). *Measuring transportation: Traffic, mobility, accessibility*. Victoria, British Columbia: Victoria Transport Policy Institute.

8. Kwan, M., & Weber, J. (2008). Scale and accessibility: Implications for the analysis of land use-travel interaction. *Applied Geography*, *28*, pp. 110–123.

9. Iacono, M., Krizek, K., & El-Genei, A. (2010). Measuring non-motorized accessibility: Issues, alternatives, and execution. *Journal of Transport Geography*, *18*, pp. 133–140.

10. Keeling, D. (2008). Transportation geography: Local challenges, global contexts. *Progress in Human Geography*, *32*, pp. 247–263.

11. Zhou, B., & Kockelman K. M. (2008). Neighborhood impacts on land use change: A multinomial logic model of spatial relationships. *Journal of Regional Science*, *42*, pp. 321–342.

12. Brömmelstroet, M. T., & Bertolin, L. (2010). Integrating land use and transport knowledge in strategy-making. *Transportation*, *37*, pp. 85–104.

13. Lehmann, S. (2006). Towards a sustainable city centre: Integrating ecologically sustainable development (ESD) principles into urban renewal. *Journal of Green Building*, *1*, pp. 83–104.

14. Burbidge, S., & Goulias, K. (2009). Active travel behavior. *Transportation Letters: The International Journal of Transportation Research, 1*, pp. 147–167.

15. *Injury Prevention & Control: Motor Vehicle Safety* (2010). Accessed at http://www.cdc.gov/Motorvehiclesafety/index.html.

16. Hasselberg, M., & Laflamme, L. (2009). How do car crashes happen among young drivers aged 18–20 years? Typical circumstances in relation to license status, alcohol impairment and injury consequences. *Accident Analysis and Prevention, 41*, pp. 734–738.
    Lee, W. Y., Cameron, P. A., & Bailey, M. J. (2006). Road traffic injuries in the elderly. *Emergency Medicine Journal, 23*, pp. 42–46.

17. Shope, J. T., & Bingham, C. R. (2008). Teen driving: Motor-vehicle crashes and factors that contribute. *American Journal of Preventive Medicine, 35*, pp. S261–S271.
    Alvarez, F. J., & Fierro, I. (2008). Older drivers, medical condition, medical impairment and crash risk. *Accident Analysis and Prevention, 40*, pp. 55–60.

18. Ponicki, W. R., Gruenewald, P. J., & LaScala, E. A. (2007). Joint impacts of minimum legal drinking age and beer taxes on U.S. youth traffic fatalities, 1975 to 2001. *Alcoholism: Clinical and Experimental Research, 31*, pp. 804–813.
    Williams, A. F. (2006). Young driver risk factors: Successful and unsuccessful approaches for dealing with them and an agenda for the future. *Injury Prevention, 12 Suppl 1*, pp. i4–i8.

19. McGwin, G., Jr., Sarrels, S. A., Griffin, R., Owsley, C., & Rue, L. W., 3rd. (2008). The impact of a vision screening law on older driver fatality rates. *Injury Prevention, 126*, pp. 1544–1547.
    Grabowski, D. C., Campbell, C. M., & Morrisey, M. A. (2004). Elderly licensure laws and motor vehicle fatalities. *JAMA, 291*, pp. 2840–6.

20. Ewing, R., & Dumbaugh, E. (2009). The built environment and traffic safety. *Journal of Planning Literature, 23*, pp. 347–367.

21. Gorrie, C. A., Brown, J., & Waite, P. M. (2008). Crash characteristics of older pedestrian fatalities: Dementia pathology may be related to 'at risk' traffic situations. *Accident Analysis and Prevention, 40*, pp. 912–919.

22. Carver, A., Timperio, A., & Crawford, D. (2008). Playing it safe: The influence of neighbourhood safety on children's physical activity. A review. *Health Place, 14*, pp. 217–227.

23. Raynault, E. (2010). *Promoting pedestrian and bicyclist safety to Hispanic audiences*. Department of Transportation. Washington, D.C.: Office of Safety Programs.

24. Costa, G., Pickup, L., & DiMarino, V. (1988). Commuting—A further stress factor for working people: evidence from the European Community. 1. A review. *International Archives of Occupational and Environmental Health, 60*, pp. 1–6.
    Koslowsky, M. (1997). Commuting stress: Problems of definition and variable identification. *Applied Psychology, 46*, pp. 153–174.
    Koslowsky, M., Kluger, A., & Reich, M. (1995). *Commuting stress: Causes, effects, and methods of coping*. New York: Plenum Press.
    Novaco, R. (1994). *Commuting stress, ridesharing, and gender: Analyses from the 1993 State of the Commute Study in Southern California*. Berkeley: The University of California Transportation Center.

25. Johnson, S., & Bowers, K. (2010). Permeability and burglary risk: Are cul-de-sacs safer? *Journal of Quantitative Criminology, 26*, pp. 89–111.

26. Frank, L. D., Saelens, B. E., Powell, K. E., & Chapman, J. E. (2007). Stepping towards causation: do built environments or neighborhood and travel preferences explain physical activity, driving, and obesity? *Social Science and Medicine, 65*, pp. 1898–1914.

27. Carver, A., Timperio, A. F., & Crawford, D. A. (2008). Neighborhood road environments and physical activity among youth: THE CLAN study. *Journal of Urban Health*, *85*, pp. 532–544.

Cozens, P., & Hillier, D. (2008). The shape of things to come: New urbanism, the grid and the cul-de-sac. *International Planning Studies*, *13*, pp. 51–73.

28. Millard, W. (2007). Suburban sprawl: Where does emergency medicine fit on the map? *Annals of Emergency Medicine*, *49*, pp. 71–74.

29. Ong, P. (2005). Spatial and transportation mismatch in Los Angeles. *Journal of Planning Education and Research*, *25*, pp. 43–56.

30. Coveney, J., & O'Dwyer, L. A. (2009). Effects of mobility and location on food access. *Health Place*, *15*, pp. 45–55.

31. Johnson, V., Currie, G., & Stanley, J. (2010). Measures of disadvantage: Is car ownership a good indicator? *Social Indicators Research*, *97*, pp. 439–450.

32. Census. (2010). *American Community Survey 2005–2010*. Washington, D.C.: U.S. Bureau of the Census.

33. Waller, P. F. (2002). Challenges in motor vehicle safety. *Annual Reviews of Public Health*, *23*, pp. 93–113.

34. Elvik, R., Hoye, A., Vaa, T., & Sorensen, M. (2009). *The handbook of road safety measures*. Bingbey, UK: Emerald Group.

35. Smith, W. A. (2006). Social marketing: An overview of approach and effects. *Injury Prevention*, *12 Suppl 1*, pp. i38–i43.

Senserrick, T. M. (2006). Reducing young driver road trauma: Guidance and optimism for the future. *Injury Prevention*, *12 Suppl 1*, pp. i56–i60.

36. Taggi, F. (2009). Cell phone and road safety. *Annali di Igiene*, *21*, pp. 3–5.

37. Loeb, P., & Clarke, W. (2008). The cell phone effect on pedestrian fatalities. *Transportation Research Part E: Logistics and Transportation Review*, *45*, pp. 284–290.

38. Kay, J. H. (1998). *Asphalt nation: How the automobile took over America, and how we can take it back*. Berkeley: University of California Press.

39. Keeler, T., & Smalls, K. (1975). *The full costs of urban transport. Part III: Automobile costs and final intermodal cost comparisons*. Berkeley: Institute of Transportation Studies. University of California. Report No.: Monograph 212.

40. Shoup, D. (2005). *The high cost of free parking*. Chicago: American Planning Association.

41. Hynes, H. P. (1999). Taking population out of the equation: Reformulating I = PAT. In: J. M. Silliman & Y. King, (Eds.), *Dangerous intersections: Feminist perspectives on population, environment, and development*. Cambridge, MA: South End Press.

42. Su, Q., & DeSalvo, J. (2008). The effect of transportation subsidies on urban sprawl. *Journal of Regional Science*, *48*, pp. 567–594.

43. Poudenx, P. (2008). The effect of transportation policies on energy consumption and greenhouse gas emission from urban passenger transportation. *Transportation Research Part A: Policy and Practice*, *42*, pp. 901–909.

44. Freemark, Y. (2010). Cars, highways, and the poor. *Dissent*, *57*, pp. 10–3.

45. Gautier, P., & Zenou Y. (2008). Car ownership and the labor market of ethnic minorities. *Journal of Urban Economics*, *67*, pp. 392–403.

46. Hott, L, Lewis, T. (1997). *Divided highways: The interstates and the transformation of American life*. A Hott Production of Florentine Films by Lawrence R. Hott and Tom Lewis. Edited by Diane Garey. A Coproduction of WETA-TV, Washington, D.C.

47. Ellis, C. (2002). Interstate highways, regional planning and the reshaping of metropolitan America. *Planning Practice and Research*, *16*, pp. 247–269.

48. Mann, E. (2004). Los Angeles bus riders derail the MTA. In R. Bullard, G. Johnson, & A. Torres (Eds.), *Highway robbery: Transportation racism and new routes to equity*. Cambridge, MA: South End Press.

    Wright, B. (1997). New Orleans neighborhoods under siege. In R. Bullard & G. Johnson (Eds.), *Just Transportation: Dismantling race and class barriers to mobility*. Stony Creek, CT: New Society Publishers.

49. Bullard, R. (2004). Addressing urban transportation equity in the United States. *Fordham Urban Law Journal, 31*, pp. 1183.

    Bullard, R., Johnson, G., & Torres, A. (2000). *Sprawl city. Race, politics and planning in Atlanta*. Washington, D.C.: Island Press.

50. Baum-Snow, N. (2007). Did highways cause suburbanization? *Quarterly Journal of Economics, 122*, pp. 775–807.

51. Foster, M. (1981). *From streetcar to superhighway: American city planners and urban transportation, 1900–1940*. Philadelphia: Temple University Press.

52. Gutfreund, O. *20th-century sprawl: Highways and the reshaping of the American landscape*. New York: Oxford University Press. (2004).

53. Freemark, *Cars, highways, and the poor*.

54. Kay, *Asphalt nation*.

55. Baxter, L. K., Clougherty, J. E., Paciorek, C. J., Wright, R. J., & Levy, J. I. (2007). Predicting residential indoor concentrations of nitrogen dioxide, fine particulate matter, and elemental carbon using questionnaire and geographic information system based data. *Atmospheric Environment, 41*, pp. 6561–6571.

    Riediker, M. (2007). Cardiovascular effects of fine particulate matter components in highway patrol officers. *Inhalation Toxicology, 19 Suppl 1*, pp. 99–105.

56. Wier, M., Sciammas, C., Seto, E., Bhatia, R., & Rivard, T. (2009). Health, traffic, and environmental justice: collaborative research and community action in San Francisco, California. *American Journal of Public Health, 99 Suppl 3*, pp. S499–S504.

57. Allen, R. W., Criqui, M. H., Diez Roux, A. V., et al. (2009). Fine particulate matter air pollution, proximity to traffic, and aortic atherosclerosis. *Epidemiology, 20*, pp. 254–264.

58. Mital, A., & Ramakrishnan, A. S. (1997). Effectiveness of noise barriers on an interstate highway: A subjective and objective evaluation. *Journal of Human Ergology (Tokyo), 26*, pp. 31–38.

59. Moudon, A. V. (2009). Real noise from the urban environment: How ambient community noise affects health and what can be done about it. *American Journal of Preventive Medicine, 37*, pp. 167–171.

60. Edwards, R. D. (2008). Public transit, obesity, and medical costs: Assessing the magnitudes. *Preventive Medicine, 46*, pp. 14–21.

    Fenton, M. (2005). Battling America's epidemic of physical inactivity: Building more walkable, livable communities. *Journal of Nutrition and Education Behavior, 37 Suppl 2*, pp. S115–S120.

    Handy, S. L., Boarnet, M. G., Ewing, R., & Killingsworth, R. E. (2002). How the built environment affects physical activity: Views from urban planning. *American Journal of Preventive Medicine, 23*, pp. 64–73.

61. Woodcock, J., Banister, D., Edwards, P., Prentice, A. M, & Roberts, I. (2007). Energy and transport. *Lancet, 370*, pp. 1078–1088.

62. Litman, T., & Burrell, D. (2006). Issues in sustainable transportation. *International Journal of Global Environmental Issues, 6*, pp. 331–347.

63. McGeehan, J., Annest, J. L., Vajani, M., Bull, M. J., Agran, P. E., & Smith, G. A. (2006). School bus-related injuries among children and teenagers in the United States, 2001–2003. *Pediatrics, 118*, pp. 1978–1984.

Emery, K. D., & Faries, S. G. (2008). The lack of motor vehicle occupant restraint use in children arriving at school. *Journal of School Health, 78*, pp. 274–279.

64. Gershon, R., Qureshi, K., Barrera, M., Erwin, M., & Goldsmith, G. (2005). Health and safety hazards associated with subways: A review. *Journal of Urban Health, 82*, pp. 10–20.

Karlsson, H., Nilsson, L., & Moller, L. (2005). Subway particles are more genotoxic than street particles and induce oxidative stress in cultured human lung cells. *Chemical Research and Toxicology, 18*, pp. 19–23.

65. Brown, J., Morris, E., & Taylor, B. (2009). Planning for cars in cities: Planners, engineers, and freeways in the 20th century. *Journal of the American Planning Association, 75*, pp. 161–177.

66. Cradock, A. L., Troped, P. J., & Fields, B., et al. (2009). Factors associated with federal transportation funding for local pedestrian and bicycle programming and facilities. *Journal of Public Health Policy, 30 Suppl 1*, pp. S38–72.

67. Plant, J. Transportation policy. In J. Rabin and A. Wachhaus (Eds.), *Encyclopedia of public administration and public policy*. Boca Raton, FL: Taylor and Francis.

68. Weiner, E. (2008). *Urban transportation planning in the United States: History, policy, and practice*. New York: Springer Science.

69. Yamaguchi, K. (2008). *Funding system and road transport: International comparative analysis*. Tokyo: Graduate School of Public Policy.

70. Sciara, G., Wachs, M. (2007). Metropolitan transportation funding: Prospects, progress, and practical considerations. *Public Works Management & Policy, 12*, pp. 379–394.

71. O'Toole, R. (2009). *Defining success: The case against rail transit*. Washington, D.C.: Cato Institute.

72. Winston, C., & Maheshr, V. (2007). On the social desirability of urban rail transit systems. *Journal of Urban Economics, 62*, pp. 362–382.

73. Burbidge, S. K. (2009). Merging long range transportation planning with public health: A case study from Utah's Wasatch Front. *Preventive Medicine, 50 Suppl 1*, pp. S6–S8.

Lemp, J. D., Zhou, B. B., Kockelman, K. M., & Parmenter, B. M. (2008). Visioning versus modeling: Analyzing the land-use-transportation futures of urban regions. *Journal of Urban Planning and Development, 134*, pp. 97–109.

74. Hess, D., & Lombardi, P. (2005). Governmental subsidies for public transit: History, current issues, and recent evidence. *Public Works Management & Policy, 10*, pp. 138–156.

75. Coverage, T., & Serials T. (2010). *What makes public transit a success? Perspectives on ridership in an era of uncertain revenues and climate change*. Transportation Research Board 89th Annual Meeting. Washington D.C.: Transportation Research Board.

76. Grengs, J. (2002). Community-based planning as a source of political change: The transit equity movement of Los Angeles' Bus Riders Union. *Journal of the American Planning Association, 68*, pp. 165–178.

77. Physical Activity Guidelines Advisory Committee report, 2008. (2009). To the Secretary of Health and Human Services. Part A: Executive summary. *Nutrition Reviews, 67*, pp. 114–120.

78. Shepard, R. (2008). Is active commuting the answer to population health? *Sports Medicine, 68*, pp. 165–178.

79. Dill, J. (2009). Bicycling for transportation and health: The role of infrastructure. *Journal of Public Health Policy*, *30*, pp. S95–S110.

80. Edwards, *Public transit, obesity, and medical costs*.

81. Martens, K. (2007). Promoting bike-and-ride: The Dutch experience. *Transportation Research Part A: Policy and Practice*, *41*, pp. 326–338.

82. Garrard, J., Rose, G., & Lo, S. K. (2008). Promoting transportation cycling for women: The role of bicycle infrastructure. *Preventive Medicine*, *46*, pp. 55–59.

83. Reynolds, C. C., Harris, M. A., Teschke, K., Cripton, P. A., & Winters, M. (2009). The impact of transportation infrastructure on bicycling injuries and crashes: Q review of the literature. *Environmental Health*, *8*, pp. 47.

84. Dill, J. (2009). Bicycling for transportation and health: The role of infrastructure. *Journal of Public Health Policy*, *30 Suppl 1*, pp. S95–S110.

85. Pucher, J., Dill, J., & Handy S. (2009). Infrastructure, programs, and policies to increase bicycling: An international review. *Preventive Medicine*, *50 Suppl 1*, pp. S106–S125.

86. Reynolds et al., *The impact of transportation infrastructure on bicycling injuries and crashes*.

87. DeMaio, P. (2009). Bike-sharing: Its history, models of provision, and future. *Journal of Public Transportation*, *12*, pp. 40–55.

88. Midgley, P. (2009). The role of smart bike-sharing systems in urban mobility. *Journies*, pp. 23–31.

89. Fenton, *Battling America's epidemic of physical inactivity*.

90. Frank et al., *Stepping towards causation*.
    Gordon-Larsen, P., Nelson, M. C., & Beam, K. (2005). Associations among active transportation, physical activity, and weight status in young adults. *Obesity Research*, *13*, pp. 868–875.
    Boarnet, M. G., Greenwald, M., & McMillan, T. E. (2008). Walking, urban design, and health. *Journal of Planning Education and Research*, *27*, pp. 341–358.
    Kochtitzky, C. S., Frumkin, H., Rodriguez, R., et al. (2006). Urban planning and public health at CDC. *MMWR Morbity and Mortality Weekly Report*, *55 Suppl 2*, pp. 34–38.
    Vaughn, A. E., Ball, S. C., Linnan, L. A., Marchetti, L. M., Hall, W. L., & Ward, D. S. (2009). Promotion of walking for transportation: A report from the Walk to School day registry. *Journal of Physical Activity & Health*, *6*, pp. 281–288.

91. Taylor, A. F., & Kuo, F. E. (2009). Children with attention deficits concentrate better after walk in the park. *Journal of Attention Disorders*, *12*, pp. 402–409.

92. *Physical Activity Guidelines Advisory Committee report*.
    Burke, N. M., Chomitz, V. R., Rioles, N. A., Winslow, S. P., Brukilacchio, L. B., & Baker, J. C. (2009). The path to active living: Physical activity through community design in Somerville, Massachusetts. *American Journal of Preventive Medicine*, *37*, pp. S386–94.
    Cerin, E., Saelens, B. E., Sallis, J. F., & Frank, L. D. (2006). Neighborhood Environment Walkability Scale: Validity and development of a short form. *Medicine and Science in Sports and Exercise*, *38*, pp. 1682–1691.

93. Handy et al., *How the built environment affects physical activity*.

94. Schuurman, N., Cinnamon, J., Crooks, V. A., & Hameed, S. M. (2009). Pedestrian injury and the built environment: An environmental scan of hotspots. *BMC Public Health*, *9*, p. 233.

95. Boarnet et al., *Walking, urban design, and health*.

96. *Then and now — Barriers and solutions.* (2010). Centers for Disease Control and Prevention. Accessed July 19, 2010, at http://www.cdc.gov/nccdphp/dnpa/kidswalk/then_and_now.htm.

97. Cooper, A., Page, A., Foster, L., & Qahwagi, D. (2003). Commuting to school: Are children who walk more physically active? *American Journal of Preventive Medicine, 25,* pp. 273–276.

98. Rodriguez, A., & Vogt, C. (2009). Demographic, environmental, access, and attitude factors that influence walking to school by elementary school-aged children. *Journal of School Health, 79,* pp. 255–261.

99. Vaughn, A. E., Ball, S. C., Linnan, L. A., Marchetti, L. M., Hall, W. L., & Ward, D. S. (2009). Promotion of walking for transportation: A report from the Walk to School day registry. *Journal of Physical Activity & Health, 6,* pp. 281–288.

100. Abbott, C., & Margheim, J. (2008). Imagining Portland's urban growth boundary: planning regulation as cultural icon. *Journal of the American Planning Association, 74,* pp. 196–208.
     Jun, M.-J. (2004). The effects of Portland's urban growth boundary on urban development patterns and commuting. *Urban Studies, 41,* pp. 13333–13349.

101. Dill, *Bicycling for Transportation and Health.*

102. Laplante, J., & McCann, B. (2008). Complete streets: We can get there from here. *ITE Journal, 2008,* pp. 21–28.

103. Geraghty, A. B., Seifert, W., Preston, T., Holm, C. V., Duarte, T. H., & Farrar, S. M. (2009). Partnership moves community toward complete streets. *American Journal of Preventive Medicine, 37,* pp. S420–S427.

104. Ibid.

105. Ewing, R., & Brown S. (2009). *U.S. traffic calming manual.* Chicago: American Planning Association.

106. Leden, L., Wikstrom P. E., Garder, P., & Rosander, P. (2006). Safety and accessibility effects of code modifications and traffic calming of an arterial road. *Accident Analysis and Prevention, 38,* pp. 455–461.
     Bunn, F., Collier, T., Frost, C., Ker, K., Roberts, I., & Wentz, R. (2003). Traffic calming for the prevention of road traffic injuries: systematic review and meta-analysis. *Injury Prevention, 9,* pp. 200–204.

107. Leape, J. (2006). The London congestion charge. *The Journal of Economic Perspectives, 29,* pp. 157–176.

108. Srinivas, M., Rys, M., & Russell, E. (2001). Environmental impact of modern roundabouts. *International Journal of Industrial Ergonomics, 38,* pp. 135–142.

109. Daniels, S., Nuyts, E., & Wets, G. (2008). The effects of roundabouts on traffic safety for bicyclists: An observational study. *Accident Analysis & Prevention, 40,* pp. 518–528.

110. Turner, S., Fitzpatrick, K., Brewer, M., & Park, E. S. (2006). Motorists yielding to pedestrians at unsignalized intersections: Findings from a national study on improving pedestrian safety. Transportation Research Record. *Journal of the Transportation Research Board, 1982,* pp. 1–12.
     Leden, L., Garder, P., Johansson, C. (2006). Safe pedestrian crossings for children and elderly. *Accident Analysis and Prevention, 38,* pp. 289–294.

Chapter Five

1. Lubove, R. (1962). *The progressives and the slums: Tenement house reform in New York City, 1890–1917*. Westport, CT: Greenwood Press.

2. Blackmar, E. (1995). Accountability for public health: Regulating the housing market in nineteenth-century New York City. In: D. Rosner, (Ed.), *Hives of sickness*. New Brunswick, NJ: Rutgers University Press.

3. Wood, E. E. (1933). A century of the housing problem. *Law and Contemporary Problems, 1*, pp. 137–47.

4. Flanagan, R. (1997). The Housing Act of 1954: The sea change in national urban policy. *Urban Affairs Review, 33*, pp. 265–76.

5. U.S. Bureau of the Census. (2007). American housing survey. Washington, D.C.: U.S. Bureau of the Census.

6. U.S. Bureau of the Census (2005). Historical census of housing tables. In *Housing and Household Economic Statistics Division*. Washington, D.C.: U.S. Bureau of the Census.

7. Fisher, J., & Quayyum, S. (2006). The great turn-of-the-century housing boom. *Economic Perspectives, 30*, pp. 19–44.

8. Ewing, R., & Rong, F. (2008). The impact of urban form on U.S. residential energy use. *Housing Policy Debate, 19*, pp. 1–30.

9. Schwartz, A. (2006). *Housing policy in the United States: An introduction*. New York: Routledge.

10. Radford, G. (2000). The federal government and housing during the Great Depression. In J. Bauman, R. Biles, & K. Szylvian (Eds.), *From tenements to the Taylor Homes: In search of an urban hosing policy in twentieth-century America*. University Park: The University of Pennsylvania Press.

11. Denton, N. (1999). Half empty or half full: Segregation and segregated neighborhoods 30 years after the Fair Housing Act. *Cityscape, 4*, pp. 107–122.

12. Hirsch, A. (2000). "Containment" on the home front. Race and federal housing policy from the New Deal to the Cold War. *Journal of Urban History, 26*, pp. 158–189.

13. Wyly, E., & Hammel, D. (1999). Islands of decay in seas of renewal: Housing policy and the resurgence of gentrification. *Housing Policy Debate, 10*, pp. 711–765.

14. Stoecker, R. (2008). The CDC model of urban redevelopment: A critique and an alternative. *Journal of Urban Affairs, 19*, pp. 1–22.

15. vanHoffman, A. (2000). A study in contradictions: The origins and legacy of the Housing Act of 1949. *Housing Policy Debate, 11*, pp. 299–326.

16. Brazley, M., & Gilderbloom, J. I. (2007). HOPE VI housing program: Was it effective? *American Journal of Economics and Sociology, 66*, pp. 433–442.

17. Rosenthal, L. (2007). *Rent reform initiatives in public housing and Section 8 voucher programs*. Berkeley, CA: Berkeley Program on Housing and Urban Policy, Institute of Business and Economic Research.

18. Research Works. (2010). *HUD user*. Washington, D.C.: U.S. Department of Housing and Urban Development., pp. 3.

19. Northridge, J., Ramirez, O. F., Stingone, J. A., & Claudio, L. (2010). The role of housing type and housing quality in urban children with asthma. *Journal of Urban Health, 87*, pp. 211–224.

20. Ventry, D. (2010). The accidental deduction: A history and critique of the tax subsidy for mortgage interest. *Law and Contemporary Problems, 72*.

21. Peirce, N., & Steinbach, C. (1987). *Corrective capitalism: The rise of America's community development corporations*. New York: Ford Foundation.

22. Gittell R. (1999). Community development corporations: Critical factors that influence success. *Journal of Urban Affairs, 21*, pp. 341–361.

23. Sahakian, N. M., Park, J. H., & Cox-Ganser, J. M. (2008). Dampness and mold in the indoor environment: Implications for asthma. *Immunology and Allergy Clinics of North America, 28*, pp. 485–505, vii.

24. Howden-Chapman, P., Saville-Smith, K., Crane, J., & Wilson, N. (2005). Risk factors for mold in housing: A national survey. *Indoor Air, 15*, pp. 469–76.

25. Miles R. (2005). Preventing asthma through housing interventions: How supportive is the U.S. policy environment? *Housing Studies, 20*, pp. 589–603.

26. Gaitens, J. M., Dixon, S. L., Jacobs, D. E., et al. (2009). Exposure of U.S. children to residential dust lead, 1999–2004: I. Housing and demographic factors. *Environmental Health Perspectives, 117*, pp. 461–467.

27. Needleman, H. (2004). Lead poisoning. *Annual Review of Medicine, 55*, pp. 209–222.

28. Lanphear, B. P., Hornung, R., & Ho, M. (2005). Screening housing to prevent lead toxicity in children. *Public Health Reports, 120*, pp. 305–10.

29. *Lead in paint, dust and soil*. (2010). Environmental Protection Agency. Accessed July 20, 2010, at http://www.epa.gov/lead/pubs/renovation.htm.

30. Chaudhuri, N. (2004). Interventions to improve children's health by improving the housing environment. *Reviews of Environmental Health, 19*, pp. 197–222.

31. Sandel, M., Phelan, K., Wright, R., Hynes, H. P., & Lanphear, B. P. (2004). The effects of housing interventions on child health. *Pediatric Annals, 33*, pp. 474–481.

32. Thomson, H., Thomas, S., Sellstrom, E., & Petticrew, M. (2009). The health impacts of housing improvement: a systematic review of intervention studies from 1887 to 2007. *American Journal of Public Health, 99 Suppl 3*, pp. S681–S692.

33. Serrell, N., Caron, R. M., Fleishman, B., & Robbins, E. D. (2009). An academic-community outreach partnership: Building relationships and capacity to address childhood lead poisoning. *Progress in Community Health Partnerships, 3*, pp. 53–59.

34. Hynes, H. P., Maxfield, R., Carroll, P., & Hillger R. (2001). Dorchester lead-safe yard project: A pilot program to demonstrate low-cost, on-site techniques to reduce exposure to lead-contaminated soil. *Journal of Urban Health, 78*, pp. 199–211.

35. *Fire Deaths and Injuries: Fact Sheet*. (2010). Accessed at http://www.cdc.gov/Homeand-RecreationalSafety/Fire-Prevention/fires-factsheet.html.

36. Ibid.
Shai, D. (2006). Income, housing, and fire injuries: A census tract analysis. *Public Health Reports, 121*, pp. 149–154.

37. DiGuiseppi, C., & Higgins, J. P. (2001). Interventions for promoting smoke alarm ownership and function. *Cochrane Database of Systemic Reviews 2001: CD002246.*

38. Ta, V. M., Frattaroli, S., Bergen, G., & Gielen, A. C. (2006). Evaluated community fire safety interventions in the United States: A review of current literature. *Journal of Community Health, 31*, pp. 176–197.

39. Butry, D. (2009). Economic performance of residential fire sprinkler systems. *Fire Technology, 45*, pp. 117–143.

40. Staunton, C. E., Frumkin, H., & Dannenberg, A. L. (2007). Changing the built environment to prevent injury. In L. S. Doll, D. A. Sleet, & S. E. Bonzo (Eds.), *Handbook of injury prevention*. New York: Springer, pp. 257–275.

41. Gillespie, L. D., Robertson, M. C., Gillespie, W. J., et al. (2009). Interventions for preventing falls in older people living in the community. *Cochrane Database of Systemic Reviews 2009: CD007146.*

42. Lyons, R. A., John, A., Brophy, S., et al. (2006). Modification of the home environment for the reduction of injuries. *Cochrane Database of Systemic Reviews 2006: CD003600.*

43. Mack, K., & Liller, K. (2010). Home injuries: Potential for prevention. *American Journal of Lifestyle Medicine, 4,* pp. 75–81.

44. Laquatra, J., Pillai, G., & Singh, A. (2008). Green and healthy housing. *Journal of Architectural Engineering, 14,* pp. 94–98.

45. Shepherd, C. A. (2006). CDC and HUD to release an updated housing inspection manual—the Healthy Housing Reference Manual. *Journal of Environmental Health, 68,* pp. 48–49.

46. *International Code Council.* Accessed at http;//www.iccsafe.org.
National Fire Protection Association. Accessed at http://www.nfpa.org.

47. Ching, F., & Winkel, S. (2007). *Building code illustrated: A guide to understanding the 2006 International Building Code.* New York: Wiley.

48. Burby R. (2005). Impacts of building code enforcement on the housing industry. In F. F. W. Wagner, E. Joder, A. J. Mumphrey, K. M. Akundi, & A. F. J. Artibise (Eds.), *Revitalizing the city: Strategies to contain sprawl and revive the core.* Armonk, NY: M.E. Sharpe.

49. *National Center for Healthy Homes.* 2010. Accessed at http://www.nchh.org/Home.aspx.

50. Zuckerman, B., Sandel, M., Lawton, E., & Morton S. (2008). Medical-legal partnerships: transforming health care. *Lancet, 372,* pp. 1615–1617.

51. Kass, D., McKelvey, W., Carlton, E., et al. (2009). Effectiveness of an integrated pest management intervention in controlling cockroaches, mice, and allergens in New York City public housing. *Environmental Health Perspectivesives, 117,* pp. 1219–1225.

52. Peters, J. L., Levy, J. I., Muilenberg, M. L., Coull, B. A., & Spengler, J. D. (2007). Efficacy of integrated pest management in reducing cockroach allergen concentrations in urban public housing. *Journal of Asthma, 44,* pp. 455–640.

53. Levy, J. I., Brugge, D., Peters, J. L., Clougherty, J. E., & Saddler, S. S. (2006). A community-based participatory research study of multifaceted in-home environmental interventions for pediatric asthmatics in public housing. *Social Science and Medicine, 63,* pp. 2191–2203.

54. Wallace, R. (1988). A synergism of plagues: Planned shrinkage, contagious housing destruction and AIDS in the Bronx. *Environmental Research, 47,* pp. 1–33.

55. Tillett, T. (2007). Beyond the bench: Clean sweep: Adopting safer urban demolition practices. *Environmental Health Perspectives, 115,* pp. A83–A84.

56. Wallace, D., & Wallace R. (1998). *A plague on your houses: How New York was burned down and national public health crumbled.* New York: Verson.

57. Hopper, K. (2003). Two genealogies of supported housing and their implications for outcome assessment. *Psychiatric Services, 54,* pp. 50–54.

58. Sylvestre, J., Nelson, G., & Sabloff, A. (2007). Housing for people with serious mental illness: A comparison of values and research. *American Journal of Behavioral Psychology, 40,* pp. 125–137.

59. National Association to End Homelessness. (2011). *State of homelessness in America.* http://www.endhomelessness.org/content/article/detail/3668.

60. Link, B. G., Susser, E., Stueve, A., Phelan, J., Moore, R. E., & Struening, E. (1994). Lifetime and five-year prevalence of homelessness in the United States. *American Journal of Public Health, 84,* pp. 1907–1112.

61. Wright, J. (2009). *Address unknown: The homeless in America*. New Brunswick, NJ: Transaction.

62. Israel, N., Toro, P. A., & Ouellette, N. (2010). Changes in the composition of the homeless population: 1992–2002. *American Journal of Community Psychology*, *46*, pp. 49–59.

    Shelton, K., Taylor, P., & Bonner, A. Risk factors for homelessness: Evidence from a population-based study. *Psychiatric Services*, *60*, pp. 465–472.

    van den Bree, M., Shelton, K., Bonner, A., Moss, S., Thomas, H., & Taylor, P. J. (2009). A longitudinal population-based study of factors in adolescence predicting homelessness in young adulthood. *Journal of Adolescent Health*, *45*, pp. 571–578.

63. Lindberg, R. A., Shenassa, E. D., Acevedo-Garcia, D., Popkin, S. J., Villaveces, A., & Morley, R. L. (2010). Housing interventions at the neighborhood level and health: A review of the evidence. *Journal of Public Health Management and Practice 16*, pp. S44–S52.

64. Sachs-Ericsson, N., Wise, E., Debrody, C. P., & Paniucki, H. B. (1999). Health problems and service utilization in the homeless. *Journal of Health Care for the Poor and Underserved*, *10*, pp. 443–452.

65. Morrison, D. S. (2009). Homelessness as an independent risk factor for mortality: Results from a retrospective cohort study. *International Journal of Epidemiology*, *38*, pp. 877–883.

    Bennett, D. E., Courval, J. M., Onorato, I., et al. (2008). Prevalence of tuberculosis infection in the United States population: The national health and nutrition examination survey, 1999–2000. *American Journal of Respiratory Critical Care Medicine*, *177*, pp. 348–355.

66. Newman, S., & Goldman, H. (2008). Putting housing first, making housing last: Housing policy for persons with severe mental illness. *American Journal of Psychiatry*, *165*, pp. 1242–1248.

    Kertesz, S. G., Crouch, K., Milby, J. B., Cusimano, R. E., & Schumacher, J. E. (2009). Housing first for homeless persons with active addiction: Are we overreaching? *Milbank Quarterly*, *87*, pp. 495–534.

67. Kertesz, S. G., & Weiner, S. J. (2009). Housing the chronically homeless: high hopes, complex realities. *JAMA*, *301*, pp. 1822–1824.

    Marcuse, P. (1997). The enclave, the citadel, and the ghetto: What has changed in the post-Fordist U.S. city. *Urban Affairs Review*, *33*, pp. 228–264.

    Harvey, D. (2003). The right to the city. *International Journal of Urban and Regional Research*, *27*, pp. 939–941.

68. Betancur, J. (2002). The politics of gentrification: The case of West Town in Chicago. *Urban Affairs Review*, *37*, pp. 780–814.

69. Lees, L., Slater, T., & Wyly, E. *Gentrification*. New York: Routledge.

70. Helms, A. (2003). Understanding gentrification: An empirical analysis of the determinants of urban housing renovation. *Journal of Urban Economics*, *54*, pp. 474–498.

    Kennedy, M., & Leonard P. (2001). *Dealing with neighborhood change: A primer on gentrification and policy choices*. Washington, D.C.: The Brookings Institute.

71. Freudenberg, N., & Galeo, S. (2008). Cities of consumption: The impact of corporate practices on the health of urban populations. *Journal of Urban Health*, *85*, pp. 462–471.

72. Gans, H. (1962). *The urban villagers: Group and class in the life of Italian-Americans*. Glencoe, NY: The Free Press.

73. Fullilove, M. (2005). *Root shock: How tearing up city neighborhoods hurts America, and what we can do about it*. New York: Random House.

    Fullilove, M., & Fullilove, R. (2000). Place matters. In R. Hofrichter (Ed.), *Reclaiming the environmental debate: The politics of health in a toxic culture*. Cambridge, MA: MIT Press.

74. Wallace, *A synergism of plagues*.

    Wallace, *A plague on your houses*.

75. *Health effects of gentrification*. (2009). CDC. Accessed January 14, 2011, at http://www.cdc .gov/healthyplaces/healthtopics/gentrification.htm.

76. Goetz, E. (2010). Gentrification in black and white: The racial impact of public housing demolition in American cities. *Urban Studies*, Online ahead of print.

77. Jackson, V., & Scott, L. (2008). Bulldozed: Innovative strategies for addressing the mental health consequences of gentrification. *Community Forum: Paper 3*.

78. Iceland, J., Weinberg, D., & Steinmetz, E. (2002). *Racial and ethnic residential segregation in the United States: 1980–2000*. Washington D.C.: U.S. Bureau of the Census.

79. Massey, D., & Denton, N. (1993). *American apartheid: Segregation and the making of the underclass*. Cambridge, MA: Harvard University Press.

80. Grant-Meyer, S. (2000). *As long as they don't move next door: Segregation and racial conflict in American neighborhoods*. Lanham, MD: Rowman & Littlefield.

81. Denton, *Half empty or half full*.

82. Redwood, Y., Schulz, A., & Israel, B. (2010). Social, economic, and political processes that create built environment inequities: Perspectives from urban African Americans in Atlanta. *Family & Community Health*, *33*, pp. 53–67.
    Collins, W., & Margo R. (2000). Residential segregation and socioeconomic outcomes: when did ghettos go bad? *Economic Letters*, *69*, pp. 239–243.
    Krivo, L., Peterson, R., Rizzo, H., Reynolds, J. (1998). Race, segregation and the concentration of disadvantage: 1980–1990. *Social Problems*, *45*, pp. 61–80.
    Yinger, J. (1997). Cash in your face: The cost of racial and ethnic discrimination in housing. *Journal of Urban Economics*, *42*, pp. 339–365.

83. Farley R. (1993). Continued racial residential segregation in Detroit: Chocolate city, vanilla suburbs: revisited. *Journal of Housing Research*, *4*, pp. 1–38.

84. Bullard, R., Mohai, P., Saha, R., & Wright, B. (2008). Toxic wastes and race at twenty: Why race still matters after all of these years. *Environmental Law*, *38*, pp. 371.

85. Acevedo-Garcia, D., & Osypuk, T. L. (2008). Invited commentary: Residential segregation and health—the complexity of modeling separate social contexts. *American Journal of Epidemiology*, *168*, pp. 1255–8.

86. Polednak, A. (1996). Segregation, discrimination and mortality in U.S. blacks. *Ethnicity and Disease*, *6*, pp. 99–107.

87. Massey & Denton, *American apartheid*.
    Peterson, R., & Krivo, L. (1999). Racial segregation, the concentration of disadvantage, and black and white homicide victimization. *Social Forum*, *14*, pp. 465–493.

88. Wood, E. E. (1919). *The housing of the unskilled wage earner*. New York: Macmillan.

89. Drewnowski, A. (2009). Obesity, diets, and social inequalities. *Nutrition Reviews*, *67 Suppl 1*, pp. S36–S39.
    Yang, T. C., & Matthews, S. A. (2010). The role of social and built environments in predicting self-rated stress: A multilevel analysis in Philadelphia. *Health Place*, *16* (5), pp. 803–810.

90. Census. (2010). *Income, poverty and health insurance coverage in the United States: 2009*. Washington, D.C.: U.S. Bureau of the Census.

91. Jacobs, D. E., Kelly, T., & Sobolewski, J. (2007). Linking public health, housing, and indoor environmental policy: Successes and challenges at local and federal agencies in the United States. *Environmental Health Perspectives*, *115*, pp. 976–982.

92. Wright, P. A., & Kloos, B. (2007). Housing environment and mental health outcomes: A levels of analysis perspective. *Journal of Environmental Psychology*, *27*, pp. 79–89.

Thomson, H., Petticrew, M., & Douglas, M. (2003). Health impact assessment of housing improvements: Incorporating research evidence. *Journal of Epidemiology and Community Health*, *57*, pp. 11–16.

Chapter Six

1. Fritz, H. M., Blount, C., Sokoloski, R., et al. (2008). Hurricane Katrina storm surge reconnaissance. *Journal of Geotechnology and Geoenvironmental Engineering*, *134*, pp. 644–656.
2. Eisenman, D. P., Cordasco, K. M., Asch, S., Golden, J. F., & Glik, D. (2007). Disaster planning and risk communication with vulnerable communities: Lessons from Hurricane Katrina. *American Journal of Public Health*, *97 Suppl 1*, pp. S109–S115.
3. Heerden, I. L., Kemp, P., Bea, R., et al. (2009). How a navigation channel contributed to most of the flooding of New Orleans during Hurricane Katrina. *Public Organization Review*, *9*, pp. 291–304.
4. Elder, K., Xirasagar, S., Miller, N., Bowen, S. A., Glover, S., & Piper, C. (2007). African Americans' decisions not to evacuate New Orleans before Hurricane Katrina: A qualitative study. *American Journal of Public Health*, *97 Suppl 1*, pp. S124–S129.
5. Littman, T. (2006). Lessons from Katrina and Rita: What major disasters can teach transportation planners. *Journal of Transportation Engineering*, *132*, pp. 11–18.
6. Costanza, R., Pérez-Maqueo, O., Martinez, M. L., Sutton, P., Anderson, S. J., & Mulder, K. (2008). The value of coastal wetlands for hurricane protection. *AMBIO: A Journal of the Human Environment*, *37*, pp. 241–248.
7. Comfort, L. K. (2006). Cities at risk. *Urban Affairs Review*, *41*, pp. 501–516.
8. Lund, J., Hannak, E., Fleenor, W., Howitt, R., Mount, J., & Moyel P. (2007). *Envisioning futures for the Sacramento-San Joaquin Delta*. San Francisco: Public Policy Institute of California.
9. Burton, C., & Cutter S. (2008). Levee failures and social vulnerability in the Sacramento-San Joaquin Delta area, California. *Natural Hazards Review*, *9*, pp. 136–149.
10. Haines, A., Kovats, R., Campbell-Lendrum, D., & Corvalan, C. (2006). Climate change and human health: Impacts, vulnerability, and mitigation. *The Lancet*, *367*, pp. 2101–2139. Aalst, M. V. (2006). The impacts of climate change on the risk of natural disasters. *Disasters*, *30*, pp. 5–18.
11. Hajat, S., Ebi, K. L., Kovats, R. S., Menne, B., Edwards, S., & Haines, A. (2005). The human health consequences of flooding in Europe: A review. In: W. Kirch, R. Bertollini, & B. Menne (Eds.), *Extreme weather events and public health responses* (pp. 185–196). Berlin: Springer-Verlag.
12. Veldhuis, J. T., Clemens, F., Sterk, G., & Berends, B. (2010). Microbial risks associated with exposure to pathogens in contaminated urban flood water. *Water Research*, *44*, pp. 2910–8291.
13. Brandt, M., Brown, C., Burkhart, J., et al. (2006). Mold prevention strategies and possible health effects in the aftermath of hurricanes and major floods. *MMWR Morbity and Mortality Weekly Report*, *55*, pp. 1–27.
14. Zareian, F., Krawinkler, H., Ibarra, L., & Lignos, D. (2009). Basic concepts and performance measures in prediction of collapse of buildings under earthquake ground motions. *The Structural Design of Tall and Special Buildings*, *19*, pp. 167–181.
15. Park, J., Towashiraporn, P., Craig, J., Goodno, B. (2009). Seismic fragility analysis of low-rise unreinforced masonry structures. *Engineering Structures*, *31*, pp. 125–137.

16. Birda, J. F., Bommerb, J. J., Crowley, H., & Pinh, R. (2005). Modelling liquefaction-induced building damage in earthquake loss estimation. *Soil Dynamics and Earthquake Engineering*, *26*, pp. 15–30.

17. Eberhart-Phillips, J., Saunders, T., Robinson, A., Hatch, D., & Parrish, R. G. (2007). Profile of mortality from the 1989 Loma Prieta Earthquake using coroner and medical examiner reports. *Disasters*, *18*, pp. 160–170.

18. Bolin, H. (1952). The Field Act of the State of California. In *Proceedings of the Symposium on Earthquake Blast Effects on Structures* (pp. 209–313). Berkeley, CA: Earthquake Engineering Research Institute.

19. Clements, B. (2009). *Disasters and public health: Planning and response.* Burlington MA: Butterworth-Heinemann.

20. Fouillet, A., Rey, G., Laurent, F., et al. (2006). Excess mortality related to the August 2003 heat wave in France. *International Archives of Occupational and Environmental Health*, *80*, pp. 16–24.

21. Klinenberg, E. (2002). *Heat wave: A social autopsy of disaster in Chicago.* Chicago: University of Chicago Press.

22. Basu R. (2009). High ambient temperature and mortality: A review of epidemiologic studies from 2001 to 2008. *Environmental Health*, *8*, pp. 40.

23. Kovats, R. S., & Hajat, S. (2008). Heat stress and public health: A critical review. *Annual Review of Public Health*, *29*, pp. 41–55.

24. Hajat, S., O'Connor, M., & Kosatsky, T. (2010). Health effects of hot weather: from awareness of risk factors to effective health protection. *Lancet*, *375*, pp. 856–863.

25. Lopez, R., & Goldoftas, B. (2009). The urban elderly in the United States: Health status and the environment. *Reviews on Environmental Health*, *24*, pp. 47–57.

26. Shusterman, D., Kaplan, J. Z., & Canabarro, C. (1993). Immediate health effects of an urban wildfire. *Western Journal of Medicine*, *158*, pp. 133–138.

27. Keeley, J., Safford, H., Fotheringham, C. J., Franklin, J., & Moritz, M. (2009). The 2007 Southern California wildfires: Lessons in complexity. *The Journal of Forestry*, *107*, pp. 287–296.
    Jakes, P., Kruger, L., Monroe, M., Nelson, K., & Sturtevant, V. (2007). Improving wildfire preparedness: Lessons from communities across the U.S. *Human Ecology*, *14*, pp. 188–197.

28. Birkland, T. (2009). Disasters, catastrophes, and policy failure in the homeland security era. *Review of Policy Research*, *26*, pp. 423–348.

29. Lein, L., Angel, R., & Bell, H. (2009). The state and civil society response to disaster: The challenge of coordination. *Organization and Environment*, *22*, pp. 448–457.

30. Schneider, S. (2005). Administrative breakdowns in the governmental response to Hurricane Katrina. *Public Administration Review*, *65*, pp. 515–516.

31. Gerber, B. (2009). Local government performance and the challenges of regional preparedness for disasters. *Public Performance and Management Review*, *32*, pp. 345–371.

32. Kapucu, N. (2007). Non-profit response to catastrophic disasters. *Disaster Prevention and Management*, *16*, pp. 551–561.

33. Steinberg T. (2006). *Acts of God: The unnatural history of natural disaster in America.* New York: Oxford University Press.

34. Rebmann, T., & Carrico R. (2008). Lessons public health professionals learned from past disasters. *Public Health Nursing*, *25*, pp. 349–352.

35. Harrald, J. (2006). Agility and discipline: Critical success factors for disaster response. *Annals of the American Academy of Political and Social Science*, *604*, pp. 256–722.

36. Fullerton, C. (2009). *Posttraumatic stress disorder: Acute and long-term responses to trauma and disaster*. Washington, D.C.: American Psychiatric Press.

    Dewo, P., Magetsari, R., & Busscher, H. (2008). Treating natural disaster victims is dealing with shortages: An orthopaedics perspective. *Technology and Health, 165*, pp. 255–259.

    Ivers, L. C., & Ryan, E. T. (2006). Infectious diseases of severe weather-related and flood-related natural disasters. *Current Opinions in Infectious Disease, 19*, pp. 408–414.

37. Mille, A., & Arquilla, B. (2008). Chronic diseases and natural hazards: impact of disasters on diabetic, renal, and cardiac patients. *Prehospital Disaster Medicine, 23*, pp. 185–194.

38. Noji, E. (2005). Public health issues in disasters. *Critical Care Medicine, 33*, pp. 1.

39. Phillips, B. (2009). *Disaster recovery*. Boca Raton, FL: Auerbach.

40. Kunreuther, H. (2006). Disaster mitigation and insurance: Learning from Katrina. *Annals of the American Academy of Political and Social Science, 604*, pp. 208–227.

41. Gotham, K., & Greenburg, M. (2009). From 9/11 to 8/29: Post-disaster recovery and rebuilding in New York and New Orleans. *Social Forces, 87*, pp. 1039–1062.

    Culpepper, D. (2008). Price gouging in the Katrina aftermath: Free markets at work. *International Journal of Social Economics, 35*, pp. 512–520.

42. Hartman, C., & Squires, G. (2006). *There is no such thing as a natural disaster: Race, class, and Hurricane Katrina*. New York: Routledge.

43. Kusumasari, B., & Alam Q. (2010). Resource capability for local government in managing disaster. *Disaster Prevention and Management, 19*, pp. 438–51.

44. Davis T. (2002). *Brownfields: A comprehensive guide to redeveloping contaminated property*. Chicago: American Bar Association.

45. *Brownfields FAQ*. (2011). Accessed January 19, 2011, at http://www.brownfieldscenter.org/big/faq.shtml.

46. Lee, C. (2002). Environmental justice: Building a unified vision of health and the environment. *Environmental Health Perspectives, 110 Suppl 2*, pp. 141–144.

47. Johnson, M. (2001). Environmental impacts of urban sprawl: A survey of the literature and proposed research agenda. *Environment and Planning A, 33*, pp. 735.

48. Ding, E. (2008). Brownfield remediation for urban health: A systematic review and case assessment of Baltimore, Maryland. *The Journal of Young Investigators, 14*.

49. Siikamaki, J. (2008). Turning brownfields into greenspaces: Examining incentives and barriers to revitalization. *Journal of Health Politics, Policy, and Law, 33*, pp. 559–593.

50. McCarthy, L. (2002). The brownfield dual land-use policy challenge: Reducing barriers to private redevelopment while connecting reuse to broader community goals. *Land Use Policy, 19*, pp. 717–733.

51. Greenberg, M., Lowrie, K., Solitare, L., & Duncan, L. (2000). Brownfields, TOADS, and the struggle for neighborhood redevelopment. *Urban Affairs Review, 35*, pp. 733.

    Engle, K. (1997). Brownfield initiatives and environmental justice: Second-class cleanups or market-based equity. *Journal of Natural Resources & Environmental Law, 13*, pp. 317.

52. Nolan, J. R. (2007). Zoning and land use planning. *Real Estate Law Journal, 36*, pp. 211–231.

    Waldner, L. (2008). Into the black hole: Do local governments implement their spatial policies? *Land Use Policy, 26*, pp. 818–827.

53. Knobloch, D. (2005). Moving a community in the aftermath of the great 1993 midwest flood. *Journal of Contemporary Water Research & Education, 130*, pp. 41–45.

54. Elmore, A. J., & Kaushal, S. S. (2008). Disappearing headwaters: patterns of stream burial due to urbanization. *Frontiers in Ecology and the Environment*, *6*, pp. 308–312.

55. Middleton, B. R. (2009). Where the river meets the city: Tracing Los Angeles' social and environmental movements. *City*, *13*, pp. 150–152.

56. Gottlieb R. *Forcing the spring: The transformation of the american environmental movement*. Washington, D.C.: Island Press. (1993).

57. Shustera, W. D., Bontab, J., Thurstona, H., Warnemuendec, E., & Smith, D. R. (2005). Impacts of impervious surface on watershed hydrology: A review. *Urban Water Journal*, *2*, pp. 263–75.

58. Kirk, K. (2006). Clean water threatened—As federal dollars decline, the cost of clean rises. *Newsletter of the Urban Water Council*.

59. American Society of Civil Engineers. (2005). *States report 2005*. Reston, VA: American Society of Civil Engineers.

60. Pagano, M., & Perry, D. (2008). Financing infrastructure in the 21st century city. *Public Works Management & Policy*, *13*, pp. 22–38.

61. Westphal, J. (2008). The politics of infrastructure. *Social Research: An International Quarterly*, *75*, pp. 793–804.

62. Adams, C. (2007). Urban governance and the control of infrastructure. *Public Works Management & Policy*, *11*, pp. 164–176.

63. Marcuson W. (2008). Fixing America's crumbling infrastructure: A call to action for all. *Public Works Management & Policy*, *12*, pp. 473–475.

64. Bedimo-Rung, A. L., Mowen, A. J., & Cohen, D. A. (2005). The significance of parks to physical activity and public health: A conceptual model. *American Journal of Preventive Medicine*, *28*, pp. 1591 1568.
    Cohen, D. A., McKenzie, T. L., Sehgal, A., Williamson, S., Golinelli, D., & Lurie, N. (2007). Contribution of public parks to physical activity. *American Journal of Public Health*, *97*, pp. 509–514.
    Grow, H. M., Saelens, B. E., Kerr, J., Durant, N. H., Norman, G. J., & Sallis, J. F. (2008). Where are youth active? Roles of proximity, active transport, and built environment. *Medicine and Science in Sports and Exercise*, *40*, pp. 2071–2079.

65. Bedimo-Rung, A. L., Mowen, A. J., & Cohen, D. A. (2005). The significance of parks to physical activity and public health: A conceptual model. *American Journal of Preventive Medicine*, *28*, pp. 159–168.

66. Grow, et al., Where are youth active?

67. Lopez, R., Campbell, R., & Jennings, J. (2008). The Boston Schoolyard Initiative: A public-private partnership for rebuilding urban play spaces. *Journal of Health Politics, Policy, and Law*, *33*, pp. 617–638.

68. Pickett, S. T. A., Cadenasso, M. L., Grove, J. M., et al. (2008). Urban ecological systems: Linking terrestrial ecological, physical, and socioeconomic components of metropolitan areas. *Annual Review of Ecology, Evolution, and Systematics*, *32*, pp. 127–157.

69. Floyd, M. F., Spengler, J. O., Maddock, J. E., Gobster, P. H., & Suau, L. J. (2008). Park-based physical activity in diverse communities of two U.S. cities. An observational study. *American Journal of Preventive Medicine*, *34*, pp. 299–305.

70. Keizer, K., Lindenberg, S., & Steg, L. (2008). The spreading of disorder. *Science*, *322*, pp. 1681–1685.
    Loukaitou-Sideris, A., & Eck, J. E. (2007). Crime prevention and active living. *American Journal of Health Promotion*, *21*, pp. 380–389, iii.

71. McCormack, G., Rock, M., & Toohey, A. (2010). Characteristics of urban parks associated with park use and physical activity: A review of qualitative research. *Health & Place, 16*, pp. 712–726.

72. Lopez, et al,. The Boston Schoolyard Initiative.

73. U.S. Consumer Product Safety Commission. (2008). *Public Playground Safety Handbook*. http://www.cpsc.gov/cpscpub/pubs/325.pdf. Washington DC: U.S. Consumer Product Safety Commission.

Chapter Seven

1. Whitmire, G., & Diver, J. (2005). Exposure assessment. In P. Wexler (Ed.), *Encyclopedia of toxicology*. San Diego: Academic Press.

2. Frank, L. D., Sallis, J. F., Conway, T. L., Chapman, J. E., Saelens, B. E., & Bachman W. (2006). Many pathways from land use to health: Associations between neighborhood walkability and active transportation, Body Mass Index, and air quality. *Journal of the American Planning Association, 72*, pp. 75–87.

3. Ringquist, E. J. (1993). Does regulation matter? Evaluating the effects of state air pollution control programs. *The Journal of Politics, 55*, pp. 1022–1045.

4. Brulle, R. J., & Pellow, D. N. (2006). Environmental justice: Human health and environmental inequalities. *Annual Reviews of Public Health, 27*, pp. 103–124.

5. Doremus, H., & Hanemann, W. M. (2008). Of babies and bathwater: Why the Clean Air Act's cooperative federalism framework Is useful for addressing global warming. *Arizona Law Review, 50*, pp. 799–834.

6. Levin, H. (1990). Critical building design factors for indoor air quality and climate: Current status and predicted trends. *Indoor Air, 1*, pp. 79–82.

7. Hubbell, B. J., Crume, R. V., Evarts, D. M., & Cohen, J. M. (2010). Regulation and progress under the 1990 Clean Air Act amendments. *Review of Environmental Economics and Policy, 4*, pp. 122–138.

8. Gilbreath, S., & Yap, P. (2008). The potential impact of residential wood burning regulations in a California region: Concurrent wintertime reductions in ambient pollution and cardiovascular mortality. *Epidemiology, 19*, p. S252.

9. Fenger, J. (2009). Air pollution in the last 50 years—from local to global. *Atmospheric Environment, 19*, pp. 43.

10. Eriksen, M. P., & Cerak, R. L. (2008). The diffusion and impact of clean indoor air laws. *Annual Reviews of Public Health, 29*, pp. 171–185.

11. Makri, A., & Stilianakis, N. I. (2008). Vulnerability to air pollution health effects. *International Journal of Hygiene and Environmental Health, 211*, pp. 326–336.

12. Araujo, J. A., & Nel, A. E. (2009). Particulate matter and atherosclerosis: Role of particle size, composition and oxidative stress. *Particle and Fibre Toxicology, 6*, p. 24.

13. Sioutas, C., Delfino, R. J., & Singh, M. (2005). Exposure assessment for atmospheric ultrafine particles (UFPs) and implications in epidemiologic research. *Environmental Health Perspectives, 113*, pp. 947–955.

14. Araujo & Nel, Particulate matter and atherosclerosis.
    Dales, R., Liu, L., Szyszkowicz, M., et al. (2007). Particulate air pollution and vascular reactivity: The bus stop study. *International Archives of Occupational and Environmental Health, 81*, pp. 159–164.

Mindell, J., Joffe, M. (2004). Predicted health impacts of urban air quality management. *Journal of Epidemiology and Community Health, 58*, pp. 103–113.

Ravindra, Mittal, A. K., Van Grieken, R. (2001). Health risk assessment of urban suspended particulate matter with special reference to polycyclic aromatic hydrocarbons: a review. *Reviews of Environmental Health, 16*, pp. 169–89.

15. Mindell & Joffe, Predicted health impacts of urban air quality management.

    Curtis, L., Rea, W., Smith-Willis, P., Fenyves, E., & Pan Y. (2006). Adverse health effects of outdoor air pollutants. *Environ Int, 32*, pp. 815–830.

16. Maricq, M. M. (2007). Chemical characterization of particulate emissions from diesel engines: A review. *Journal of Aerosol Science, 38*, pp. 1079–1118.

17. Houston, D., Krudysz, M., & Winer, A. (2008). Diesel truck traffic in low-income and minority communities adjacent to ports: Environmental justice implications of near-roadway land use conflicts. *Transportation Research Record: Journal of the Transportation Research Board, 2067*, pp. 38–46.

18. Brown, P., Mayer, B., Zavestoski, S., Luebke, T., Mandelbaumc, J., & McCormick, S. (2003). The health politics of asthma: Environmental justice and collective illness experience in the United States. *Social Science and Medicine, 57*, pp. 453–464.

19. Appleton, J. D. (2007). Radon: Sources, health risks, and hazard mapping. *Ambio, 36*, pp. 85–89.

20. Gadgil, A. J. (1992). Models of radon entry. *Radiation Protection Dossimetry, 45*, pp. 373–379.

21. U.S. Environmental Protection Agency. (2010). *Radon*. Washington, D.C.: U.S. Environmental Protection Agency.

22. U.S. Environmental Protection Agency. (2010). *A citizen's guide to radon*. Washington, D.C.: U.S. Environmental Protection Agency.

23. Nazaroff, W. W., & Nero, A. V. (1988). *Radon and its decay products in indoor air*. New York: Wiley.

24. Brown, S. K., Sim, M. R., Abramson, M. J., & Gray, C. N. (2008). Concentrations of volatile organic compounds in indoor air—A review. *Indoor Air, 4*, pp. 123–134.

25. Mitchell, C. S., Zhang, J. J., Sigsgaard, T., et al. (2007). Current state of the science: health effects and indoor environmental quality. *Environmental Health Perspectives, 115*, pp. 958–964.

26. Jones, A. P. (2000). Asthma and the home environment. *Journal of Asthma, 37*, pp. 103–124.

27. Lupoli, T. A., Ciaccio, C. E., & Portnoy, J. M. (2009). Home and school environmental assessment and remediation. *Current Allergy & Asthma Reports, 9*, pp. 419–425.

28. Corn, J. K., & Starr, J. (1987). Historical perspective on asbestos: Policies and protective measures in World War II shipbuilding. *American Journal of Industrial Medicine, 11*, pp. 359–373.

29. Garfinkel, L. (1984). Asbestos: Historical perspective. *CA: A Cancer Journal for Clinicians, 34*, pp. 44–47.

30. Brody, A. R. (1993). Asbestos-induced lung disease. *Environmental Health Perspectives, 100*, pp. 21–30.

    Lasky, J. A., Bonner, J. C., & Brody, A. R. (1991). The pathobiology of asbestos-induced lung disease: A proposed role for macrophage-derived growth factors. *Annals of the New York Academy of Science, 643*, pp. 239–244.

31. Matrat, M., Pairon, J. C., Paolillo, A. G., et al. (2004). Asbestos exposure and radiological abnormalities among maintenance and custodian workers in buildings with friable

asbestos-containing materials. *International Archives of Occupational and Environmental Health*, *77*, pp. 307–312.

Gaensler, E. A. (1992). Asbestos exposure in buildings. *Clinics in Chest Medicine*, *13*, pp. 231–242.

32. Bang, K. M., Pinheiro, G. A., Wood, J. M., & Syamlal, G. (2006). Malignant mesothelioma mortality in the United States, 1999–2001. *International Journal of Occupational Environmental Health*, *12*, pp. 9–15.

33. U.S. Environmental Protection Agency. (2010). *Asbestos*. http//www.epa.gov/asbestos/. Washington, D.C.: U.S. Environmental Protection Agency.

34. Nriagu, J. (1990). The rise and fall of leaded gasoline. *Science of the Total Environment*, *92*, pp. 13–28.

    Rosner, D., & Markowitz, G. (2007). The politics of lead toxicology and the devastating consequences for children. *American Journal of Industrial Medicine*, *50*, pp. 740–756.

35. Lewis, J. (1985). Lead poisoning: A historical perspective. *Journal of the Environmental Protection Agency*, *11*, pp. 15–20.

36. Rogan, W. J., & Ware, J. H. (2003). Exposure to lead in children—how low is low enough? *New England Journal of Medicine*, *348*, pp. 1515–1516.

    Warniment, C., Tsang, K., & Galazka, S. S. (2010). Lead poisoning in children. *American Family Physician*, *81*, pp. 751–757.

37. Bell, M. L., Peng, R. D., Dominici, F., & Samet, J. M. (2009). Emergency hospital admissions for cardiovascular diseases and ambient levels of carbon monoxide: Results for 126 United States urban counties, 1999–2005. *Circulation*, *120*, pp. 949–955.

    Samoli, E., Touloumi, G., Schwartz, J., et al. (2007). Short-term effects of carbon monoxide on mortality: An analysis within the APHEA project. *Environmental Health Perspectives*, *115*, pp. 1578–1583.

    Graber, J. M., Macdonald, S. C., Kass, D. E., Smith, A. E., & Anderson, H. A. (2007). Carbon monoxide: The case for environmental public health surveillance. *Public Health Reports*, *122*, pp. 138–144.

38. Centers for Disease Control and Prevention. (2008). Nonfatal, unintentional, non-fire-related carbon monoxide exposures—United States, 2004–2006. *MMWR Morbity and Mortality Weekly Report*, *57*, pp. 896–899.

39. Dales, R., Liu, L., Wheeler, A. J., Gilbert, N. L. (2008). Quality of indoor residential air and health. *CMAJ*, *179*, pp. 147–152.

40. Brooks, N., & Sethi, R. (1997). The distribution of pollution: Community characteristics and exposure to air toxics. *Journal of Environmental Economics and Management*, *32*, pp. 233–50.

    National air toxics assessment. (2001). Environmental Protection Agency. Accessed November 6, 2002, at http://www.epa.gov/ttn/atw/nata/natsalim2.html.

41. Lopez, R. (2002). Segregation and black/white differences in exposure to air toxics in 1990. *Environmental Health Perspectivesives*, *110*, pp. 289–295.

    Morello-Frosch, R., Pastor, M., & Sadd, J. (2001). The distribution of air toxics exposures and health risks among diverse communities. *Urban Affairs Review*, *36*, pp. 551–578.

42. Peden, D. (2002). Pollutants and asthma: Role of air toxics. *Environmental Health Perspectives*, *110*, pp. 565–568.

    Rosenbaum, A., Axelrad, D., Woodruff, T., Wei, Y., Ligocki, M., & Cohen, J. (1999). National estimates of outdoor air toxics concentrations. *Journal of the Air and Waste Management Association*, *49*, pp. 1138–1152.

43. National air toxics assessment.

Woodruff, T., Axelrad, D., Caldwell, J., Morello-Frosch, R., & Rosenbaum, A. (1998). Public health implications of 1990 air toxics concentrations across the United States. *Environmental Health Perspectivesives*, *106*, pp. 245–251.

Wu, C., & Pratt, G. (2001). Analysis of air toxics emission inventory: inhalation toxicity-based ranking. *Journal of the Air Waste Management Association*, *51*, pp. 1129–1141.

44. Godwin, C., & Batterman, S. (2007). Indoor air quality in Michigan schools. *Indoor Air*, *17*, pp. 109–121.

Petronella, S. A., Thomas, R., Stone, J. A., Goldblum, R. M., & Brooks, E. G. (2005). Clearing the air: A model for investigating indoor air quality in Texas schools. *Journal of Environmental Health*, *67*, pp. 35–42.

45. Daisey, J., Angell, W., & Apte, M. (2003). Indoor air quality, ventilation and health symptoms in schools: An analysis of existing information. *Indoor Air*, *13*, pp. 53–64.

46. U.S. Environmental Protection Agency. (2010). *IAQ — Tools for Schools Program*. Washington, D.C.: U.S. Environmental Protection Agency.

47. Yolton, K., Dietrich, K., Auinger, P., Lanphear, B., & Hornung, R. (2005). Exposure to environmental tobacco smoke and cognitive abilities among U.S. children and adolescents. *Environmental Health Perspectivesives*, *113*, pp. 98–103.

Jefferis, B. J., Thomson, A. G., Lennon, L. T., et al. (2009). Changes in environmental tobacco smoke (ETS) exposure over a 20-year period: cross-sectional and longitudinal analyses. *Addiction*, *104*, pp. 496–503.

48. Stolzenberg, L., & D'Alessio, S. J. (2007). Is nonsmoking dangerous to the health of restaurants? The effect of California's indoor smoking ban on restaurant revenues. *Evaluation Review*, *31*, pp. 75–92.

Wakefield, M., Roberts, L., & Miller, C. (1999). Perceptions of the effect of an impending restaurant smoking ban on dining-out experience. *Preventive Medicine*, *29*, pp. 53–56.

49. McMillen, R. .C, Winickoff, J. P., Klein, J. D., & Weitzman, M. (2003). U.S. adult attitudes and practices regarding smoking restrictions and child exposure to environmental tobacco smoke: Changes in the social climate from 2000–2001. *Pediatrics*, *112*, pp. e55–e60.

Muilenburg Legge, J., Latham, T., Annang, L., et al. (2009). The home smoking environment: Influence on behaviors and attitudes in a racially diverse adolescent population. *Health Education & Behavior*, *36*, pp. 777–793.

50. Franchini, M., & Mannucci, P. M. (2009). Particulate air pollution and cardiovascular risk: short-term and long-term effects. *Seminars in Thrombosis and Hemostasis*, *35*, pp. 665–670.

51. Laumbach, R. J. (2010). Patient information: Outdoor air pollution and your health. *American Family Physician*, *81*, pp. 181.

52. Link, M. S., & Dockery, D. W. (2010). Air pollution and the triggering of cardiac arrhythmias. *Current Opinions in Cardiology*, *25*, pp. 16–22.

Peters, A., Dockery, D. W., Muller, J. E., & Mittleman, M. A. (2001). Increased particulate air pollution and the triggering of myocardial infarction. *Circulation*, *103*, pp. 2810–2815.

53. U.S. Environmental Protection Agency. (2009). Integrated Science Assessment for Particulate Matter (External Review Draft). Research Triangle Park. http://cfpub.epa.gov/ncea/isa/recordisplay.cfm?deid=201805.

54. Woodruff, T. J., Grillo, J., & Schoendorf, K. C. (1997). The relationship between selected causes of postneonatal infant mortality and particulate air pollution in the United States. *Environmental Health Perspectives*, *105*, pp. 608–612.

55. Dannenberg, A. L., Jackson, R. J., Frumkin, H., et al. (2003). The impact of community design and land-use choices on public health: A scientific research agenda. *American Journal of Public Health*, *93*, pp. 1500–1508.

56. Gee, G. C., & Payne-Sturges, D. C. (2004). Environmental health disparities: A framework integrating psychosocial and environmental concepts. *Environmental Health Perspectives*, *112*, pp. 1645–1653.

57. Gern, J. E., Visness, C. M., Gergen, P. J., et al. (2009). The urban environment and childhood asthma (URECA) birth cohort study: Design, methods, and study population. *BMC Pulmonary Medicine*, *9*, p. 17.

58. Patel, M. M., & Miller, R. L. (2009). Air pollution and childhood asthma: Recent advances and future directions. *Current Opinion in Pediatrics*, *21*, pp. 235–242.
    Neidell, M. J. (2004). Air pollution, health, and socio-economic status: The effect of outdoor air quality on childhood asthma. *Journal of Health and Economics*, *23*, pp. 1209–1236.
    Salvi, S. (2003). Ambient particulate air pollution and childhood asthma exacerbations. *Annals of Allergy and Asthma Immunology*, *91*, pp. 321–323.

59. Salo, P. M., Sever, M. L., & Zeldin, D. C. (2009). Indoor allergens in school and day care environments. *Journal of Allergy and Clinical Immunology*, *124*, pp. 185–92, e1–e9 (quiz 93–4).
    Northridge, J., Ramirez, O. F., Stingone, J. A., & Claudio, L. (2010). The role of housing type and housing quality in urban children with asthma. *Journal of Urban Health*, *87*, pp. 211–224.
    Rosenbaum, E. (2008). Racial/ethnic differences in asthma prevalence: The role of housing and neighborhood environments. *Journal of Health and Social Behavior*, *49*, pp. 131–145.
    Frisk, M., Arvidsson, H., Kiviloog, J., Ivarsson, A. B., Kamwendo, K., & Stridh, G. (2006). An investigation of the housing environment for persons with asthma and persons without asthma. *Scandinavian Journal of Occupational Therapy*, *13*, pp. 4–12.

60. Hahn, E. J., Ashford, K. B., Okoli, C. T., Rayens, M. K., Ridner, S. L., & York, N. L. (2009). Nursing research in community-based approaches to reduce exposure to secondhand smoke. *Annual Review of Nursing Research*, *27*, pp. 365–391.

61. Hynes, H. P., Brugge, D., Osgood, N. D., Snell, J., Vallarino, J., & Spengler, J. (2004). Investigations into the indoor environment and respiratory health in Boston public housing. *Reviews of Environmental Health*, *19*, pp. 271–289.

62. Williams, D., Portnoy, J. M., & Meyerson, K. (2010). Strategies for improving asthma outcomes: A case-based review of successes and pitfalls. *Journal of Managed Care Pharmacology*, *16*, pp. S3–14 (quiz S6–7).

63. Straus, D. C. (2009). Molds, mycotoxins, and sick building syndrome. *Toxicology and Industrial Health*, *25*, pp. 617–635.
    Norback, D. (2009). An update on sick building syndrome. *Current Opinion in Allergy and Clinical Immunology*, *9*, pp. 55–59.
    Fisk, W. J., Mirer, A. G., & Mendell, M. J. (2009). Quantitative relationship of sick building syndrome symptoms with ventilation rates. *Indoor Air*, *19*, pp. 159–165.

64. Lee, T. G. (2009). Mold remediation in a hospital. *Toxicology & Industrial Health*, *25*, pp. 723–730.

65. Haverinen-Shaughnessy, U., Hyvarinen, A., Putus, T., & Nevalainen, A. (2008). Monitoring success of remediation: Seven case studies of moisture and mold damaged buildings. *Science of the Total Environment*, *399*, pp. 19–27.

66. Wah, C., & Kim, J. (2010). Building pathology, investigation of sick buildings—VOC emissions. *Indoor and Built Environment*, *19*, pp. 30–39.

Chapter Eight

1. Haller, L., Hutton, G., & Bartram, J. (2007). Estimating the costs and health benefits of water and sanitation improvements at global level. *Journal of Water and Health*, *5*, pp. 467–480.
   Pruss, A., Kay, D., Fewtrell, L., & Bartram, J. (2002). Estimating the burden of disease from water, sanitation, and hygiene at a global level. *Environmental Health Perspectives*, *110*, pp. 537–542.
2. Melosi, M. (2008). *The sanitary city: Environmental services in urban America from colonial times to the present*. Pittsburgh, PA: University of Pittsburgh Press.
   Melosi, M. (2001). *Effluent America: Cities, industry, energy, and the environment*. Pittsburgh, PA: University of Pittsburgh Press.
   Andreen W. (2004). Water quality today—Has the Clean Water Act been a success? *Alabama Law Review*, *55*, pp. 537–594.
3. Tarr, J. (1989). Infrastructure and city-building in the nineteenth and twentieth century. In S. Hayes (Ed.), *City at the point: Essays in the social history of Pittsburgh*. Pittsburgh: University of Pittsburgh Press.
4. Lang, R. (2003). Open spaces, bounded places: Does the American West's arid landscape yield dense metropolitan growth? *Housing Policy Debate*, *13*, pp. 758–778.
5. Tiemann, M. (2001). Environmental laws: Safe Drinking Water Act. In V. A. Silyok (Ed.), *Summaries of statutes administered by the Environmental Protection Agency*. Huntington, NY: Nova Science Press.
6. Copeland, C. (2001). Clean Water Act. In V. A. Silyok (Ed.), *Summaries of statutes administered by the Environmental Protection Agency*. Huntington, NY: Nova Science Press.
7. Adler R. (2009). Institutions affecting the urban water environment. In L. Baker (Ed.), *The water environment of cities*. New York: Springer.
8. Ibid.
9. Johnson, S. (2006). *The ghost map*. New York: Riverhead Books.
10. Tarr, J. (1984). The evolution of urban infrastructure in the nineteenth and twentieth centuries. In R. Hanson (Ed.), *Perspectives on urban infrastructure*. Washington, D.C.: National Academies Press.
11. Schultz, S., & McShane, C. (1976). To engineer the metropolis: Sewers, sanitation, and city planning in late-nineteenth-century America. *The Journal of American History*, *65*, pp. 389–411.
12. Marcuson, W. (2008). Fixing America's crumbling infrastructure: A call to action for all. *Public Works Management & Policy*, *12*, pp. 473–435.
    Pagano, M., & Perry, D. (2008). Financing infrastructure in the 21st century city. *Public Works Management & Policy*, *13*, pp. 22–38.
    Westphal, J. (2008). The politics of infrastructure. *Social Research: An International Quarterly*, *75*, pp. 793–804.
13. Rosen, G. (1993). *A history of public health*. Baltimore, MD: Johns Hopkins University Press.

14. Szreter, S., & Mooney, G. (1998). Urbanization, mortality, and the standard of living debate: New estimates of the expectation of life at birth in nineteenth century British cities. *Economic History Review*, *51*, pp. 84–92.

15. McGuire, M. (2006). Eight revolutions in the history of U.S. drinking water disinfection. *AWWA Journal*, *98*, pp. 123–149.

16. MacKenzie, W. R., Schell, W. L., Blair, K. A., et al. (1995). Massive outbreak of waterborne cryptosporidium infection in Milwaukee, Wisconsin: Recurrence of illness and risk of secondary transmission. *Clinical Infectious Disease*, *21*, pp. 57–62.

17. Adams, B., & Foster S. (2007). Land-surface zoning for groundwater protection. *Water and Environment Journal*, *6*, pp. 312–319.

18. Ward, L. A., Cain, O. L., Mullally, R. A., et al. (2009). Health beliefs about bottled water: A qualitative study. *BMC Public Health*, *9*, pp. 196.

19. Arnold, E. (2006). Bottled water: Pouring resources down the drain. Washington, D.C.: Earth Policy Institute.

20. Gleick, P. H., & Cooley, H. S. (2009). Energy implications of bottled water. *Environmental Research Letters*, *4*, pp. 1–6.

21. Napier, G. L., & Kodner, C. M. (2008). Health risks and benefits of bottled water. *Primary Care*, *35*, pp. 789–802.

22. Parag, Y., Roberts, J. T. (2009). A battle against the bottles: Building, claiming, and regaining tap-water trustworthiness. *Society and Natural Resources*, *22*, pp. 625–636.

23. Cech, T. V. (2003). *Principles of water resources: History, development, management, and policy.* Hoboken NJ: Wiley.

24. Duhigg, C. (2010, March 22). U.S. bolsters chemical restrictions for water. *New York Times.*

25. Proctor, M. E., Blair, K. A., Davis, J. P. (1998). Surveillance data for waterborne illness detection: An assessment following a massive waterborne outbreak of Cryptosporidium infection. *Epidemiology and Infection*, *120*, pp. 43–54.

26. Morris, R. (2007). *Blue death: True tales of disease, disaster, and the water we drink.* New York: HarperCollins.

27. Ibid.

28. Duhigg, C. (2009 December 7). Millions in U.S. drink dirty water, records show. *New York Times.*

29. Gray, N. F. (2008). Drinking water quality: Problems and solutions. Cambridge, UK: Cambridge University Press.

30. Asano, T., Burton, F., Leverenz, H., Tsuchihashi, R., & Tchobanoglous, G. (2006). *Water reuse: Issues, technologies, and applications.* New York: McGraw-Hill.

31. Hayes, T., Wilson, R., & Hansen, E. (2006). GIS streamlines recycled water management. *OPFlow*, *32*, pp. 20–23.

32. Hartley, T. (2004). Public perception and participation in water reuse. *Desalination*, *187*, pp. 115–126.

33. Miller, W. (2004). Integrated concepts in water reuse: Managing global water needs. *Desalination*, *187*, pp. 65–75.

34. Khawaji, A. D., Kutubkhanah, I. K., & Wie, J.-M. (2007). Advances in seawater desalination technologies. *Desalination*, *221*, pp. 47–69.

35. Fritzmann, C., Löwenberg, J., Wintgens, T., & Melin T. (2007). State-of-the-art of reverse osmosis desalination. *Desalination*, *216*, pp. 1–76.

Lattemann, S., & Höpner T. (2008). Environmental impact and impact assessment of seawater desalination. *Desalination, 220*, pp. 1–15.

36. Heisler, J., Glibert, P. M., Burkholder, J. M., et al. (2008). Eutrophication and harmful algal blooms: A scientific consensus. *Harmful Algae, 8*, pp. 3–13.

37. Jarvie, H. P., Neal, C., & Withers, P. J. A. (2006). Sewage-effluent phosphorus: A greater risk to river eutrophication than agricultural phosphorus? *Science of the Total Environment, 360*, pp. 246–253.

38. Gay, J., Webster, R., Roberts, D., & Trett, M. (2007). Environmental implications of treatment of coastal sewage discharges. *Water and Environment Journal, 5*, pp. 573–580.

39. McLellan, S. L., Hollis, E. J., Depas, M. M., Dyke, M. V., Harris, J., & Scopel, C. O. (2007). Distribution and fate of Escherichia coli in Lake Michigan following contamination with urban stormwater and combined sewer overflows. *Journal of Great Lakes Research, 33*, pp. 565–580.

40. Hall, J. E. (2007). Sewage sludge production, treatment and disposal in the European Union. *Water and Environment Journal, 9*, pp. 335–343.

41. McGrath, S. P., Knight, B., Killham, K., Preston, S., & Paton, G. I. (2009). Assessment of the toxicity of metals in soils amended with sewage sludge using a chemical speciation technique and a lux-based biosensor. *Environmental Toxicology and Chemistry, 18*, pp. 659–683.

42. Cantor, K. P. (1997). Drinking water and cancer. *Cancer Causes Control, 8*, pp. 292–308.
    Aggazzotti, G., Righi, E., Fantuzzi, G., et al. (2004). Chlorination by-products (CBPs) in drinking water and adverse pregnancy outcomes in Italy. *Journal of Water and Health, 2*, pp. 233–247.
    Bove, F., Shim, Y., & Zeitz P. (2002). Drinking water contaminants and adverse pregnancy outcomes: a review. *Environmental Health Perspectives, 110 Suppl 1*, pp. 61–74.

43. Fiss, E. M., Rule, K. L., & Vikesland, P. J. (2007). Formation of chloroform and other chlorinated byproducts by chlorination of triclosan-containing antibacterial products. *Environmental Science and Technology, 41*, pp. 2387–2394.
    Gopal, K., Tripathy, S. S., Bersillon, J. L., & Dubey, S. P. (2007). Chlorination byproducts, their toxicodynamics and removal from drinking water. *Journal of Hazardous Materials, 140*, pp. 1–6.
    Nieuwenhuijsen, M. J., Toledano, M. B., Eaton, N. E., Fawell, J., & Elliott P. (2000). Chlorination disinfection byproducts in water and their association with adverse reproductive outcomes: A review. *Occupational and Environmental Medicine, 57*, pp. 73–85.

44. Edwards, M., Triantafyllidou, S., & Best, D. (2009). Elevated blood lead in young children due to lead-contaminated drinking water: Washington, D.C., 2001-2004. *Environmental Science and Technology, 43*, pp. 1818–1823.

45. U.S. Environmental Protection Agency. (2010). *Actions you can take to reduce lead in drinking water*. Washington, D.C.: U.S. Environmental Protection Agency.

46. Maas, R. P., Patch, S. C., Morgan, D. M., & Pandolfo, T. J. (2005). Reducing lead exposure from drinking water: Recent history and current status. *Public Health Reports, 120*, pp. 316–321.

47. Chalupka, S. (2005). Tainted water on tap: What to tell patients about preventing illness from drinking water. *American Journal of Nursing, 105*, pp. 40–52. (quiz 3).
    Guidotti, T. L., & Ragain, L. (2007). Protecting children from toxic exposure: Three strategies. *Pediatric Clinics of North America, 54*, pp. 227–235, vii.

48. Comerton, A. M., Andrews, R. C., & Bagley, D. M. (2009). Practical overview of analytical methods for endocrine-disrupting compounds, pharmaceuticals and personal care products in water and wastewater. *Philosophical Transactions Series A: Mathematical, Physical and Engineering Sciences*, *367*, pp. 3923–3939.

Rahman, M. F., Yanful, E. K., & Jasim, S. Y. (2009). Endocrine disrupting compounds (EDCs) and pharmaceuticals and personal care products (PPCPs) in the aquatic environment: Implications for the drinking water industry and global environmental health. *Journal of Water and Health*, *7*, pp. 224–243.

49. Heberer, T. (2002). Occurrence, fate, and removal of pharmaceutical residues in the aquatic environment: a review of recent research data. *Toxicological Letters*, *131*, pp. 5–17.

Glassmeyer, S. T., Hinchey, E. K., Boehme, S. E., et al. (2008). Disposal practices for unwanted residential medications in the United States. *Environment International*, *35*, pp. 566–572.

50. Cutter, W. B. (2007). Valuing groundwater recharge in an urban context. *Land Economics*, *83*, pp. 234–252.

51. Carrera-Hernández, J. J., & Gaskin, S. J. (2009). Water management in the Basin of Mexico: Current state and alternative scenarios. *Hydrogeology Journal*, *17*, pp. 1483–1494.

52. Shoham, T. (2006). *Groundwater decline and the preservation of property in Boston*. Cambridge, MA: Massachusetts Institute of Technology.

53. Schnoor, J. L. (2010). Three myths about water. *Environmental Science and Technology*, *44*, pp. 1516–1517.

54. Sophocleous, M. (2005). Groundwater recharge and sustainability in the High Plains aquifer in Kansas, U.S.A. *Hydrogeology Journal*, *13*, pp. 351–365.

55. Iveya, J. L., Loë, R. D., Kreutzwisera, R., & Ferreyra, C. (2006). An institutional perspective on local capacity for source water protection. *Geoforum*, *37*, pp. 944–957.

56. Halich, G., & Stephenson, K. (2009). Effectiveness of residential water-use restrictions under varying levels of municipal effort. *Land Economics*, *85*, pp. 614–626.

57. Ilha, M., & Oliveira, L., Gonçalves, O. (2009). Environmental assessment of residential buildings with an emphasis on water conservation. *Building Services Engineering Research and Technology*, *30*, pp. 15–26.

58. Aitken, C. K., McMahon, T. A., Wearing, A. J., & Finlayson, B. L. (2006). Residential water use: Predicting and reducing consumption. *Journal of Applied Social Psychology*, *24*, pp. 136–158.

59. Michelsen, A. M., McGuckin, J. T., & Stumpf, D. (1999). Nonprice water conservation programs as a demand management tool. *Journal of the American Water Resources Association*, *35*, pp. 593–602.

60. Sovocool, K., Morgan, M., & Bennett, D. (2006). An in-depth investigation of xeriscape as a water conservation measure. *Journal of the American Water Resources Association*, *98*, pp. 82–93.

61. McKenney, C., & Terry R. (1995). The effectiveness of using workshops to change audience perception of and attitudes about xeriscaping. *HortTechnology*, *5*, pp. 327–329.

62. Ismail, Z., & Puad, W.F.W.A. (2007). Non-revenue water losses: A case study. *Environment and Energy Sciences*, *4*, pp. 113–117.

63. Knutson, C. L. (2008). The role of water conservation in drought planning. *Journal of Soil and Water Conservation*, *63*, pp. 159A–160A.

64. Hunaidi, O., & Wang, A. (2006). A new system for locating leaks in urban water distribution pipes. *Management of Environmental Quality*, *17*, pp. 450–466.

65. Mansur, E. T., & Olmstead, S. M. (2003). *The value of scarce water: Measuring the inefficiency of municipal regulations*. Working Paper W13513. Cambridge, MA: National Bureau of Economic Research.

66. Dowd, B. M., Press, D., Huertos, M. L. (2008). Agricultural nonpoint source water pollution policy: The case of California's Central Coast. *Agriculture Ecosystems and Environment*, *128*, pp. 151–161.
    Carpenter, S. R., Caraco, N. F., Correll, D. L., Howarth, R. W., Sharpley, A. N., & Smith V. H. (1998). Nonpoint pollution of surface waters with phosphorus and nitrogen. *Ecological Applications*, *8*, pp. 559–568.

67. Hardy, S., & Koontz T. (2008). Reducing nonpoint source pollution through collaboration: policies and programs across the U.S. States. *Environmental Management*, *41*, pp. 308–310.

68. Chin, D. (2010). Linking pathogen sources to water quality in small urban streams. *Journal of Environmental Engineering*, *136*, pp. 249–523.

69. Pereira, T. (2009). Sustainability: An integral engineering design approach. *Renewable and Sustainable Energy Reviews*, *13*, pp. 1133–1137.

70. Germer, J., Boh, M. Y., Schoeffler, M., & Amoah, P. (2010). Temperature and deactivation of microbial faecal indicators during small scale co-composting of faecal matter. *Waste Management*, *30*, pp. 185–191.

71. Hotta, S., & Funamizu, N. (2007). Biodegradability of fecal nitrogen in composting process. *Bioresource Technology*, *98*, pp. 3412–3414.

72. Cordovaa, A., & Knuth, B. A. (2005). Barriers and strategies for dry sanitation in large-scale and urban settings. *Urban Water Journal*, *2*, pp. 245–262.

Chapter Nine

1. Gardner, D. S., & Rhodes, P. (2009). Developmental origins of obesity: Programming of food intake or physical activity? *Advances in Experimental Medicine and Biology*, *646*, pp. 83–93.

2. Ershow, A. G. (2009). Environmental influences on development of type 2 diabetes and obesity: Challenges in personalizing prevention and management. *Journal of Diabetes Science and Technology*, *3*, pp. 727–734.

3. Pritchett, L. (1997). Divergence, big time. *The Journal of Economic Perspectives*, *11*, pp. 3–17.

4. Chyau, J. (2009). Casting a global safety net—a framework for food safety in the age of globalization. *Food Drug Law Journal*, *64*, pp. 313–334.

5. Hussein, H. S. (2007). Prevalence and pathogenicity of Shiga toxin-producing Escherichia coli in beef cattle and their products. *Journal of Animal Science*, *85*, pp. E63–E72.

6. Oldfield, E. C., III. (2001). Emerging foodborne pathogens: Keeping your patients and your families safe. *Reviews in Gastrointestinal Disorders*, *1*, pp. 177–186.

7. Doyle, M. P., & Erickson, M. C. (2008). Summer meeting 2007—the problems with fresh produce: an overview. *Journal of Applied Microbiology*, *105*, pp. 317–330.

8. *Food-related diseases*. (2010). Centers for Disease Control and Prevention. Accessed July 15, 2010, at http://www.cdc.gov/ncidod/diseases/food/index.htm.

9. Thorns, C. J. (2000). Bacterial food-borne zoonoses. *Revue Scientifique et Technique*, *19*, pp. 226–239.

10. Fischer, A. R., de Jong, A. E., de Jonge, R., Frewer, L. J., & Nauta, M. J. (2005). Improving food safety in the domestic environment: The need for a transdisciplinary approach. *Risk Analysis*, *25*, pp. 503–517.

11. Dodd, C. I., & Powell, D. (2009). Regulatory management and communication of risk associated with Escherichia coli O157:H7 in ground beef. *Foodborne Pathogens and Disease*, *6*, pp. 743–747.

12. Albrecht, J. A., & Nagy-Nero, D. (2009). Position of the American Dietetic Association: Food and water safety. *Journal of the American Dietetic Association*, *109*, pp. 1449–1460.

13. Stevens, C. A. (2010). Exploring food insecurity among young mothers (15–24 years). *Journal for Specialists in Pediatric Nursing*, *15*, pp. 163–171.

14. Rose, D. (2010). Access to healthy food: S key focus for research on domestic food insecurity. *The Journal of Nutrition*, *140*, pp. 1167–1169.

15. Block, D., & Kouba, J. (2006). A comparison of the availability and affordability of a market basket in two communities in the Chicago area. *Public Health Nutrition*, *9*, pp. 837–845.

16. Moore, L. V., & Diez Roux, A. V. (2006). Associations of neighborhood characteristics with the location and type of food stores. *American Journal of Public Health*, *96*, pp. 325–331. Cummins, S., & Macintyre, S. (2006). Food environments and obesity—Neighbourhood or nation? *International Journal of Epidemiology*, *35*, pp. 100–104.

17. Seligman, H. K., Laraia, B. A., & Kushel, M. B. (2010). Food insecurity is associated with chronic disease among low-income NHANES participants. *The Journal of Nutrition*, *140*, pp. 304–310. Gao, X., Scott, T., Falcon, L. M., Wilde, P. E., & Tucker, K. L. (2009). Food insecurity and cognitive function in Puerto Rican adults. *The American Journal of Clinical Nutrition*, *89*, pp. 1197–1203.

18. Drewnowski, A. (2009). Obesity, diets, and social inequalities. *Nutrition Reviews*, *67 Suppl 1*, pp. S36–S39.

19. Rank, M. R., & Hirschl, T. A. (2009). Estimating the risk of food stamp use and impoverishment during childhood. *Archives of Pediatric and Adolescent Medicine*, *163*, pp. 994–999.

20. Kaiser, L. (2008). Why do low-income women not use food stamps? Findings from the California Women's Health Survey. *Public Health Nutrition*, *11*, pp. 1288–1295.

21. Goodman, A. (2009). President Obama's health plan and community-based prevention. *American Journal of Public Health*, *99*, pp. 1736–1738.

22. Devaney, B. L., Ellwood, M. R., & Love, J. M. (1997). Programs that mitigate the effects of poverty on children. *Future Child*, *7*, pp. 88–112.

23. Owen, A. L., & Owen, G. M. (1997). Twenty years of WIC: A review of some effects of the program. *Journal of the American Dietetic Association*, *97*, pp. 777–782.

24. Hoisington, A., Shultz, J. A., & Butkus, S. (2002). Coping strategies and nutrition education needs among food pantry users. *Journal of Nutrition and Education Behavior*, *34*, pp. 326–333.

25. Biel, M., Evans, S. H., & Clarke, P. (2009). Forging links between nutrition and healthcare using community-based partnerships. *Family and Community Health*, *32*, pp. 196–205.

26. Daponte, B. O., & Bade S. (2006). How the private food assistance network evolved: Interactions between public and private responses to hunger. *Nonprofit and Voluntary Sector Quarterly*, *35*, pp. 668–690.

27. Martin, K. S., Cook, J. T., Rogers, B. L., & Joseph, H. M. (2003). Public versus private food assistance: Barriers to participation differ by age and ethnicity. *Journal of Nutrition and Education Behavior*, *35*, pp. 249–254.

28. Levine, S. (2008). *School lunch politics: The surprising history of America's favorite welfare program*. Princeton, NJ: Princeton University Press.

29. Hastert, T. A., & Babey, S. H. (2009). School lunch source and adolescent dietary behavior. *Prevention of Chronic Disease*, *6*, p. A117.

Condon, E. M., Crepinsek, M. K., & Fox, M. K. (2009) School meals: Types of foods offered to and consumed by children at lunch and breakfast. *Journal of the American Dietetic Association, 109*, pp. S67–S78.

30. Nollen, N. L., Befort, C. A., Snow, P., Daley, C. M., Ellerbeck, E. F., & Ahluwalia, J. S. (2007). The school food environment and adolescent obesity: Qualitative insights from high school principals and food service personnel. *International Journal Behavior, Nutrition, and Physical Activity, 4*, p. 18.

31. Cho, H., & Nadow, M. Z. (2004). Understanding barriers to implementing quality lunch and nutrition education. *Journal of Community Health, 29*, pp. 421–435.

32. Story, M., Nanney, M. S., & Schwartz, M. B. (2009). Schools and obesity prevention: Creating school environments and policies to promote healthy eating and physical activity. *Milbank Quarterly, 87*, pp. 71–100.

33. Izumi, B. T., Alaimo, K., & Hamm, M. W. (2010). Farm-to-school programs: Perspectives of school food service professionals. *Journal of Nutrition and Education Behavior, 42*, pp. 83–91. Vallianatos, M., Gottlieb, R., & Haase, M. A. (2004). Farm-to-school. *Journal of Planning Education and Research, 23*, pp. 414–423.

34. Bagdoni, J. M., Hinrichs, C., & Schafft, K. A. (2009). The emergence and framing of farm-to-school initiatives: Civic engagement, health and local agriculture. *Agriculture and Human Values, 26*, pp. 107–1319.

35. Suarez-Balcazar, Y., Redmond, L., Kouba, J., et al. (2007). Introducing systems change in the schools: The case of school luncheons and vending machines. *American Journal of Community Psychology, 39*, pp. 335–45.

36. French, S. A., Story, M., Fulkerson, J. A., & Gerlach, A. F. (2003). Food environment in secondary schools: A la carte, vending machines, and food policies and practices. *American Journal of Public Health, 93*, pp. 1161–1167.

37. Kaufmann, L. J. (2003). Vending machines and competitive foods in schools. *NCSL Legisbrief, 11*, pp. 1–2.

38. Kubik, M. Y., Lytle, L. A., Farbakhsh, K., Moe, S., & Samuelson, A. (2009). Food use in middle and high school fundraising: Does policy support healthful practice? Results from a survey of Minnesota school principals. *Journal of the American Dietetic Association, 109*, pp. 1215–1219.

39. Cullen, K. W., & Watson, K. B. (2009). The impact of the Texas public school nutrition policy on student food selection and sales in Texas. *American Journal of Public Health, 99*, pp. 706–712.

40. Bendelius, J. (2004). Vending machines in schools: What are we to do? *School Nurse News, 21*, pp. 20–21.

41. McAleese, J. D., & Rankin, L. L. (2007). Garden-based nutrition education affects fruit and vegetable consumption in sixth-grade adolescents. *Journal of the American Dietetic Association, 107*, pp. 662–665.

42. Graham, H., Beall, D., Lussier, M., McLaughlin, P., & Zidenberg-Cherr, S. (2009). Use of school gardens in academic instruction. *Journal of Nutrition Education and Behavior, 37*, pp. 147–151.

43. White, M. (2007). Food access and obesity. *Obesity Review, 8 Suppl 1*, pp. 99–107.

44. Bodor, J. N., Rice, J. C., Farley, T. A., Swalm, C. M., & Rose, D. (2010). Disparities in food access: Does aggregate availability of key foods from other stores offset the relative lack of supermarkets in African-American neighborhoods? *Preventive Medicine, 51*, pp. 63–67.

45. Walker, R. E., Keane, C. R., & Burke, J. G. (2010). Disparities and access to healthy food in the United States: A review of food deserts literature. *Health Place, 16*, pp. 876–884.

46. Lovasi, G. S., Hutson, M. A., Guerra, M., & Neckerman, K. M. (2009). Built environments and obesity in disadvantaged populations. *Epidemiological Review, 31*, pp. 7–20.

47. Rose, D., Bodor, J. N., Hutchinson, P. L., & Swalm, C. M. (2010). The importance of a multi-dimensional approach for studying the links between food access and consumption. *The Journal of Nutrition, 140*, pp. 1170–1174.

48. Galvez, M. P., Morland, K., Raines, C., et al. Race and food store availability in an inner-city neighbourhood. *Public Health Nutrition*, (2008). *11*, pp. 624–31.

49. Zenk, S. N., Schulz, A. J., Israel, B. A., James, S. A., Bao, S., & Wilson, M. L. (2005). Neighborhood racial composition, neighborhood poverty, and the spatial accessibility of supermarkets in metropolitan Detroit. *American Journal of Public Health, 95*, pp. 660–667.

50. Lopez, R. P. (2007). Neighborhood risk factors for obesity. *Obesity, 15*, pp. 2111–2119.

51. Wendt, M., Kinsey, J., & Kaufman, P. (2008). *Food accessibility in the inner city: What have we learned? A literature review 1963–2007*. St. Paul, MN: The Food Industry Center.

52. Karpyn, A., Manon, M., Treuhaft, S., Giang, T., Harries, C., & McCoubrey, K. (2010). Policy solutions to the "grocery gap." *Health Affairs (Millwood), 29*, pp. 473–480.

53. Gittelsohn, J., Song, H. J., Suratkar, S., et al. (2010). An urban food store intervention positively affects food-related psychosocial variables and food behaviors. *Health Education and Behavior, 37*, pp. 390–402.

54. Sturm, R., & Cohen, D. A. (2009). Zoning for health? The year-old ban on new fast-food restaurants in South LA. *Health Affairs (Millwood), 28*, pp. w1088–w1097.
    Creighton, R. (2009). Cheeseburgers, race, and paternalism. Los Angeles' ban on fast food restaurants. *Journal of Legal Medicine, 30*, pp. 249–267.

55. Fleischhacker, S. E., Evenson, K. R., Rodriguez, D. A., & Ammerman, A. S. A systematic review of fast food access studies. *Obesity Review, 12*, pp. e46–e471.

56. Allena, P., Dusena, D. V., Lundya, J., & Gliessman, S. (1991). Integrating social, environmental, and economic issues in sustainable agriculture. *American Journal of Alternative Agriculture, 6*, pp. 34–39.
    Smolika, J. D., Dobbsa, T. L., & Rickerl, D. H. (1995). The relative sustainability of alternative, conventional, and reduced-till farming systems. *American Journal of Alternative Agriculture, 10*, pp. 25–35.
    Aneja, V. P., Schlesinger, W. H., & Erisman, J. W. (2008). Farming pollution. *Nature Geoscience, 1*, pp. 409–411.

57. Sneeringer, S. (2009). Does animal feeding operation pollution hurt public health? A national longitudinal study of health externalities identified by geographic shifts in livestock production. *American Journal of Agricultural Economics, 91*, pp. 124–137.

58. Heederik, D., Sigsgaard, T., Thorne, P. S., et al. (2007). Health effects of airborne exposures from concentrated animal feeding operations. *Environmental Health Perspectives, 115*, pp. 298–302.

59. Burkholder, J., Libra, B., Weyer, P., et al. (2007). Impacts of waste from concentrated animal feeding operations on water quality. *Environmental Health Perspectives, 115*, pp. 308–312.

60. Wing, S., Cole, D., & Grant, G. (2000). Environmental injustice in North Carolina's hog industry. *Environmental Health Perspectives, 108*, pp. 225–31.

61. Donham, K. J., Wing, S., Osterberg, D., et al. (2007). Community health and socioeconomic issues surrounding concentrated animal feeding operations. *Environmental Health Perspectives, 115*, pp. 317–320.

62. Pimentel, D., Hanson, J., Seidel, R., Douds, D., & Hepperly, P. (2005). Environmental, energetic, and economic comparisons of organic and conventional farming systems. *Bioscience, 55*, pp. 573–582.

63. Mepharn, T. B. (2000). The role of food ethics in food policy. *Proceedings of the Nutrition Society, 59*, pp. 609–611.

64. Allen, P. (2010). Realizing justice in local food systems. *Cambridge Journal of Regions, Economy and Society, 3*, pp. 255–308.

65. Charney, M. (2009). FoodRoutes Network and the Local Food Movement. *Agricultural and Food Information, 10*, pp. 173–181.

    Coit, M. (2008). Jumping on the next bandwagon: An overview of the policy and legal aspects of the local food movement. *Journal of Food Law and Policy, 4*, pp. 45–70.

66. Engelhaupt, E. (2008). Do food miles matter? *Environmental Science and Technology, 42*, p. 3482.

67. Coley, D., & Howard, M. (2005). Local food, food miles and carbon emissions: A comparison of farm shop and mass distribution approaches. *Food Policy, 34*, pp. 150–155.

68. Holben, D. H. (2010). Farmers' markets: fertile ground for optimizing health. *Journal of the American Dietetic Association, 110*, pp. 364–365.

69. McCormack, L. A., Laska, M. N., Larson, N. I., & Story, M. (2010). Review of the nutritional implications of farmers' markets and community gardens: A call for evaluation and research efforts. *Journal of the American Dietetic Association, 110*, pp. 399–408.

70. Boehmer, T. K., Brownson, R. C., Haire-Joshu, D., & Dreisinger, M. L. (2007). Patterns of childhood obesity prevention legislation in the United States. *Prevention of Chronic Disease, 4*, pp. A56.

71. Larsen, K., & Gilliland, J. (2009). A farmers' market in a food desert: Evaluating impacts on the price and availability of healthy food. *Health Place, 15*, pp. 1158–1162.

72. Lang, K. (2011). The changing face of community-supported agriculture. *Culture and Agriculture, 32*, pp. 17–26.

73. Centner, T. (2007). Governments and unconstituional takings: When do right-to-farm laws go too far. *Boston College Environmental Law Affairs Review, 33*, pp. 87–148.

74. Brodt, S., Feenstra, G., Kozloff, R., Klonsky, K., & Tourte, L. (2006). Farmer-community connections and the future of ecological agriculture in California. *Agriculture and Human Values, 23*, pp. 75–81.

75. Hynes, H. P. (1996). *A patch of Eden: America's inner-city gardeners*. White River Junction, VT: Chelsea Green.

76. Pudup, M. B. (2008). It takes a garden: Cultivating citizen-subjects in organized garden projects *Geoforum, 39*, pp. 1228–1240.

    Alaimo, K., Packnett, E., Miles, R. A., & Kruger, D. J. (2008). Fruit and vegetable intake among urban community gardeners. *Journal of Nutrition Education and Behavior, 40*, pp. 94–101.

    Sallis, J. F., & Glanz, K. (2006). The role of built environments in physical activity, eating, and obesity in childhood. *Future Child, 16*, pp. 89–108.

77. Leake, J. R., Adam-Bradford, A., & Rigby, J. E. (2009). Health benefits of "grow your own" food in urban areas: Implications for contaminated land risk assessment and risk management? *Environmental Health, 8 Suppl 1*, pp. S6.

78. Schillinga, J., Logan, J. (2008). Greening the rust belt: A green infrastructure model for right sizing America's shrinking cities. *Journal of the American Planning Association, 74*, pp. 451–466.

79. Foster, S. (2006–2007). The city as an ecological space: Social capital and urban land use. *Notre Dame Law Review, 62*, pp. 527–582.

80. Meehan, A. (2007). *Community in the garden in the community: The development of an open space resource in Boston's South End*. Cambridge: Massachusetts Institute of Technology.

Chapter Ten

1. Villerme, L. R. (1830). *De la mortalité dans les divers quartiers de la ville de Paris*. Paris.

2. Marmot, M. (2007). Achieving health equity: From root causes to fair outcomes. *Lancet, 370*, pp. 1153–1163.

3. Gee, G., & Payne-Sturges, D. (2004). Environmental health disparities: A framework integrating psychosocial and environmental concepts. *Environmental Health Perspectivesives, 112*, pp. 1645–1653.

4. Hynes, H., & Lopez, R. (2007). Cumulative risk and a call for action in environmental justice communities. *Journal of Health Disparities Research and Practice, 1*, pp. 29–58.

5. Geronimus, A. T., Hicken, M., Keene, D., & Bound, J. (2006). "Weathering" and age patterns of allostatic load scores among blacks and whites in the United States. *American Journal of Public Health, 96*, pp. 826–833.

6. Gehlert, S., Sohmer, D., Sacks, T., Mininger, C., McClintock, M., & Olopade, O. (2008). Targeting health disparities: A model linking upstream determinants to downstream interventions. *Health Affairs (Millwood), 27*, pp. 339–349.

7. Morello-Frosch, R., & Lopez, R. (2006). The riskscape and the color line: Examining the role of segregation in environmental health disparities. *Environmental Research, 102*, pp. 181–196.

8. Pacione, M. (2003). Quality-of-life research in urban geography. *Urban Geography, 243*, pp. 314–339.

9. Cohen, D., Farley, T., & Mason, K. (2003). Why is poverty unhealthy? Social and physical mediators. *Social Science and Medicine, 57*, pp. 1631–1641.

10. Bullard, R. (1996). Environmental justice: It's more than waste facility siting. *Social Science Quarterly, 77*, pp. 493–499.

11. Cunningham, G. O., & Michael, Y. L. (2004). Concepts guiding the study of the impact of the built environment on physical activity for older adults: A review of the literature. *American Journal of Health Promotion, 18*, pp. 435–443.

12. Gordon-Larsen, P., Nelson, M., Page, P., & Popkin, B. (2006). Inequality in the built environment underlies key health disparities in physical activity and obesity. *Pediatrics, 117*, pp. 417–424.

13. Bassett, M. T. (2000). The pursuit of equity in health: Reflections on race and public health data in Southern Africa. *American Journal of Public Health, 90*, pp. 1690–1693.

14. Caulfield, T., Fullerton, S. M., Ali-Khan, S. E., et al. (2009). Race and ancestry in biomedical research: Exploring the challenges. *Genome Medicine, 1*, p. 8.
Sankar, P. (2003). MEDLINE definitions of race and ethnicity and their application to genetic research. *Nature Genetics, 34*, pp. 119, (discussion 20).

15. Herman, A. A. (1996). Toward a conceptualization of race in epidemiologic research. *Ethnicity and Disease, 6*, pp. 7–20.

16. Flores, G. (2010). Technical report—racial and ethnic disparities in the health and health care of children. *Pediatrics, 125*, pp. e979–e1020.

17. Landrine, H., Corral, I. (2009). Separate and unequal: Residential segregation and black health disparities. *Ethnicity and Disease, 19*, pp. 179–184.

18. Grieco, E. (2000). *Overview of race and Hispanic origin.* Washington D.C.: U.S. Bureau of the Census.

19. Ford, M. E., & Kelly, P. A. (2005). Conceptualizing and categorizing race and ethnicity in health services research. *Health Services Research, 40*, pp. 1658–1675.

20. Griffith, D. M., Johnson, J., Ellis, K. R., & Schulz, A. J. (2010). Cultural context and a critical approach to eliminating health disparities. *Ethnicity and Disease, 20*, pp. 71–76.

21. Chang, V. W., Hillier, A. E., & Mehta, N. K. (2009). Neighborhood racial isolation, disorder and obesity. *Soc Forces, 87*, pp. 2063–2092.

22. Massey, D. (2004). Segregation and stratification: A biosocial perspective. *Du Bois Review, 1*, pp. 1–19.
    Massey, D., & Denton, N. (1993). *American apartheid: Segregation and the making of the underclass.* Cambridge, MA: Harvard University Press.

23. Lopez, R. (2002). Segregation and black/white differences in exposure to air toxics in 1990. *Environmental Health Perspectives, 110*, pp. 289–295.

24. Cunningham et al., Concepts guiding the study of the impact of the built environment on physical activity for older adults.

25. Yu, S. M., Huang, Z. J., & Singh, G. K. (2010). Health status and health services access and utilization among Chinese, Filipino, Japanese, Korean, South Asian, and Vietnamese children in California. *American Journal of Public Health, 100*, pp. 823–830.

26. Alexander, G. R., Wingate, M. S., Bader, D., & Kogan, M. D. (2008). The increasing racial disparity in infant mortality rates: Composition and contributors to recent U.S. trends. *American Journal of Obstetrics & Gynecology, 198*, pp. 51 e1–e9.
    Hearst, M. O., Oakes, J. M., & Johnson, P. J. (2008). The effect of racial residential segregation on black infant mortality. *American Journal of Epidemiology, 168*, pp. 1247–1254.

27. Akinbami, L. J., Moorman, J. E., Garbe, P. L., & Sondik, E. J. (2009). Status of childhood asthma in the United States, 1980–2007. *Pediatrics, 123 Suppl 3*, pp. S131–S145.
    Landrigan, P. J., Rauh, V. A., & Galvez, M. P. (2010). Environmental justice and the health of children. *Mt. Sinai Journal of Medicine, 77*, pp. 178–187.

28. Vega, W. A., Rodriguez, M. A., & Gruskin, E. (2009). Health disparities in the Latino population. *Epidemiological Review, 31*, pp. 99–112.

29. MacDorman, M. F., Callaghan, W. M., Mathews, T. J., Hoyert, D. L., & Kochanek, K. D. (2007). Trends in preterm-related infant mortality by race and ethnicity, United States, 1999–2004. *International Journal of Health Services, 37*, pp. 635–641.

30. Morales, L. S., Lara, M., Kington, R. S., Valdez, R. O., & Escarce, J. J. (2002). Socioeconomic, cultural, and behavioral factors affecting Hispanic health outcomes. *Journal of Health Care for the Poor and Underserved, 13*, pp. 477–503.

31. McKinnon, J. (2001). *The black population: 2000.* Washington, D.C.: Bureau of the Census.

32. Heynen, N. (2006). Green urban political ecologies: Toward a better understanding of inner-city environmental change. *Environment and Planning A*, 499–516.

33. Bullard, R. (1990). *Dumping in Dixie: Race, class, and environmental quality.* Boulder, CO: Westview Press.

34. Guzman, B. (2001 May). *The Hispanic population.* Census 2000 Brief. Washington D.C.: U.S. Department of Commerce Economics and Statistics Division U.S. Bureau of the Census.

35. Carlson, S. A., Brooks, J. D., Brown, D. R., & Buchner, D. M. (2010). Racial/ethnic differences in perceived access, environmental barriers to use, and use of community parks. *Prevention of Chronic Disease, 7*, pp. A49.

36. Barnes, J., & Bennett, C. (2001 February). *The Asian population: 2000.* Census 2000 Brief. Washington D.C.: U.S. Department of Commerce Economics and Statistics Division U.S. Bureau of the Census.

37. Morello-Frosch & Lopez, The riskscape and the color line.

38. Bullard, R., & Johnson, G. (2000). Environmental justice: Grassroots activism and its impact on public policy decision making. *Journal of Social Issues, 56*, pp. 555–574.

39. Brulle R. J., & Pellow, D. N. (2006). Environmental justice: Human health and environmental inequalities. *Annual Reviews of Public Health, 27*, pp. 103–124.

40. Rust, G., & Cooper, L. A. (2007). How can practice-based research contribute to the elimination of health disparities? *Journal of the American Board of Family Medicine,* pp. 105–114.

41. Shaya, F. T., Gu, A., & Saunders, E. (2006). Addressing cardiovascular disparities through community interventions. *Ethnicity and Disease, 16*, pp. 138–144.

42. Ochoa, E. R., Jr., & Nash, C. (2009). Community engagement and its impact on child health disparities: Building blocks, examples, and resources. *Pediatrics, 124 Suppl 3*, pp. S237–45.

43. Report of the National Advisory Commission on Civil Disorders. (1968). Washington, D.C.: Government Printing Office.

44. Massey & Denton, American apartheid.

45. Massey, D., & Fischer, M. (2000). Does rising income bring integration? New results for Blacks, Hispanics and Asians in 1990. *Social Science Research, 28*, pp. 316–326.

46. Polednak, A. (1996). Segregation, discrimination and mortality in U.S. blacks. *Ethnicity and Disease, 6*, pp. 99–107.

47. Polednak, A. (1997). *Segregation, poverty, and mortality in urban African Americans.* New York: Oxford University Press.

48. Morello-Frosch, R., Pastor, M., & Sadd, J. (2001). The distribution of air toxics exposures and health risks among diverse communities. *Urban Affairs Review, 36*, pp. 551–578.

49. Primack, B. A., Bost, J. E., Land, S. R., & Fine, M. J. (2007). Volume of tobacco advertising in African American markets: Systematic review and meta-analysis. *Public Health Reports, 122*, pp. 607–615.

50. Carlson et al., Racial/Ethnic differences in perceived access, environmental barriers to use, and use of community parks.
    Powell, L. M., Han, E., & Chaloupka, F. J. (2010). Economic contextual factors, food consumption, and obesity among U.S. adolescents. *The Journal of Nutrition, 140*, pp. 1175–1180.
    Sager, A. (1983). Why urban voluntary hospitals close. *Health Services Research, 18*, pp. 451–481.

51. Graham, J. D., Chang, B. H., & Evans, J. S. (1992). Poorer is riskier. *Risk Analysis, 12*, pp. 333–337.

52. Duncan, G. J. (1996). Income dynamics and health. *International Journal of Health Services, 26*, pp. 419–444.

53. Conroy, K., Sandel, M., & Zuckerman, B. (2010). Poverty grown up: How childhood socioeconomic status impacts adult health. *Journal of Developmental and Behavioral Pediatrics, 31*, pp. 154–160.

54. Berkman, L. F. (2009). Social epidemiology: Social determinants of health in the United States: are we losing ground? *Annual Reviews of Public Health, 30*, pp. 27–41.

55. Wallace, R. (1988). A synergism of plagues: Planned shrinkage, contagious housing destruction and AIDS in the Bronx. *Environmental Research, 47*, pp. 1–33.

56. Victora, C. G., Wagstaff, A., Schellenberg, J. A., Gwatkin, D., Claeson, M., & Habicht, J. P. (2003). Applying an equity lens to child health and mortality: More of the same is not enough. *Lancet, 362*, pp. 233–241.

57. Kawachi, I., & Kennedy, B. (1997). The relationship of income inequality to mortality: Does the choice of indicator matter? *Social Science and Medicine, 45*, pp. 121–127.
    Marmot, M. (2001). Income inequality, social environment and inequities in health. *Journal of Policy Analysis and Management, 20*, pp. 156–159.
    Subramanian, S., & Kawachi, I. (2004). Income inequality and health: What have we learned so far? *Epidemiological Reviews, 26*, pp. 78–91.

58. Lopez, R. (2004). Income inequality and self-rated health in U.S. metropolitan areas: a multi-level analysis. *Social Science and Medicine, 59*, pp. 2409–2419.

59. Kawachi, I., Kennedy, B., Lochner, K., Prothow-Stith, D. (1997). Social capital, income inequality, and mortality. *American Journal of Public Health, 87*, pp. 1491–1498.

60. Birchfield, V. L. (2008). *Income inequality in capitalist democracies: The interplay of values and institutions*. University Park, PA: Penn State Press.

61. Srinivasan, S., O'Fallon, L., & Dearry, A. (2003). Creating healthy communities, healthy homes, healthy people: Initiating a research agenda on the built environment and public health. *American Journal of Public Health, 93*, pp. 1446–1450.

62. Baker, E. A., Schootman, M., Barnidge, E., & Kelly, C. (2006). The role of race and poverty in access to foods that enable individuals to adhere to dietary guidelines. *Prevention of Chronic Disease, 3*, p. A76.

63. Flores, G., & Vega, L. R. (1998). Barriers to health care access for Latino children: S review. *Family Medicine, 30*, pp. 196–205.

64. Green, C., Ndao-Brumblay, S., West, B., & Washington, T. (2005). Differences in prescription opioid analgesic availability: Comparing minority and white pharmacies across Michigan. *Journal of Pain, 6*, pp. 689–699.

65. Accordino, J., & Johnson, G. (2000). Addressing the vacant and abandoned property problem. *Journal of Urban Affairs, 22*, pp. 301–315.
    Keating, W. (2010). Redevelopment of vacant land in the blighted neighbourhoods of Cleveland, Ohio, resulting from the housing foreclosure crisis. *Journal of Urban Regeneration and Renewal, 4*, pp. 39–52.

66. Baker et al., The role of race and poverty in access to foods.
    Bedimo-Rung, A. L., Mowen, A. J., & Cohen, D. A. (2005). The significance of parks to physical activity and public health: A conceptual model. *American Journal of Preventive Medicine, 28*, pp. 159–168.

67. Lopez, R. P. (2007). Neighborhood risk factors for obesity. *Obesity, 15*, pp. 2111–2119.
    Lovasi, G. S., Hutson, M. A., Guerra, M., & Neckerman, K. M. (2009). Built environments and obesity in disadvantaged populations. *Epidemiological Review, 31*, pp. 7–20.
    Pearce, J., Witten, K., & Bartie, P. (2006). Neighbourhoods and health: A GIS approach to measuring community resource accessibility. *Journal of Epidemiology and Community Health, 60*, pp. 389–395.

68. Johnson, N., & Collins, C. (2010). *State tax changes in response to the recession.* Washington, D.C.: Center on Budget and Policy Priorities.
69. Acevedo-Garcia, D., Lochner, K. A., Osypuk, T. L., & Subramanian, S. V. (2003). Future directions in residential segregation and health research: A multilevel approach. *American Journal of Public Health, 93*, pp. 215–221.
70. Browning, C., & Cagney, K. (2003). Moving beyond poverty: Neighborhood structure, social processes, and health. *Journal of Health and Social Behavior, 44*, pp. 552–557.
71. Cohen et al., Why is poverty unhealthy?
72. Laveist, T. A. (1993). Segregation, poverty, and empowerment: Health consequences for African Americans. *Milbank Quarterly, 71*, pp. 41–64.
73. Curley, A. (2005). Theories of urban poverty and implications for public housing policy. *Journal of Sociology and Social Welfare, 32*, pp. 97–119.
74. Kain, J. (1992). The spatial mismatch hypothesis: Three decades later. *Housing Policy Debate, 3*, pp. 371–460.
75. Kochtitzky, C. S., Frumkin, H., Rodriguez, R., et al. (2006). Urban planning and public health at CDC. *MMWR Morbity and Mortality Weekly Report, 55 Suppl 2*, pp. 34–38.
    Martin, R. (1997). Job decentralization with suburban housing discrimination: An urban equilibrium model of spatial mismatch. *Journal of Housing Economics, 6*, pp. 293–317.
    Martin, R. (2001). Spatial mismatch and costly suburban commutes: Can commuting subsidies help? *Urban Studies, 38*, pp. 1305–1318.
    Meurs, H., & Haaijer, R. (2001). Spatial structure and mobility. *Transportation Research Part D: Transport and Environment, 6*, pp. 429–446.
76. Bearer, C. F. (1995). How are children different from adults? *Environmental Health Perspectives, 103 Suppl 6*, pp. 7–12.
77. Landrigan, P. J. (1998). Environmental hazards for children in U.S.A. *International Journal of Occupational Medicine and Environmental Health, 11*, pp. 189–194.
78. Schoeters, G., Den Hond, E., Dhooge, W., van Larebeke, N., & Leijs, M. (2008). Endocrine disruptors and abnormalities of pubertal development. *Basic and Clinical Pharmacology Toxicology, 102*, pp. 168–175.
79. Loukaitou-Sideris, A., & Eck, J. E. (2007). Crime prevention and active living. *American Journal of Health Promotion, 21*, pp. 380–9, iii.
80. Needleman, H. (2004). Lead poisoning. *Annual Review of Medicine, 55*, pp. 209–222.
81. Trasande, L., & Thurston, G. D. (2005). The role of air pollution in asthma and other pediatric morbidities. *Journal of Allergy and Clinical Immunology, 115*, pp. 689–699.
82. Israel, B. A., Parker, E. A., Rowe, Z., et al. (2005). Community-based participatory research: Lessons learned from the Centers for Children's Environmental Health and Disease Prevention Research. *Environmental Health Perspectives, 113*, pp. 1463–1471.
83. Ochoa et al., Community engagement and its impact on child health disparities.
    Lupoli, T. A., Ciaccio, C. E., & Portnoy, J. M. (2009). Home and school environmental assessment and remediation. *Current Allergy and Asthma Reports, 9*, pp. 419–425.
    Makri, A., & Stilianakis, N. I. (2008). Vulnerability to air pollution health effects. *International Journal of Hygiene and Environmental Health, 211*, pp. 326–336.
    Molnar, D., & Livingstone, B. (2000). Physical activity in relation to overweight and obesity in children and adolescents. *European Journal of Pediatrics, 159*, pp. S45–S55.
    Potwarka, L. R., Kaczynski, A. T., & Flack, A. L. (2008). Places to play: Association of park space and facilities with healthy weight status among children. *Journal of Community Health, 33*, pp. 344–350.

84. Lopez, R., & Goldoftas, B. (2009). The urban elderly in the United States: Health status and the environment. *Reviews on Environmental Health, 24*, pp. 47–57.

Schumucker, D. (2001). Liver function and phase 1 drug metabolism in the elderly: A paradox. *Drugs and Aging, 18*, pp. 837–845.

Symanski, E., & Hertz-Picciotto, I. (1995). Blood lead levels in relation to menopause, smoking, and pregnancy history. *American Journal of Epidemiology, 141*, pp. 1047–1058.

85. Li, F., Fisher, K. J., Brownson, R. C., & Bosworth, M. (2005). Multilevel modelling of built environment characteristics related to neighbourhood walking activity in older adults. *Journal of Epidemiology and Community Health, 59*, pp. 558–564.

86. Erickson, M., Robison, J., Ewen, H., Kraut, J. (2006). Should I stay or should I go? Moving plans of older adults. *Journal of Housing for the Elderly, 20*, pp. 5–22.

87. Lopez, R. P., & Hynes, H. P. (2006). Obesity, physical activity, and the urban environment: Public health research needs. *Environmental Health, 5*, pp. 25.

88. Evans, S. (2009). *Community and ageing: Maintaining quality of life in housing with care settings.* Portland, OR: The Policy Press.

89. Leden, L., Garder, P., Johansson, C. (2006). Safe pedestrian crossings for children and elderly. *Accident Analysis and Prevention, 38*, pp. 289–294.

90. Lopez & Goldoftas, The urban elderly in the United States.

91. Hennessy, C. H. (2010). Aging and place: Situating lives and care in the community. *Gerontologist, 50* (4), pp. 564–568.

92. Lau, D. T., Scandrett, K. G., Jarzebowski, M., Holman, K., & Emanuel, L. (2007). Health-related safety: A framework to address barriers to aging in place. *Gerontologist, 47*, pp. 830–837.

93. Cannuscio, C., Block, J., & Kawachi, I. (2003). Social capital and successful aging: The role of senior housing. *Annals of Internal Medicine, 139*, pp. 395–399.

94. Fuhrman, M. P. (2009). Home care for the elderly. *Nutrition in Clinical Practice 24*, pp. 196–205.

95. Kirchner, C. E., Gerber, E. G., & Smith, B. C. (2008). Designed to deter: Community barriers to physical activity for people with visual or motor impairments. *American Journal of Preventive Medicine, 34*, pp. 349–352.

96. Spivock, M., Gauvin, L., & Brodeur, J. M. (2007). Neighborhood-level active living buoys for individuals with physical disabilities. *American Journal of Preventive Medicine, 32*, pp. 224–30.

97. Clarke, P., Ailshire, J. A., Bader, M., Morenoff, J. D., & House, J. S. (2008). Mobility disability and the urban built environment. *American Journal of Epidemiology, 168*, pp. 506–513.

98. Clarke, P., Ailshire, J. A., & Lantz, P. (2009). Urban built environments and trajectories of mobility disability: Findings from a national sample of community-dwelling American adults (1986–2001). *Social Science and Medicine, 69*, pp. 964–970.

99. Iwarsson, S., & Stahl, A. (2003). Accessibility, usability and universal design—Positioning and definition of concepts describing person-environment relationships. *Disability and Rehabilitation, 25*, pp. 57–66.

100. *Universal design principles.* (2010). Accessed June 18, 2010, at http://www.design.ncsu.edu/cud/about_ud/udprincipleshtmlformat.html#top.

101. Ho, P. S., Kroll, T., Kehn, M., Anderson, P., & Pearson, K. M. (2007). Health and housing among low-income adults with physical disabilities. *Journal of Health Care for the Poor and Underserved, 18*, pp. 902–915.

Zola, I. K. (1989). Toward the necessary universalizing of a disability policy. *Milbank Quarterly 67 Suppl 2* Pt 2, pp. 401–428.

102. Chan, E., & Lee, G. (2009). Universal design for people with disabilities: A study of access provisions in public housing estates. *Property Management, 27*, pp. 138–146.

Chapter Eleven

1. Burnet, J. & Robert, E. (2008). Park and the Chicago School of Sociology: A centennial tribute. *Canadian Journal of Sociology, 1*, pp. 156–164.

2. Cloward, R. (1959). Illegitimate means: Anomie and deviant behavior. *American Sociological Review, 24*, pp. 164–176.

3. Merton, R. (1938). Social structure and anomie. *American Sociological Review, 3*, pp. 672–682.

4. Crocker, R. (1992). Social work and social order: The Settlement Movement in two industrial cities 1889–1930. Champaign: University of Illinois Press.

5. Berry, J. W. (2008). Globalization and acculturation. *International Journal of Intercultural Relations, 32*, pp. 328–336.

6. Hunt, L. M., Schneider, S., & Comer, B. (2004). Should "acculturation" be a variable in health research? A critical review of research on U.S. Hispanics. *Social Science and Medicine, 59*, pp. 973–986.

7. Ali, J. S., McDermott, S., & Gravel, R. G. (2004). Recent research on immigrant health from statistics Canada's population surveys. *Canadian Journal of Public Health, 95*, pp. I9–I13.

8. Sanders, A. E. (2010). A Latino advantage in oral health-related quality of life is modified by nativity status. *Social Science and Medicine, 71*, pp. 205–211.

9. Oudenhoven, J. P. V., Ward, C., & Masgoret, A.-M. (2008). Patterns of relations between immigrants and host societies. *International Journal of Intercultural Relations 32*, pp. 328–336.

10. Frumkin, H. (2001). Beyond toxicity: Human health and the natural environment. *American Journal of Preventive Medicine, 20*, pp. 234–240.

11. Bolunda, P., & Hunhammar, S. (1999). Ecosystem services in urban areas. *Ecological Economics, 29*, pp. 293–301.

12. Wilson, E. O. (1986). *Biophilia*. Cambridge, MA: Harvard University Press.

13. Ulrich, R. (1984). View through a window may influence recovery from surgery. *Science, 224*, pp. 420–421.

14. Ulrich, R. S., Simons, R. F., Losito, B. D., Fiorito, E., Miles, M. A., & Zelson, M. (1991). Stress recovery during exposure to natural and urban environments. *Journal of Environmental Psychology, 11*, pp. 201–230.
Jackson, L. (2003). The relationship of urban design to human health and condition. *Landscape and Urban Planning, 64*, pp. 191–200.

15. Kuo, F. E., & Sullivan, W. C. (2001). Environment and crime in the inner city. *Environment and Behavior, 33*, pp. 343–367.

16. Louv, R. (2008). *Last child in the woods: Saving our children from nature-deficit disorder*. Chapel Hill, NC: Algonquin Books.

17. Szreter, S., & Mooney, G. (1998). Urbanization, mortality, and the standard of living debate: New estimates of the expectation of life at birth in nineteenth century British cities. *Economic History Review, 51*, pp. 84–92.

18. Higgs, G. (1999). Investigating trends in rural health outcomes: A research agenda. *Geoforum, 30*, pp. 203–21.

19. Paykel, E. S., Abbott, R., Jenkins, R., Brugha, T. S., & Meltzer, H. (2000). Urban-rural mental health differences in great Britain: Findings from the national morbidity survey. *Psychological Medicine, 30*, pp. 269–80.

20. Vlahov, D., Galea, S., & Freudenberg, N. (2005). The urban health "advantage." *Journal of Urban Health, 82*, pp. 1–4.
    Vlahov, D., Gibble, E., Freudenberg, N., Galea, S. (2004). Cities and health: History, approaches, and key questions. *Academic Medicine, 79*, pp. 1133–1138.

21. Sharkey, J. R., Johnson, C. M., & Dean, W. R. (2010). Food access and perceptions of the community and household food environment as correlates of fruit and vegetable intake among rural seniors. *BMC Geriatrics, 10*, pp. 32.
    Hart-Hester, S., & Thomas, C. (2003). Access to health care professionals in rural Mississippi. *Southern Medical Journal, 96*, pp. 149–154.

22. Frost, S. S., Goins, R. T., Hunter, R. H., et al. (2010). Effects of the built environment on physical activity of adults living in rural settings. *American Journal of Health Promotion, 24*, pp. 267–283.
    Ossenbruggen, P., Pendhankar, J., & Ivan, J. (2001). Roadway safety in rural and small urbanized areas. *Accident Analysis and Prevention, 33*, pp. 485–498.

23. Chadwick, E., & Flinn, M. W. (1965). *Report on the sanitary condition of the labouring population of Great Britain.* Edinburgh: Edinburgh University Press.
    Shattuck, L. (1850). *Report of the Sanitary Commission of Massachusetts 1850.* Boston: Dutton and Wentworth, State Printers.
    Shaw, G. (1924). Housing problems in Philadelphia. *American Journal of Public Health, 14*, pp. 401–403.

24. Calhoun, J. (1962). Population density and social pathology. *Scientific American, 206*, pp. 139–148.
    Calhoun, J. (1962). A behavioral sink. In E. Bliss (Ed.), *Roots of behavior.* New York: Harper.

25. Hall, E. T. (1969). *The hidden dimension.* New York: Anchor Books.

26. Greenbie, B. (1971). What can we learn from other animals? Behavioral biology and the ecology of cities. *Journal of the American Planning Association, 37*, pp. 162–168.

27. Gillis, A. R. (1983). Strangers next door: An analysis of density, diversity, and scale in public housing projects. *Canadian Journal of Sociology, 8*, pp. 1–20.

28. Mitchell, R. E. (1971). Some social implications of high density housing. *American Sociological Review, 36*, pp. 18–29.

29. Choidin, H. (1978). Urban density and pathology. *Annual Review of Sociology, 4*, pp. 91–113.

30. LeCorbusier. (1923). *Towards a new architecture.* New York: Dover.
    LeCorbusier. (1929). *The city of to-morrow.* Cambridge MA: MIT Press.

31. Jacobs, J. (1961). *The death and life of great American cities.* New York: Vintage Books.

32. Kunstler, J. H., & Salngaros, N. (2007). The end of tall buildings. In A. Chavan, C. Peralta, & C. Steins (Eds.), *Planetizen contemporary debates in urban planning.* Washington, D.C.: Island Press.

33. Gifford, R. (2007). The consequences of living in high-rise buildings. *Architectural Science Review, 50*, pp. 2–17.

34. Newman, O. (1972). *Defensible space: Crime prevention through urban design.* New York City: Macmillan.

35. Vale, L. (1999). The future of planned poverty: Redeveloping America's most distressed public housing projects. *Journal of Housing and the Built Environment, 14*, pp. 13–31.

36. Crowe, T. (2000). *Crime prevention through environmental design*. Woburn, MA: Butterworth-Heinemann.

37. Seeman, T., Epel, E., Gruenewald, T., Karlamangla, A., & McEwen, B. S. (2010). Socio-economic differentials in peripheral biology: Cumulative allostatic load. *Annals of the New York Academy of Science, 1186*, pp. 223–239.

38. Morello-Frosch, R., & Shenassa, E. D. (2006). The environmental "riskscape" and social inequality: Implications for explaining maternal and child health disparities. *Environmental Health Perspectives, 114*, pp. 1150–1153.

39. Dowd, J. B., Simanek, A. M., & Aiello, A. E. (2009). Socio-economic status, cortisol and allostatic load: A review of the literature. *International Journal of Epidemiology, 38*, pp. 1297–1309.

40. Virtue, S., Vidal-Puig, A. (2010). Adipose tissue expandability, lipotoxicity and the metabolic syndrome—An allostatic perspective. *Biochimica et Biophysica Acta, 1801*, pp. 338–349.

41. Logan, J. G., & Barksdale, D. J. (2008). Allostasis and allostatic load: Expanding the discourse on stress and cardiovascular disease. *Journal of Clinical Nursing, 17*, pp. 201–208.

42. Fullilove, M. (2005). *Root shock: How tearing up city neighborhoods hurts America, and what we can do about it*. New York: Random House.

    Fullilove, M., & Fullilove, R. (2000). Place matters. In R. Hofrichter (Ed.), *Reclaiming the environmental debate: The politics of health in a toxic culture*. Cambridge, MA: MIT Press.

    Fried, M. (1966). Grieving for a lost home: Psychological costs of relocation. In J. Q. Wilson (Ed.), *Urban renewal: The record and the controversy*. Cambridge, MA: MIT Press.

43. Lopez, R. (2009). Public health, the APHA, and urban renewal. *American Journal of Public Health, 99*, pp. 1603–1611.

44. Kennedy, M., & Leonard, P. (2001 April). *Dealing with neighborhood change: A primer on gentrification and policy choices*. Washington, D.C.: The Brookings Institute.

45. Wallace, D., & Wallace, R. (1998). *A plague on your houses: How New York was burned down and national public health crumbled*. New York: Verson.

    Wallace, R. (1988). A synergism of plagues: Planned shrinkage, contagious housing destruction and AIDS in the Bronx. *Environmental Research, 47*, pp. 1–33.

46. Smith, N. (1996). *The new urban frontier: Gentrification and the revanchist city*. New York: Routledge.

47. Helms, A. (2003). Understanding gentrification: An empirical analysis of the determinants of urban housing renovation. *Journal of Urban Economics, 54*, pp. 474–98.

    Marcuse, P. (1999). Comment on Elvin K. Wyly & Daniel J. Hammel's "Islands of decay in seas of renewal: Housing policy and the resurgence of gentrification." *Housing Policy Debate, 10*, pp. 780–797.

    Wyly, E., & Hammel, D. (1999). Islands of decay in seas of renewal: housing policy and the resurgence of gentrification. *Housing Policy Debate, 10*, pp. 711–765.

48. McCurdy, L. E., Winterbottom, K. E., Mehta, S. S., & Roberts, J. R. (2010). Using nature and outdoor activity to improve children's health. *Current Problems in Pediatric and Adolescent Health Care, 40*, pp. 102–117.

    Kruger, J., Nelson, K., Klein, P., McCurdy, L. E., Pride, P., & Carrier Ady, J. (2009). Building on partnerships: Reconnecting kids with nature for health benefits. *Health Promotion Practice, 11*, pp. 340–346.

49. Taylor, A. F., & Kuo, F. E. (2009). Children with attention deficits concentrate better after walk in the park. *Journal of Attention Disorders, 12*, pp. 402–409.

50. Evans, G. (2003). The built environment and mental health. *Journal of Urban Health, 80*, pp. 536–555.

51. Babisch, W. (2006). Transportation noise and cardiovascular risk: Updated review and synthesis of epidemiological studies indicate that the evidence has increased. *Noise Health, 8*, pp. 1–29.

52. Babisch, W., & Kamp, I. (2009). Exposure-response relationship of the association between aircraft noise and the risk of hypertension. *Noise Health, 11*, pp. 161–168.

53. Babisch, W., Neuhauser, H., Thamm, M., & Seiwert, M. (2009). Blood pressure of 8–14-year-old children in relation to traffic noise at home—Results of the German Environmental Survey for Children (GerES IV). *Science of the Total Environment, 407*, pp. 5839–5843.

    Nilsson, M. E., Andehn, M., & Lesna, P. (2008). Evaluating roadside noise barriers using an annoyance-reduction criterion. *Journal of the Acoustical Society of America, 124*, pp. 3561–3567.

54. Nielsen, P. V. (2009). Control of airborne infectious diseases in ventilated spaces. *Journal of the Royal Society Interface, 6 Suppl 6*, pp. S747–S755.

55. van de Glind, I., de Roode, S., & Goossensen, A. (2007). Do patients in hospitals benefit from single rooms? A literature review. *Health Policy, 84*, pp. 153–161.

56. Reiling, J. (2006). Safe design of healthcare facilities. *Quality and Safety in Health Care, 15 Suppl 1*, pp. i34–i40.

57. Montague, K. N., Blietz, C. M., & Kachur, M. (2009). Ensuring quieter hospital environments. *American Journal of Nursing, 109*, pp. 65–67.

58. Joseph, A., & Rashid, M. (2007). The architecture of safety: Hospital design. *Current Opinion in Critical Care, 13*, pp. 714–719.

59. Stichler, J. F. (2007). Enhancing safety with facility design. *Journal of Nursing Administration, 37*, pp. 319–323.

    Stichler, J. F. (2007). Using evidence-based design to improve outcomes. *Journal of Nursing Administration, 37*, pp. 1–4.

60. Ulrich, R. S., Craig Zimring, P., Zhu, X., et al. (2008). A review of the research literature on evidence-based healthcare design. *Health Environments Research and Design, 1*, pp. 101–165.

61. Harris, D., Joseph, A., Becker, F., Hamilton, K., Zimring, C., & Shepley, M. (2008). *A practitioner's guide to evidence-based design*. Concord, CA: Center for Healthcare Design.

Chapter Twelve

1. Clark, A. M., DesMeules, M., Luo, W., Duncan, A. S., & Wielgosz, A. (2009). Socioeconomic status and cardiovascular disease: Risks and implications for care. *Nature Reviews: Cardiology, 6*, pp. 712–722.

    Schaap, M. M., & Kunst, A. E. (2009). Monitoring of socio-economic inequalities in smoking: Learning from the experiences of recent scientific studies. *Public Health, 123*, pp. 103–109.

2. Kandel, D. B., Griesler, P. C., & Schaffran, C. (2009). Educational attainment and smoking among women: Risk factors and consequences for offspring. *Drug and Alcohol Dependence, 104 Suppl 1*, pp. S24–S33.

    Khan, N., Afaq, F., & Mukhtar, H. (2010). Lifestyle as risk factor for cancer: Evidence from human studies. *Cancer Letters, 293*, pp. 133–143.

3. Peet, R. (1985). The social origins of environmental determinism. *Annals of the Association of American Geographers, 75*, pp. 309–333.

4. Hayden, D. (2003). *Building suburbia: Green fields and urban growth, 1820–2000*. New York: Vintage Books.

5. Bandura, A. (2004). Health promotion by social cognitive means. *Health Education and Behavior, 31*, pp. 143–164.

6. Ewing, R. (2005). Can the physical environment determine physical activity levels? *Exercise and Sport Sciences Review, 33*, pp. 69–75.

7. Portes, A. (1998). Social capital: Its origins and applications in modern sociology. *Annual Review of Sociology, 24*, pp. 1–24.

8. Brehm, J., & Rahn, W. (1997). Individual-level evidence for the causes and consequences of social capital. *American Journal of Political Science, 41*, pp. 999–1023.

9. Portes, A. (2000). The two meanings of social capital. *Social Forces, 15*, pp. 1–12.

10. Dasgupta, P., & Serageldin, I. (2000). *Social capital: A multifaceted perspective*. Washington, D.C.: World Bank.

11. Kawachi, I., Kennedy, B. P., & Glass, R. (1999). Social capital and self-rated health: A contextual analysis. *American Journal of Public Health, 89*, pp. 1187–1193.

12. Lochner, K., Kawachi, I., & Kennedy, B. P. (1999). Social capital: A guide to its measurement. *Health Place, 5*, pp. 259–270.

13. Lomas, J. (1998). Social capital and health: Implications for public health and epidemiology. *Social Science and Medicine, 47*, pp. 1181–1188.
    Keele, L. (2007). Social capital and the dynamics of trust in government. *American Journal of Political Science, 51*, pp. 241–254.

14. Lin, N., Fu Y.-C., & Hsung, R.-M. (2006). The position generator: Measurement techniques for investigations of social capital. In R. Burt, K. Cook, & N. Lin (Eds.), *Social capital: Theory and research*. New Brunswick, NJ: Transaction.

15. Helliwell, J. (2005). *Well-being, social capital and public policy: What's new?* Cambridge, MA: National Bureau of Economic Research.

16. McPherson, M., Smith-Lovin, L., & Brashears, M. E. (2009). Models and marginals: Using survey evidence to study social networks. *American Sociological Review, 74*, pp. 670–680.

17. Paxton, P. (2007). Association memberships and generalized trust: A multilevel model across 31 countries. *Social Forces, 86*, pp. 47–76.

18. Rupasingha, A., Goetz, S., & Freshwate, D. (2006). The production of social capital in U.S. counties. *Journal of Socio-Economics, 35*, pp. 83–101.

19. Putnam, R. (2001). *Bowling alone: The collapse and revival of American community*. New York: Simon & Schuster.

20. Paxton, P. (1999). Is social capital declining in the United States? A multiple indicator assessment. *American Journal of Sociology, 105*, pp. 88–127.

21. Duany, A., Plater-Zyberk, E., & Speck, J. (2000). *Suburban nation*. New York: North Point Press.
    Kunstler, J. (1993). *The geography of nowhere: The rise and decline of America's man-made landscape*. New York: Simon & Schuster.

22. Jacobs, J. (1961). *The death and life of great American cities*. New York: Vintage Books.
    Mumford, L. (1962 December 1). Mother Jacobs' home remedies. *The New Yorker*, pp. 148–179.

23. Smith, M. H., Beaulieu, L. J., & Seraphine, A. (2010). Social capital, place of residence, and college attendance. *Rural Sociology, 60*, pp. 363–380.

24. DeFilippis, J. (2001). The myth of social capital in community development. *Housing Policy Debate, 12*, pp. 781–806.

25. Saegert, S., Thompson, P., & Warren, M. (2000). *Social capital and poor communities*. New York: Russell Sage Foundation.

26. Wacquant, L. (1998). Negative social capital: State breakdown and social destitution in America's urban core. *Journal of Housing and the Built Environment, 12*, pp. 25–40.

27. Adler, P., & Kwon S-W. (2000). Social capital: The good, the bad, and the ugly. In E. L. Lesser (Ed.), *Knowledge and social capital*. Woburn, MA: Butterworth-Heinemann.

28. Grant-Meyer, S. (2000). *As long as they don't move next door: Segregation and racial conflict in American neighborhoods*. Lanham, MD: Rowman & Littlefield.

29. Rubio, M. (1997). Perverse social capital—some evidence from Colombia. *Journal of Economic Issues, 31*, pp. 805–816.

30. Wakefield, S. E., Poland, B. (2005). Family, friend or foe? Critical reflections on the relevance and role of social capital in health promotion and community development. *Social Science and Medicine, 60*, pp. 2819–2832.

31. Coffé, H., Geys, B. (2007). Toward an empirical characterization of bridging and bonding social capital. *Nonprofit and Voluntary Sector Quarterly, 36*, pp. 121–139.

32. Kawachi, I., Kim, D., Coutts, A., & Subramanian, S. V. (2004). Commentary: Reconciling the three accounts of social capital. *International Journal of Epidemiology, 33*, pp. 682–690, (discussion 700–4).

33. Kim, D., Subramanian, S. V., & Kawachi, I. (2006). Bonding versus bridging social capital and their associations with self rated health: A multilevel analysis of 40 U.S. communities. *Journal of Epidemiology and Community Health, 60*, pp. 116–122.

34. Sorensen, G., Emmons, K., Hunt, M. K., et al. (2003). Model for incorporating social context in health behavior interventions: Applications for cancer prevention for working-class, multiethnic populations. *Preventive Medicine, 37*, pp. 188–197.
    Kawachi, I., & Berkman, L. F. (2001). Social ties and mental health. *Journal of Urban Health, 78*, pp. 458–467.
    Berkman, L. F. (2000). Social support, social networks, social cohesion and health. *Social Work and Health Care, 31*, pp. 3–14.
    Berkman, L. F. (1995). The role of social relations in health promotion. *Advances in Psychosomatic Medicine, 57*, pp. 245–524.

35. Lindstrom, M. (2010). Social capital, economic conditions, marital status and daily smoking: A population-based study. *Public Health, 124*, pp. 71–77.
    Long, J. A., Field, S., Armstrong, K., Chang, V. W., & Metlay, J. P. Social capital and glucose control. *Journal of Community Health, 35* (5), pp. 519–526.
    Moffat, T., Galloway, T., & Latham, J. (2005). Stature and adiposity among children in contrasting neighborhoods in the city of Hamilton, Ontario, Canada. *American Journal of Human Biology, 17*, pp. 355–367.

36. Garcia, M., & McDowell, T. (2010). Mapping social capital: A critical contextual approach for working with low-status families. *Journal of Marital and Family Therapy, 36*, pp. 96–107.

37. Srinivasan, S., O'Fallon, L., & Dearry, A. (2003). Creating healthy communities, healthy homes, healthy people: Initiating a research agenda on the built environment and public health. *American Journal of Public Health, 93*, pp. 1446–1450.

38. Leyden, K. (2003). Social capital and the built environment: The importance of walkable neighborhoods. *American Journal of Public Health, 93*, pp. 1546–1551.

39. Jackson, R. (2003). The impact of the built environment on health: An emerging field. *American Journal of Public Health, 93*, pp. 1382–1384.

40. Alinsky, S. (1971). *Rules for radicals*. New York: Vintage Books.

41. Gittell, R., & Vidal, A. (1998). *Community organizing: Building social capital as a development strategy*. Thousand Oaks, CA: Sage.

42. Campbell, C., & MacPhail, C. (2002). Peer education, gender and the development of critical consciousness: Participatory HIV prevention by South African youth. *Social Science and Medicine, 55*, pp. 331–345.

43. Medoff, P., & Sklar, H. (1994). *Streets of hope*. Boston: South End Press.

44. Hynes, H., & Lopez, R. (2007). Cumulative risk and a call for action in environmental justice communities. *Journal of Health Disparities Research and Practice, 1*, pp. 29–58.

45. Gutman, M. A., Barker, D. C., Samples-Smart, F., & Morley, C. (2009). Evaluation of active living research progress and lessons in building a new field. *American Journal of Preventive Medicine, 36*, pp. S22–S33.

46. Becker, A. B., Israel, B. A., Schulz, A. J., Parker, E. A., & Klem, L. (2002). Predictors of perceived control among African American women in Detroit: Exploring empowerment as a multilevel construct. *Health Education and Behavior, 29*, pp. 699–715.

47. Wilkinson, D. (2007). The multidimensional nature of social cohesion: Psychological sense of community, attraction, and neighboring. *American Journal of Community Psychology, 40*, pp. 214–229.

48. Braunack-Mayer, A., & Louise, J. (2008). The ethics of community empowerment: Tensions in health promotion theory and practice. *Promotion and Education, 15*, pp. 5–8.

49. Ohmer, M. L., & Korr, W. (2006). The effectiveness of community practice interventions: A review of the literature. *Research on Social Work Practice, 16*, pp. 132–145.

50. Yoo, S., Butler, J., Elias, T. I., & Goodman, R. M. (2009). The 6-step model for community empowerment: Revisited in public housing communities for low-income senior citizens. *Health Promotion and Practice, 10*, pp. 262–275.

51. Griffith, D. M., Allen, J. O., DeLoney, E. H., et al. (2010). Community-based organizational capacity building as a strategy to reduce racial health disparities. *Journal of Primary Prevention, 31*, pp. 31–39.

52. Tang, H., Abramsohn, E., Park H. Y., Cowling, D. W., & Al-Delaimy, W. K. (2010). Using a cessation-related outcome index to assess California's cessation progress at the population level. *Tobacco Control, 19 Suppl 1*, pp. i56–i61.

53. Hipwell, A. E., Keenan, K., Loeber, R., & Battista, D. (2010). Early predictors of sexually intimate behaviors in an urban sample of young girls. *Developmental Psychology, 46*, pp. 366–378.

54. Rhodes, S. D., Hergenrather, K. C., Griffith, D. M., et al. (2009). Sexual and alcohol risk behaviours of immigrant Latino men in the South-eastern U.S.A. *Culture, Health and Sexuality, 11*, pp. 17–34.
Abad, N. S., & Sheldon, K. M. (2008). Parental autonomy support and ethnic culture identification among second-generation immigrants. *Journal of Family Psychology, 22*, pp. 652–657.

55. Wilson, J., & Kelling, G. (1982). Broken windows. *Atlantic Monthly, 249*, pp. 29–38.

56. Keizer, K., Lindenberg, S., & Steg, L. (2008). The spreading of disorder. *Science, 322*, pp. 1681–1685.
Melendez, L. (2005). Disease and "broken windows." *Environmental Health Perspectives, 113*, pp. A657, (author reply A.).

57. Cohen, D., Spear, S., Scribner, R., Kissinger, P., Mason, K., & Wildgen, J. (2000). "Broken windows" and the risk of gonorrhea. *American Journal of Public Health, 90*, pp. 230–236.

58. Franco Suglia, S., Duarte, C. S., Sandel, M. T., & Wright, R. J. (2009). Social and environmental stressors in the home and childhood asthma. *Journal of Epidemiology and Community Health, 64*, pp. 636–642.

59. Cerda, M., Tracy, M., Messner, S. F., Vlahov, D., Tardiff, K., & Galea, S. (2009). Misdemeanor policing, physical disorder, and gun-related homicide: A spatial analytic test of "broken-windows" theory. *Epidemiology, 20*, pp. 533–541.

60. Pellow, D. N. (2004). The politics of illegal dumping: An environmental justice framework *Qualitative Sociology, 27*, pp. 511–525.

61. Primack, B. A., Bost, J. E., Land, S. R., & Fine, M. J. (2007). Volume of tobacco advertising in African American markets: Systematic review and meta-analysis. *Public Health Reports, 122*, pp. 607–615.

62. Mead, M. (1928). *Coming of age in Samoa: A psychological study of primitive youth for western civilisation*. New York: Morrow.
    Lewis, O. (1959). *Five families: Mexican case studies in the culture of poverty*. New York: Basic Books.
    Gans, H. (1962). *The urban villagers: Group and class in the life of Italian-Americans*. Glencoe, NY: The Free Press.

63. Patterson, J. (1981). *America's struggle against poverty, 1900–1980*. Cambridge, MA: Harvard University Press.

64. Roach, J. L., & Gursslin, O. R. (1967). An evaluation of the concept "culture of poverty." *Social Forces, 45*, pp. 383–392.

65. Welshman, J. (2006). Searching for social capital: Historical perspectives on health, poverty and culture. *Journal of the Royal Society for the Promotion of Health, 126*, pp. 268–274.
    Pearson, L. J. (2003). Understanding the culture of poverty. *Journal for Nurse Practitioners, 28*, pp. 6.

66. Cellini, S., McKernan, S., & Ratcliffe, C. (2008). The dynamics of poverty in the United States: A review of data, methods, and findings. *Journal of Policy Analysis and Management, 27*, pp. 577–605.

67. Curley, A. (2005). Theories of urban poverty and implications for public housing policy. *Journal of Sociology and Social Welfare, 32*, pp. 97–119.

68. Goetz, E. (2003). *Clearing the way: Deconcentrating the poor in urban America*. Washington, D.C.: The Urban Institute Press.

69. Patel, S., d'Cruz, C,. & Burra, S. (2002). Beyond evictions in a global city: People-managed resettlement in Mumbai. *Environment and Urbanization, 14*, pp. 159–172.

70. Sanbonmatsu, L., Kling, J. R., Duncan, G. J., & Brooks-Gunn, J. (2006). Neighborhoods and academic achievement: Results from the Moving to Opportunity Experiment. *Journal of Human Resources, 41*, pp. 649–691.

71. Clark, W. A. (2008). Reexamining the moving to opportunity study and its contribution to changing the distribution of poverty and ethnic concentration. *Demography, 45*, pp. 515–535.
    Leventhal, T., Fauth, R. C., & Brooks-Gunn, J. (2005). Neighborhood poverty and public policy: A 5-year follow-up of children's educational outcomes in the New York City moving to opportunity demonstration. *Developmental Psychology, 41*, pp. 933–952.
    Leventhal, T., & Brooks-Gunn, J. (2003). Moving to opportunity: An experimental study of neighborhood effects on mental health. *American Journal of Public Health, 93*, pp. 1576–1582.

Chapter Thirteen

1. Bullard, R. (1994). Environmental justice for all: It's the right thing to do. *Journal of Environmental Law and Litigation, 9*, pp. 281–308.
2. Bullard, R., & Johnson, G. (2000). Environmental justice: Grassroots activism and its impact on public policy decision making. *Journal of Social Issues, 56*, pp. 555–574.
3. Cole, L. W., & Foster, S. R. (2001). *From the ground up: Environmental racism and the rise of the environmental justice movement*. New York: NYU Press.
4. Bullard, R. (1993). *Confronting environmental racism: Voices from the grassroots*. Boston: South End Press.
5. Taylor, D. (2000). The rise of the environmental justice paradigm. *American Behavioral Scientist, 43*, pp. 508–580.
6. Nash, L. (2004). The fruits of ill-health: Pesticides and workers' bodies in post–World War II California. *Osiris, 19*, pp. 203–219.
7. Bullard, R. (1990). *Dumping in Dixie: Race, class, and environmental quality*. Boulder, CO: Westview Press.
8. McGurty, E. M. (2000). Warren County, NC, and the emergence of the environmental justice movement: Unlikely coalitions and shared meanings in local collective action. *Society and Natural Resources, 13*, pp. 373–387.
9. Bailey, C., Faupel, C., Alley, K. (1995). Environmental Justice: Mobilization of a grassroots social movement. *Journal of Agricultural & Food Information, 2*, pp. 3–21.
10. Lee, C. (2002). Environmental justice: Building a unified vision of health and the environment. *Environmental Health Perspectives, 110 Suppl 2*, pp. 141–144.
11. Ishiyama, N. (2002). Environmental justice and American Indian tribal sovereignty: Case study of a land–use conflict in Skull Valley, Utah. *Antipode, 35*, pp. 119–139.
12. Platt, K. (1997). Chicana strategies for success and survival: Cultural poetics of environmental justice from the mothers of East Los Angeles. *Frontiers: A Journal of Women Studies, 18*, pp. 48–72.
13. Brown, P., Mayer, B., Zavestoski, S., Luebke, T., Mandelbaum, J., & McCormick, S. (2003). The health politics of asthma: Environmental justice and collective illness experience in the United States. *Social Science and Medicine, 57*, pp. 453–464.
14. O'Fallon, L. R., & Dearry, A. (2002). Community-based participatory research as a tool to advance environmental health sciences. *Environmental Health Perspectives, 110 Suppl 2*, pp. 155–159.
15. Shepard, P., Northridge, M., Prakash, S., & Stover, G. (2002). Advancing environmental justice through community-based participatory research. *Environmental Health Perspectivesives, 110*, pp. 139–40.
16. United Church of Christ. (1987). *Toxic waste and race in the United States: A national report on the racial and socioeconomic characteristics of communities with hazardous waste sites*. New York: United Church of Christ.
17. Rivers, F. R. (2009). The black-green-white divide: The impact of diversity in environmental nonprofit organizations. *William & Mary Environmental Law and Policy Review, 33*, pp. 449.
18. Gottlieb, R. (1993). *Forcing the spring: The transformation of the American environmental movement*. Washington, D.C.: Island Press.
19. Liu, F. (2001). *Environmental justice analysis: Theories, methods, and practice*. Boca Raton, FL: CRC Press.

20. Coburn, J. (2002). *Street science: The fusing of local and professional knowledge in environmental policy*. Cambridge: Massachusetts Institute of Technology.
21. First People of Color Environmental Leadership Summit. (1991). *Principles of Environmental Justice*. www.ejnet.org/ej/principles.html.
22. Hernandez, W. (1995). Environmental justice: Looking beyond executive order no. 12,898. *UCLA Journal of Environmental Law and Policy, 14*, pp. 181.
23. Murphy–Greene, C., Leip, L. (2002). Assessing the effectiveness of executive order 12898: Environmental justice for all? *Public Administration Review, 62*, pp. 679–687.
24. Brulle, R. J., & Pellow, D. N. (2006). Environmental justice: Human health and environmental inequalities. *Annual Reviews of Public Health, 27*, pp. 103–124.
25. Bullard, R. (1999). Dismantling environmental racism in the U.S.A. *Local Environment, 4*, pp. 5–19.
26. Agyeman, J., Bullard, R., Evans, B. (2002). Exploring the nexus: Bringing together sustainability, environmental justice and equity. *Space and Polity, 6*, pp. 77–90.
27. Floyd, M., Johnson, C. (2002). Coming to terms with environmental justice in outdoor recreation: A conceptual discussion with research implications. *Leisure Sciences, 24*, pp. 59–77.
    Floyd, M. F., Taylor, W. C., Whitt-Glover, M. (2009). Measurement of park and recreation environments that support physical activity in low-income communities of color: Highlights of challenges and recommendations. *American Journal of Preventive Medicine, 36*, pp. S156–S160.
28. Cintron, A., & Morrison, R. S. (2006). Pain and ethnicity in the United States: A systematic review. *Journal of Palliative Medicine, 9*, pp. 1454–1473.
    Sager, A. (1983). Why urban voluntary hospitals close. *Health Services Research, 18*, pp. 451–481.
29. Bullard, R. (2004). Addressing urban transportation equity in the United States. *Fordham Urban Law Journal, 31*, pp. 1183.
30. Brown et al., *The health politics of asthma*.
31. Cutter, S. (1995). Race, class and environmental justice. *Progress in Human Geography, 19*, pp. 111–122.
32. Bowen W. (2001). *Environmental justice through research-based decision-making*. New York: Garland.
33. Evans, G. W., & Marcynyszyn, L. A. (2004). Environmental justice, cumulative environmental risk, and health among low- and middle-income children in upstate New York. *American Journal of Public Health, 94*, pp. 1942–1944.
34. Northridge, M. E., Stover, G. N., Rosenthal, J. E., & Sherard, D. (2003). Environmental equity and health: Understanding complexity and moving forward. *American Journal of Public Health, 93*, pp. 209–214.
35. Morello-Frosch, R., Pastor, M., Porras, C., & Sadd, J. (2002). Environmental justice and regional inequality in Southern California: Implications for future research. *Environmental Health Perspectives, 110*, pp. 149–154.
36. Laskowski, R., Bednarska, A. J., Kramarz, P. E., et al. Interactions between toxic chemicals and natural environmental factors—A meta-analysis and case studies. *Science of the Total Environment, 408* (18), pp. 3763–7437.
37. Salmon, A. G. (2009). Do standard risk assessment procedures adequately account for cumulative risks? An exploration of the possibilities using California's Air Toxics Hot Spots guidelines. *International Journal of Toxicology 29*, pp. 65–70.

38. Jardine, C., Hrudey, S., Shortreed, J., et al. (2003). Risk management frameworks for human health and environmental risks. *Journal of Toxicology and Environmental Health B: Critical Reviews, 6*, pp. 569–720.

39. Lucchini, R., & Zimmerman, N. (2009). Lifetime cumulative exposure as a threat for neurodegeneration: Need for prevention strategies on a global scale. *Neurotoxicology, 30*, pp. 1144–1148.

40. Anderton, D., Anderson, A., Oakes, J., & Fraser, M. (1994). Environmental equity: The demographics of dumping. *Demography, 31*, pp. 229–248.
    Anderton, D., Anderson, A., Rossi, P., Oakes, J., Fraser, M., Weber, E. (1994). "Environmental equity" issues in metropolitan areas. *Evaluation Review, 18*, pp. 123–142.
    Ibid., pp. 123–140.
    Anderton, D., Oakes, J., & Egan, K. (1997). Environmental equity in Superfund. Demographics of discovery and prioritization of abandoned toxic sites. *Evaluation Review, 21*, pp. 2–26.
    Davidson, P., & Anderton, D. (2000). Demographics of dumping II: A national environmental equity survey and the distribution of hazardous materials handlers. *Demography, 37*, pp. 481–486.
    Lopez, R. (2002). Segregation and black/white differences in exposure to air toxics in 1990. *Environmental Health Perspectivesives, 110*, pp. 289–295.

41. Cutter, *Race, class and environmental justice*.
    Cutter, S., Holm, D., & Clark, L. (1996). The role of geographic scale in monitoring environmental justice. *Risk Analysis, 16*, pp. 517–524.

42. Agyeman et al., *Exploring the nexus*.
    Brown, P. (1995). Race, class and environmental health: A review and systematization of the literature. *Environmental Research, 69*, pp. 15–30.

43. Scammell, M. K., Senier, L., Darrah-Okike, J., Brown, P., & Santos, S. (2009). Tangible evidence, trust and power: Public perceptions of community environmental health studies. *Social Science and Medicine, 68*, pp. 143–53.

44. Mennis, J. (2002). Using geographic information systems to create and analyze statistical surfaces of population and risk for environmental justice analysis. *Social Science Quarterly, 83*, pp. 281–297.

45. Mohai, P., & Saha, R. (2006). Reassessing racial and socioeconomic disparities in environmental justice research. *Demography, 43*, pp. 383–399.

46. Nuckols, J. R., Ward, M. H., & Jarup, L. (2004). Using geographic information systems for exposure assessment in environmental epidemiology studies. *Environmental Health Perspectives, 112*, pp. 1007–1015.

47. Bowen, W. (2002). An analytical review of environmental justice research: What do we really know? *Environmental Management, 29*, pp. 3–15.

48. Hynes, H. P., & Brugge, D. (2005). Science with the people. In D. Brugge & H. P. Hynes (Eds.), *Community research in environmental health: Studies in science, advocacy, and ethics*. Burlington VT: Ashgate.

49. Bowen, *Environmental justice through research-based decision-making*.

50. Pulido, L. (2006). A critical review of the methodology of environmental racism research. *Antipode, 28*, pp. 142–159.

51. Massey, D., & Denton, N. (1993). *American apartheid: Segregation and the making of the underclass*. Cambridge, MA: Harvard University Press.

52. Pastor, M., Sadd, J., & Hipp, J. (2001). Which came first? Toxic facilities, minority move-in, and environmental justice. *Journal of Urban Affairs, 22*, pp. 1–21.

53. Bass, R. (1996). Evaluating environmental justice under the national environmental policy act. *Environmental Impact Assessment Review, 18*, pp. 83–92.

54. Lazarus, R. J., & Tai, S. (1999). Integrating environmental justice into EPA permitting authority. *Ecology Law Quarterly, 26*. pp. 617–678.

55. Elliott, M. R., Wang, Y., Lowe, R. A., & Kleindorfer, P. R. (2004). Environmental justice: frequency and severity of U.S. chemical industry accidents and the socioeconomic status of surrounding communities. *Journal of Epidemiology and Community Health, 58*, pp. 24–30.

56. Kuehn, R. (1996). The limits of devolving enforcement of federal environmental laws. *Tulane Law Review, 20*, pp. 2373.

57. Wilson, S., Wilson, O., Heaney, C., & Cooper, J. (2007). Use of EPA collaborative problem-solving model to obtain environmental justice in North Carolina. *Progress in Community Health Partnerships: Research, Education, and Action, 1*, pp. 327–337.

58. Ringquist, E. (1998). A question of justice: Equity in environmental litigation, 1974–1991. *Journal of Politics, 60*, pp. 1148–1165.

59. Lynch, M., Stretesky, P., & Burns, R. (2004). Determinants of environmental law violation fines against petroleum refineries: Race, ethnicity, income, and aggregation effects. *Society & Natural Resources, 17*, pp. 333–347.

60. Wilson, S. M., Wilson, O. R., Heaney, C. D., & Cooper, J. (2007). Use of EPA collaborative problem-solving model to obtain environmental justice in North Carolina. *Progress in Community Health Partnerships: Research, Education, and Action, 1*, pp. 327–337.

61. Fisher, M. (1998). Environmental racism claims brought under Title VI of the Civil Rights Act. *Environmental Law, 25*, pp. 285.

62. Agyeman, J., Bullard, R., & Evans, B. (2003). *Just sustainabilities: Development in an unequal world*. Cambridge, MA: MIT Press.

63. Heiman, M. (1994). Race, waste, and class: New perspectives on environmental justice. *Antipode, 28*, pp. 111–121.

64. Shapiro, M. (2005). Equity and information: Information regulation, environmental justice, and risks from toxic chemicals. *Journal of Policy Analysis and Management, 24*, pp. 373–938.

65. McCallion, K., & Sharma, H. 1999). Environmental justice without borders: The need for an international court of the environment to protect fundamental environmental rights. *George Washington International Law Review, 32*, p. 351.

Chapter Fourteen

1. Forsberg, A., & Malmborg, F. V. (2004). Tools for environmental assessment of the built environment. *Building and Environment, 39*, pp. 223–228.

2. Stokey, E., & Zeckhauser, R. (1978). *A primer for policy analysis*. New York: Norton.

3. Nilsson, M., Jordan, A., Turnpenny, J., Hertin, J., Nykvist, B., & Russe, D. (2008). The use and non-use of policy appraisal tools in public policy making: An analysis of three European countries and the European Union. *Policy Sciences, 41*, pp. 335–355.

4. Scammell, M. K., Senier, L., Darrah-Okike, J., Brown, P., & Santos, S. (2009). Tangible evidence, trust and power: Public perceptions of community environmental health studies. *Social Science and Medicine, 68*, pp. 143–153.

5. Jaya, S., Jones, C., Slinnc, P., & Wood, C. (2006). Environmental impact assessment: Retrospect and prospect. *Environmental Impact Assessment Review, 27*, pp. 287–300.

6. O'Faircheallaigh, C. (2010). Public participation and environmental impact assessment: Purposes, implications, and lessons for public policy making. *Environmental Impact Assessment Review, 30*, pp. 19–27.

7. Matthews, W. (2009). Objective and subjective judgements in environmental impact analysis. *Environmental Conservation, 27*, pp. 287–300.

8. Jaya et al., Environmental impact assessment.

9. Collins, J., & Koplan, J. P. (2009). Health impact assessment: A step toward health in all policies. *JAMA, 302*, pp. 315–317.

10. Bhatia, R., & Wernham, A. (2009). Integrating human health into environmental impact assessment: an unrealized opportunity for environmental health and justice. *Cien Saude Colet, 14*, pp. 1159–1175.

    Dannenberg, A. L., Bhatia, R., Cole, B. L., Heaton, S. K., Feldman, J. D., & Rutt, C. D. (2008). Use of health impact assessment in the U.S.: 27 case studies, 1999–2007. *American Journal of Preventive Medicine, 34*, pp. 241–256.

    Bhatia, R. (2007). Protecting health using an environmental impact assessment: A case study of San Francisco land use decision making. *American Journal of Public Health, 97*, pp. 406–413.

    Dannenberg, A. L., Bhatia, R., Cole, B. L., et al. (2006). Growing the field of health impact assessment in the United States: An agenda for research and practice. *American Journal of Public Health, 96*, pp. 262–270.

11. Dannenberg, et al., *Use of health impact assessment in the U.S.*

12. *Oak to Ninth Avenue health impact assessment*. (2006). Accessed at http://ehs.sph.berkeley.edu/hia/O2N.HIA.C7.pdf.

13. Parry, J., & Stevens, A. (2001). Prospective health impact assessment: Pitfalls, problems, and possible ways forward. *BMJ, 323*, pp. 1177–1182.

14. Lhachimi, S. K., Nusselder, W. J., Boshuizen, H. C., & Mackenbach, J. P. (2010). Standard tool for quantification in health impact assessment: A review. *American Journal of Preventive Medicine, 38*, pp. 78–84.

15. Knol, A. B., Slottje, P., van der Sluijs, J. P., & Lebret, E. (2010). The use of expert elicitation in environmental health impact assessment: A seven-step procedure. *Environmental Health 9*, p. 19.

16. Active Living Research. (2010). *Neighborhood Environment Walkability Survey (NEWS) & Neighborhood Environment Walkability Survey—Abbreviated (NEWS-A)*. www.activelivingresearch.org/node/10649.

17. Shigematsu, R., Sallis, J. F., Conway, T. L., et al. (2009). Age differences in the relation of perceived neighborhood environment to walking. *Medicine and Science in Sports and Exercise, 41*, pp. 314–321.

18. Adams, M. A., Ryan, S., Kerr, J., et al. (2009). Validation of the Neighborhood Environment Walkability Scale (NEWS) items using geographic information systems. *Journal of Physical Activity & Health, 6 Suppl 1*, pp. S113–S123.

    Rosenberg, D., Ding, D., Sallis, J. F., et al. (2009). Neighborhood Environment Walkability Scale for Youth (NEWS-Y): Reliability and relationship with physical activity. *Preventive Medicine, 49*, pp. 213–218.

Frank L. D., Sallis, J. F., Saelens, B. E., et al. (2010). The development of a walkability index: Application to the Neighborhood Quality of Life Study. *British Journal of Sports Medicine, 13*, pp. 924–933.

Cerin, E., Saelens, B. E., Sallis, J. F., & Frank, L. D. (2006). Neighborhood Environment Walkability Scale: Validity and development of a short form. *Medicine and Science in Sports and Exercise, 38*, pp. 1682–1691.

19. Pearce, J., Witten, K., & Bartie, P. (2006). Neighbourhoods and health: A GIS approach to measuring community resource accessibility. *Journal of Epidemiology and Community Health, 60*, pp. 389–395.

20. Foody, G. M. (2006). GIS: Health implications. *Progress in Physical Geography, 30*, pp. 691–695.

21. Nykiforuk, C. I., & Flaman, L. M. (2009). Geographic Information Systems (GIS) for health promotion and public health: A review. *Health Promotion Practice,*

22. Maantay, J., Maroko, A. (2009). Mapping urban risk: Flood hazards, race, and environmental justice in New York. *Applied Geography, 29*, pp. 111–124.

23. Lightstone, A. S., Dhillon, P. K., Peek-Asa, C., & Kraus, J. F. (2001). A geographic analysis of motor vehicle collisions with child pedestrians in Long Beach, California: Comparing intersection and midblock incident locations. *Injury Prevention, 7*, pp. 155–160.

24. O'Dwyer, L. A., & Burton, D. L. (2008). Potential meets reality: GIS and public health research in Australia. *Australian and New Zealand Journal of Public Health, 22*, pp. 819–823.

25. Boone, J. E., Gordon-Larsen, P., Stewart, J. D., & Popkin, B. M. (2008). Validation of a GIS facilities database: Quantification and implications of error. *Annals of Epidemiology, 18*, pp. 371–377.

26. Jeffery, C., Ozonoff, A. L., White, L. F., Nuno, M., & Pagano, M. (2009). Power to detect spatial disturbances under different levels of geographic aggregation. *Journal of the American Medical Informatics Association, 16*, pp. 847–854.

27. Dark, S. J., & Bram, D. (2007). The modifiable areal unit problem (MAUP) in physical geography. *Progress in Physical Geography, 31*, pp. 471–479.

28. Stafford, M., Duke-Williams, O., & Shelton, N. (2008). Small area inequalities in health: Are we underestimating them? *Social Science and Medicine, 67*, pp. 891–899.

29. Atkinson, G., & Mourato, S. (2008). Environmental cost-benefit analysis. *Annual Review of Environment and Resources, 33*, pp. 317–394.

30. Boarnet, M. G., Greenwald, M., & McMillan, T. E. (2008). Walking, urban design, and health. *Journal of Planning Education and Research, 27*, pp. 341–358.

31. Hahn, R. W., & Dudley, P. M. (2007). How well does the U.S. government do benefit-cost analysis? *Review of Environmental Economics and Policy, 1*, pp. 192–211.

32. Driesen, D. M. (2006). Is cost-benefit analysis neutral? *University of Colorado Law Review, 77*.

33. Hansson, S. O. (2007). Philosophical problems in cost benefit analysis. *Economics and Philosophy, 23*, pp. 163–183.

34. Sunstein, C. R., & Rowell, A. (2007). On discounting regulatory benefits: Risk, money, and intergenerational equity. *The University of Chicago Law Review, 74*, pp. 171–208.

35. Lind, R. (1995). Intergenerational equity, discounting, and the role of cost-benefit analysis in evaluating global climate policy. *Energy Policy, 23*, pp. 379–389.

36. Bourguignon, F., Ferreira, F., Walton, M. (2007). Equity, efficiency and inequality traps: A research agenda. *Journal of Economic Inequality, 5*, pp. 235–56.

37. Levy, J. I., Wilson, A. M., & Zwack, L. M. (2007). Quantifying the efficiency and equity implications of power plant air pollution control strategies in the United States. *Environmental Health Perspectives, 115*, pp. 743–750.

Quah, E. (2006). Cost-benefit analysis and the problem of locating environmentally noxious facilities. *Journal of International Development, 6*, pp. 79–92.

38. Saris, W. H. (1985). The assessment and evaluation of daily physical activity in children. A review. *Acta Paediatrica Scandinavica Suppl, 318*, pp. 37–48.

39. Ainsworth, B. E., Macera, C. A., Jones, D. A., et al. (2006). Comparison of the 2001 BRFSS and the IPAQ Physical Activity Questionnaires. *Medicine and Science in Sports and Exercise, 38*, pp. 1584–1592.

40. Bauman, A., Ainsworth, B. E., Bull, F., et al. (2009). Progress and pitfalls in the use of the International Physical Activity Questionnaire (IPAQ) for adult physical activity surveillance. *Journal of Physical Activity & Health, 6 Suppl 1*, pp. S5–S8.

41. Thacker, E. L., Chen, H., Patel, A. V., et al. (2008). Recreational physical activity and risk of Parkinson's disease. *Movement Disorders, 23*, pp. 69–74.

42. Nelson, N. M., & Woods, C. B. (2010). Neighborhood perceptions and active commuting to school among adolescent boys and girls. *Journal of Physical Activity & Health, 7*, pp. 257–266.

43. Hagstromer, M., Oja, P., & Sjostrom, M. (2006). The International Physical Activity Questionnaire (IPAQ): A study of concurrent and construct validity. *Public Health Nutrition, 9*, pp. 755–762.
Mader, U., Martin BW, Schutz, Y., & Marti, B. (2006). Validity of four short physical activity questionnaires in middle-aged persons. *Medicine and Science in Sports and Exercise, 38*, pp. 1255–1266.

44. McKenzie, T. L., Cohen, D. A., Sehgal, A., Williamson, S., & Golinell, D. (2006). System for Observing Play and Recreation in Communities (SOPARC): Reliability and feasibility measures. *Journal of Physical Activity and Health, 3*, pp. S208–S222.

45. Shores, K. A., & West, S. T. (2010). Rural and urban park visits and park-based physical activity. *Preventive Medicine, 50 Suppl 1*, pp. S13–S17.

46. Fukuoka, Y., Vittinghoff, E., Jong, S. S., & Haskell, W. (2010). Innovation to motivation-pilot study of a mobile phone intervention to increase physical activity among sedentary women. *Preventive Medicine, 51*. pp. 287–289.

47. Troiano, R. P., Berrigan, D., Dodd, K. W., Masse, L. C., Tilert, T., & McDowell, M. (2008). Physical activity in the United States measured by accelerometer. *Medicine and Science in Sports and Exercise, 40*, pp. 181–188.

48. Kelly, E. B., Parra-Medina, D., Pfeiffer, K. A., et al. (2010). Correlates of physical activity in black, Hispanic, and white middle school girls. *Journal of Physical Activity & Health, 7*, pp. 184–193.

49. Jago, R., Macdonald-Wallis, K., Thompson, J. L., Page, A. S., Brockman, R., & Fox, K. R. (2010). Better with a buddy: The influence of best friends on children's physical activity. *Medicine and Science in Sports and Exercise, 43*, pp. 259–265.

50. Rowlands, A. V. (2007). Accelerometer assessment of physical activity in children: An update. *Pediatric Exercise Science, 19*, pp. 252–266.

51. Tudor-Locke, C. E., & Myers, A. M. (2001). Challenges and opportunities for measuring physical activity in sedentary adults. *Sports Medicine, 31*, pp. 91–100.

52. CDC. (2010). *National Health and Nutrition Examination Survey.* www.cdc.gov/nchs/nhanes.htm.

53. CDC. (2000). *Behavioral risk factor surveillance system survey data.* Atlanta, GA: U.S. Department of Health and Human Services, Centers for Disease Control and Prevention.

54. CDC, *National Health Interview Survey.*

55. CDC. (2010). *Youth Behavioral Risk Factor Surveillance System.* www.cdc.gov/yrbs.

56. Cambridge Health Alliance (2010). *National Latino and Asian American survey.* www .multiculturalmentalhealth.org/nlaas.asp.

57. Berrigan, D., & Troiano, R. (2002). The association between urban form and physical activity in U.S. adults. *American Journal of Preventive Medicine, 23*, pp. 74–79.

58. Ewing, R., Schmid, T., Killingsworth, R., Zlot, A., & Raudenbush, S. (2003). Relationship between urban sprawl and physical activity, obesity, and morbidity. *American Journal of Health Promotion, 18*, pp. 47–57.

59. Brownson, R. C., Hoehner, C. M., Day, K., Forsyth, A., & Sallis, J. F. (2009). Measuring the built environment for physical activity: State of the science. *American Journal of Preventive Medicine, 36*, pp. S99–S123 e12.

60. Morello-Frosch, R., Pastor, M., Porras, C., & Sadd, J. (2002). Environmental justice and regional inequality in Southern California: Implications for future research. *Environmental Health Perspectivesives, 110*, pp. 149–154.

61. Perkinsa, D. D., Larsenb, C., & Brown, B. B. Mapping urban revitalization: Using GIS spatial analysis to evaluate a new housing policy. *Prevention and Intervention in the Community, 37*, pp. 48–65.

Chapter Fifteen

1. Frank, L. D., & Kavage, S. (2008). Urban planning and public health: A story of separation and reconnection. *Journal of Public Health Management and Practice, 14*, pp. 214–220.

2. Corburn, J. (2004). Confronting the challenges in reconnecting urban planning and public health. *American Journal of Public Health, 94*, pp. 541–546.

3. Maantay, J. (2001). Zoning, equity, and public health. *American Journal of Public Health, 91*, pp. 1033–1041.

4. De Ville, K. A., & Sparrow, S. E. (2008). Zoning, urban planning, and the public health practitioner. *Journal of Public Health Management and Practice, 14*, pp. 313–316.

5. Kochtitzky, C. S., Frumkin, H., Rodriguez, R., et al. (2006). Urban planning and public health at CDC. *MMWR Morbity and Mortality Weekly Report, 55 Suppl 2*, pp. 34–38.

6. Burke, N. M., Chomitz, V. R., Rioles, N. A., Winslow, S. P., Brukilacchio, L. B., & Baker, J. C. (2009). The path to active living: Physical activity through community design in Somerville, Massachusetts. *American Journal of Preventive Medicine, 37*, pp. S386–S394.

7. Moore, S. E., Harris, C., & Wimberly, Y. (2010). Perception of weight and threat to health. *Journal of the National Medical Association, 102*, pp. 119–124.
   Kersey, M., Lipton, R., Quinn, M. T., & Lantos, J. D. (2010). Overweight in Latino preschoolers: Do parental health beliefs matter? *American Journal of Health Behavior, 34*, pp. 340–348.

8. Cawley, J. (2006). Markets and childhood obesity policy. *Future Child, 16*, pp. 69–88.

9. Karsten, L. (2007). Housing as a way of life: Towards an understanding of middle-class families' preference for an urban residential location. *Housing Studies, 22*, pp. 83–98.

10. Lopez, R. (2009). Public health, the APHA, and urban renewal. *American Journal of Public Health, 99*, pp. 1603–1611.
    Myers, D., & Gearin, E. (2001). Current preferences and future demand for denser residential environments. *Housing Policy Debate, 12*, pp. 633–659.

11. Fenton, M. (2005). Battling America's epidemic of physical inactivity: Building more walkable, livable communities. *Journal of Nutrition and Education Behavior, 37 Suppl 2*, pp. S115–S120.

12. Klein, J. D., & Dietz W. (2010). Childhood obesity: The new tobacco. *Health Affairs (Millwood), 29*, pp. 388–392.

13. Stokes, R. J., MacDonald, J., & Ridgeway, G. (2008). Estimating the effects of light rail transit on health care costs. *Health Place, 14*, pp. 45–58.

14. Finegood, D. T., Karanfil, O., & Matteson, C. L. (2008). Getting from analysis to action: Framing obesity research, policy and practice with a solution-oriented complex systems lens. *Healthcare Papers, 9*, pp. 36–41, (discussion 62–7).

15. Deshpande, A. D., Dodson, E. A., Gorman, I., & Brownson, R. C. (2008). Physical activity and diabetes: Opportunities for prevention through policy. *Physical Therapy, 88*, pp. 1425–1435.
    Goodman, R. M., Larsen, B. A., Marmet, P. F., et al. (2008). The public health role in the primary prevention of diabetes: Recommendations from the chronic disease directors' project. *Journal of Public Health Management and Practice, 14*, pp. 15–25.

16. Dobson, N. G., & Gilroy, A. R. (2009). From partnership to policy: The evolution of active living by design in Portland, Oregon. *American Journal of Preventive Medicine, 37*, pp. S436–S444.

17. Blackwell, A. G. (2009). Active living research and the movement for healthy communities. *American Journal of Preventive Medicine, 36*, pp. S50–S52.

18. Buchner, D. M., & Schmid, T. (2009). Active living research and public health: Natural partners in a new field. *American Journal of Preventive Medicine, 36*, pp. S44–S46.

19. Sallis, J. F., Linton, L. S., Kraft, M. K., et al. (2009). The Active Living Research program: Six years of grantmaking. *American Journal of Preventive Medicine, 36*, pp. S10–S21.

20. Burbidge, S. K. (2009). Merging long range transportation planning with public health: A case study from Utah's Wasatch Front. *Preventive Medicine, 50 Suppl 1*, pp. S6–S8.
    Schilling, J. M., Giles-Corti, B., & Sallis, J. F. (2009). Connecting active living research and public policy: Transdisciplinary research and policy interventions to increase physical activity. *Journal of Public Health Policy, 30 Suppl 1*, pp. S1–S15.

21. Gutman, M. A., Barker, D. C., & Morley, C. (2009). Evaluation of Active Living Research progress and lessons in building a new field. *American Journal of Preventive Medicine, 36*, pp. S22–S33.

22. Ottoson, J. M., Green, L. W., Beery, W. L., et al. (2009). Policy-contribution assessment and field-building analysis of the Robert Wood Johnson Foundation's Active Living Research Program. *American Journal of Preventive Medicine, 36*, pp. S34–S43.

23. Drewnowski, A. (2009). Obesity, diets, and social inequalities. *Nutrition Reviews, 67 Suppl 1*, pp. S36–S39.

24. Hynes, H., & Lopez, R. (2007). Cumulative risk and a call for action in environmental justice communities. *Journal of Health Disparities Research and Practice, 1*, pp. 29–58.

25. Bassett, E. M., & Glandon, R. P. (2008). Influencing design, promoting health. *Journal of Public Health Management and Practice, 14*, pp. 244–254.

26. Collie-Akers, V., Schultz, J. A., Carson, V., Fawcett, S. B., & Ronan, M. (2009). Evaluating mobilization strategies with neighborhood and faith organizations to reduce risk for health disparities. *Health Promotion Practice, 10*, pp. 118S–127S.

27. Story, M., Nanney, M. S., & Schwartz, M. B. (2009). Schools and obesity prevention: Creating school environments and policies to promote healthy eating and physical activity. *Milbank Quarterly, 87*, pp. 71–100.

    Kubik, M. Y., Story, M., & Davey, C. (2007). Obesity prevention in schools: Current role and future practice of school nurses. *Preventive Medicine, 44*, pp. 504–507.

28. Brownell, K. D., Schwartz, M. B., Puhl, R. M., Henderson, K. E., & Harris, J. L. (2009). The need for bold action to prevent adolescent obesity. *Journal of Adolescent Health, 45*, pp. S8–S17.

29. Haire-Joshu, D., Elliott, M., Schermbeck, R., Taricone, E., Green, S., & Brownson, R. C. (2010). Surveillance of obesity-related policies in multiple environments: The Missouri Obesity, Nutrition, and Activity Policy Database, 2007–2009. *Prevention of Chronic Disease, 7*, p. A80.

    Pomeranz, J. L., Teret, S. P., Sugarman, S. D., Rutkow, L., & Brownell, K. D. (2009). Innovative legal approaches to address obesity. *Milbank Quarterly, 87*, pp. 185–213.

30. Greves, H. M., & Rivara, F. P. (2006). Report card on school snack food policies among the United States' largest school districts in 2004–2005: Room for improvement. *International Journal of Behavioral Nutrition and Physical Activity, 3*, p. 1.

31. Zenzen, W., & Kridli, S. (2009). Integrative review of school-based childhood obesity prevention programs. *Journal of Pediatric Health Care, 23*, pp. 242–258.

32. Benjamin, S. E., Cradock, A., Walker, E. M., Slining, M., & Gillman, M. W. (2008). Obesity prevention in child care: A review of U.S. state regulations. *BMC Public Health, 8*, pp. 188.

33. Barroso, C. S., Kelder, S. H., Springer, A. E., et al. (2009). Senate Bill 42: Implementation and impact on physical activity in middle schools. *Journal of Adolescent Health, 45*, pp. S82–S90.

    Kelder, S. H., Springer, A. S., Barroso, C. S., et al. (2009). Implementation of Texas Senate Bill 19 to increase physical activity in elementary schools. *Journal of Public Health Policy, 30 Suppl 1*, pp. S221–S247.

34. O'Connor, T. M., Jago, R., & Baranowski, T. (2009). Engaging parents to increase youth physical activity: A systematic review. *American Journal of Preventive Medicine, 37*, pp. 141–149.

35. Nihiser, A. J., Lee, S. M., Wechsler, H., et al. (2009). BMI measurement in schools. *Pediatrics, 124 Suppl 1*, pp. S89–S97.

36. Ryan, K. W. (2009). Surveillance, screening, and reporting children's BMI in a school-based setting: A legal perspective. *Pediatrics, 124 Suppl 1*, pp. S83–S88.

    Gibbs, L., O'Connor, T., Waters, E., et al. (2007). Addressing the potential adverse effects of school-based BMI assessments on children's well-being. *International Journal of Pediatric Obesity*, pp. 1–7.

    Kubik, M. Y., Story, M., & Rieland, G. (2007). Developing school-based BMI screening and parent notification programs: Findings from focus groups with parents of elementary school students. *Health Education Behavior, 34*, pp. 622–633.

37. Lopez, R., Campbell, R., & Jennings, J. (2008). The Boston Schoolyard Initiative: A public-private partnership for rebuilding urban play spaces. *Journal of Health Politics, Policy, and Law, 33*, pp. 617–638.

38. Lopez, R., Jennings, J., & Campbell, R. (2008). *Schoolyard improvements and standardized test scores: An ecologic analysis.* Boston: Mauricio Gaston Institute.

39. Cohen, A. (2010). Achieving healthy school siting and planning policies: Understanding shared concerns of environmental planners, public health professionals, and educators. *New Solutions, 20*, pp. 49–72.

40. Marshall, J. D., Wilson, R. D., Meyer, K. L., Rajangam, S. K., McDonald, N. C., & Wilson, E. J. (2010). Vehicle emissions during children's school commuting: Impacts of education policy. *Environmental Science and Technology, 44*, pp. 1537–1543.
    Potera, C. (2008). Children's health: School siting poses particulate problem. *Environmental Health Perspectives, 116*, p. A474.

41. Lees, E., Salvesen, D., & Shay, E. (2008). Collaborative school planning and active schools: A case study of Lee County, Florida. *Journal of Health Politics, Policy and Law, 33*, pp. 595–615.

42. Rinaldi, M. J. (2010). Taxing sugar-sweetened beverages. *New England Journal of Medicine, 362*, p. 369.
    Brownell, K. D., Farley, T., Willett, W. C., et al. (2009). The public health and economic benefits of taxing sugar-sweetened beverages. *New England Journal of Medicine, 361*, pp. 1599–1605.

43. Ashe, M., Jernigan, D., Kline, R., & Galaz, R. (2003). Land use planning and the control of alcohol, tobacco, firearms, and fast-food restaurants. *American Journal of Public Health, 93*, pp. 1401–1408.

44. Perdue, W., Gostin, L., & Stone, L. (2003). Public health and the built environment: Historical, empirical, and theoretical foundations for an expanded role. *Journal of Law, Medicine and Ethics, 31*, pp. 557–566.

45. Kelley, E. (2009). *Community planning: An introduction to the comprehensive plan.* Washington D.C.: Island Press.

46. *Richmond general plan health element.* (2010). Healthy Communities by Design. (Accessed June 22, 2010, at http://www.healthycommunitiesbydesign.org/Content/10021/richmondgeneralplanhealthelement.html.)

47. Geraghty, A. B., Seifert, W., Preston, T., Holm, C. V., Duarte, T. H., & Farrar, S. M. (2009). Partnership moves community toward complete streets. *American Journal of Preventive Medicine, 37*, pp. S420–S427.

Chapter Sixteen

1. Hunter, D. (2006). Using a theory of change approach to build organizational strength, capacity and sustainability with not-for-profit organizations in the human services sector. *Evaluation and Program Planning, 29*, pp. 193–200.

2. Agyeman, J., Bullard, R., Evans, B. (2003). *Just sustainabilities: Development in an unequal world.* Cambridge, MA: MIT Press.
   Agyeman, J., & Evans, T. (2003). Toward just sustainability in urban communities: Building equity rights with sustainable solutions. *Annals of the American Academy of Political and Social Science, 590*, pp. 35–53.

3. Padilla, E. (2002). Intergenerational equity and sustainability. *Ecological Economics, 41*, pp. 69–83.

4. Wackernagel, M., & Rees, W. (1997). Perceptual and structural barriers to investing in natural capital: Economics from an ecological footprint perspective. *Ecological Economics, 20*, pp. 3–24.

5. Jones, P., Patterson, J., Lannon, S. (2007). Modelling the built environment at an urban scale—Energy and health impacts in relation to housing. *Landscape and Urban Planning, 83,* pp. 39–49.

6. Hudson, R. (2007). Region and place: Devolved regional government and regional economic success? *Progress in Human Geography, 31,* pp. 827–836.

7. Colvin, V. (2003). The potential environmental impact of engineered nanomaterials. *Nature Biotechnology, 21,* pp. 1166–1170.

8. Friedrichs, J. (2010). Global energy crunch: How different parts of the world would react to a peak oil scenario. *Energy Policy, 38,* pp. 4562–4569.
Verbruggen, A. (2008). Renewable and nuclear power: A common future? *Energy Policy, 36,* pp. 4036–4047.

9. Younger, M., Morrow-Almeida, H. R., Vindigni, S. M., & Dannenberg, A. L. (2008). The built environment, climate change, and health: Opportunities for co-benefits. *American Journal of Preventive Medicine, 35,* pp. 517–526.

10. United Nations. (1987). *Report of the World Commission on Environment and Development.* http://www.un.org/documents/ga/res/42/ares42–187.htm.

11. Marcuse, P. (1998). Sustainability is not enough. *Environment and Urbanization, 10,* pp. 103–112.

12. Saha, D., & Patterson, R. (2008). Local government efforts to promote the "Three Es" of sustainable development: Survey in medium to large cities in the United States. *Journal of Planning Education and Research, 28,* pp. 21–37.

13. Agyeman & Evans, Toward just sustainability in urban communities.
Agyeman, J., Bullard, R., & Evans, B. (2002). Exploring the nexus: Bringing together sustainability, environmental justice and equity. *Space and Polity, 6,* pp. 77–90.

14. Wackernagel, M., & Rees W. (1996). *Our ecological footprint: Reducing human impact on the earth.* Gabriola Island, BC: New Society Publishers.

15. Bell, S., & Morse, S. (1999). *Sustainability indicators: Measuring the immeasurable?* London: Earthscan.

16. Wilson, J., Tyedmers, P., & Pelot, R. (2007). Contrasting and comparing sustainable development indicator metrics. *Ecological Indicators, 7,* pp. 299–314.

17. White, T. (2000). Diet and the distribution of environmental impact. *Ecological Economics, 34,* pp. 145–153.

18. Wiedmann, T., Minx, J. (2008). A definition of "carbon footprint." In C. C. Pertsova (Ed.), *Ecological economics research trends.* Hauppage, NY: Nova Science Press.

19. Venetoulis, J., & Talberth, J. (2008). Refining the ecological footprint. *Environment, Development and Sustainability, 10,* pp. 441–469.

20. Wackernagel, M., Monfred, C., Schulz, N. B., Erb K.-H., Haberl, H., & Krausmann, F. (2004). Calculating national and global ecological footprint time series: Resolving conceptual challenges. *Land Use Policy, 21,* pp. 271–278.

21. Dietz, T., Rosa, E., York, R. (2007). Driving the human ecological footprint. *Frontiers in Ecology and the Environment, 5,* pp. 13–18.

22. Fiala, N. (2008). Measuring sustainability: Why the ecological footprint is bad economics and bad environmental science. *Ecological Economics, 67,* pp. 519–525.

23. Barretta, J., Bircha, R., Cherretta, N., & Wiedmann, T. (2005). Exploring the application of the ecological footprint to sustainable consumption policy. *Journal of Environmental Policy and Planning, 7,* pp. 303–316.

24. Owen, D. (2009). *Green metropolis: Why living smaller, living closer, and driving less are the keys to sustainability*. New York: Penguin.

25. Sarkissian, W., Hofe, N., Vajda, S., Shore, Y., & Wilkinson, C. (2008). *Kitchen table sustainability: Practical recipes for community engagement with sustainability*. London: Earthscan.

26. Freeman, C. (1996). Local government and emerging models of participation in the Local Agenda 21 process. *Journal of Environmental Planning and Management, 39*, pp. 65–78.

27. *Welcome to Sustainable Seattle*. (2010). Sustainable Seattle. Accessed June 30, 2010, at http://sustainableseattle.org/.

28. Saha & Patterson, Local government efforts to promote the "three es" of sustainable development.

29. Saha, D. (2009). Factors influencing local government sustainability efforts. *State and Local Government Review, 41*, pp. 39–48.

30. McHarg, I. (1969). *Design with nature*. Hoboken, NJ: Wiley.

31. Blakely, E., & Leigh, N. (2009). *Planning local economic development: Theory and practice*. Thousand Oaks, CA: Sage.

32. Beatley, T., & Manning, K. (1997). *The ecology of place: Planning for environment, economy, and community*. Washington, D.C.: Island Press.

33. Slocombe, D. (1993). Environmental planning, ecosystem science, and ecosystem approaches for integrating environment and development. *Environmental Management, 17*, pp. 289–303.

34. Maikov, K., Bell, S., & Sepp, K. (2008). Designing with nature in landscape architecture. *WIT Transactions on Ecology and the Environment, 1*.

35. David Rudlin, N. F. (1999). *Sustainable urban neighbourhood: Building the 21st century home*. Burlington, MA: Architecture Press.

36. Daniels, T., & Lapping, M. (2005). Land preservation: An essential ingredient in smart growth. *Journal of Planning Literature, 19*, pp. 316–329.

37. Pendal, R., Martin, J., & Fulton, W. (2002). *Holding the line: Urban containment in the United States*. Washington D.C.: Brookings Institute.

38. Amati, M. (2008). *Urban green belts in the twenty-first century*. Burlington, VT: Ashgate.

39. Abbott, C., & Margheim, J. (2008). Imagining Portland's urban growth boundary: Planning regulation as cultural icon. *Journal of the American Planning Association, 74*, pp. 196–208.

40. O'Toole, R. (2003). *San Jose demonstrates the limits of urban growth boundaries and urban rail*. Washington D.C.: Reason Institute.

41. O'Toole, R. (2007). The planning tax: The case against regional growth-management planning. Washington, D.C.: Cato Institute. *Report No.: Cato Policy Analysis Series, No. 606*. Kahn, M. (2001). Does sprawl reduce the black/white housing consumption gap? *Housing Policy Debate, 17*, pp. 349–355.

42. Mohamed, R. (2008). Who would pay for rural open space preservation and inner-city redevelopment? Identifying support for policies that can contribute to regional land use governance. *Urban Studies, 45*, pp. 2783–2803.

43. Jun, M.-J. (2004). The effects of Portland's urban growth boundary on urban development patterns and commuting. *Urban Studies, 41*, pp. 1333–1349.

44. Arnfield, A. (2003). Two decades of urban climate research: A review of turbulence, exchanges of energy and water, and the urban heat island. *International Journal of Climatology, 23*, pp. 1–26.

45. Takebayashi, H., Moriyama, M. (2007). Surface heat budget on green roof and high reflection roof for mitigation of urban heat island. *Building and Environment, 42*, pp. 2972–2979.

46. Carter, T., & Fowler, L. (2008). Establishing green roof infrastructure through environmental policy instruments. *Environmental Management, 42*, pp. 151–164.

47. Dvorak, B., & Volder, A. (2010). Green roof vegetation for North American ecoregions: A literature review. *Landscape and Urban Planning, 96*, pp. 197–215.

48. Suehrcke, H., Peterson, E., & Selby, N. (2008). Effect of roof solar reflectance on the building heat gain in a hot climate. *Energy and Buildings, 40*, pp. 2224–2235.

49. Landry, S., & Chakraborty, J. (2009). Street trees and equity: Evaluating the spatial distribution of an urban amenity. *Environment and Planning A, 41*, pp. 2651–2670.

50. Felson, A. (2009). The Million Trees Project: An initiative to transform New York City parkland into long-term ecological research sites on urban reforestation. In *Ecological society of America.* Albuquerque, NM. http://eco.confex.com/eco/2009/techprogram/P15696.HTM62.
    Climate action plan. (2010). Accessed June 30, 2010, at http://www.ci.la.ca.us/ead/ead_climatechange.htm.

51. Bertin, R. I., Manner, M. E., Larrow, B. F., Cantwell, T. W., & Berstene, E. M. (2005). Norway maple (Acer platanoides) and other non-native trees in urban woodlands of central Massachusetts. *The Journal of the Torrey Botanical Society, 132*, pp. 225–235.

52. Wilson, J. S., & Lindsey, G. H. (2009). Identifying urban neighborhoods for tree canopy restoration through community participation, In J. D. Gatrell and R. R. Jensen (Eds.), *Planning and socioeconomic applications.* New York: Springer.

53. Zahran, S., Grover, H., Brody, S., & Vedlitz, A. (1998). Risk, stress, and capacity: Explaining metropolitan commitment to climate protection. *Urban Affairs Review, 43*, pp. 447–474.

54. McHale, M., McPherson, E. G., & Burke, I. (2007). The potential of urban tree plantings to be cost effective in carbon credit markets. *Built Environment, 33*, pp. 115–139.

55. Paul, W., & Taylor, P. (2008). A comparison of occupant comfort and satisfaction between a green building and a conventional building. *Building and Environment, 43*, pp. 1858–1870.

56. Bunz, K., Henze, G., & Tiller, D. (2006). Survey of sustainable building design practices in North America, Europe, and Asia. *Journal of Architectural Engineering, 12*, pp. 33–62.

57. Retzlaff, R. (2008). Green building assessment systems: A framework and comparison for planners. *Journal of the American Planning Association, 74*, pp. 505–519.

58. Ahn, Y. H., & Pearce, A. R. (2007). Green construction: Contractor experiences, expectations, and perceptions. *Journal of Green Building, 2*, pp. 105–122.

59. Sartori, I., & Hestnes, A. (2007). Energy use in the life cycle of conventional and low-energy buildings: A review article. *Energy and Buildings, 39*, pp. 249–257.

60. *LEED rating systems.* (2010). U.S. Green Building Council. Accessed June 30, 2010, at http://www.usgbc.org/DisplayPage.aspx?CMSPageID=222.

61. Williams, L. (2010). The pragmatic approach to green design: Achieving LEED certification from an architect's perspective. *Journal of Green Building, 5*, pp. 3–12.

62. Newsham, G. R., Mancini, S., & Birt, S.M., (2009). Do LEED-certified buildings save energy? Yes, but . . . *Energy and Buildings, 41*, pp. 897–905.

63. Haapio, A., & Viitaniem, P. (2008). A critical review of building environmental assessment tools. *Environmental Impact Assessment Review, 28*, pp. 469–482.

64. Gregg, T., Strub, D., & Gross, D. (2007). Water efficiency in Austin, Texas, 1983–2005: An historical perspective. *Journal of the American Water Works Association, 99*, pp. 76–86.

65. Sovocool, K., Morgan, M., & Bennett, D. (2006). An in-depth investigation of xeriscape as a water conservation measure. *Journal of the American Water Works Association, 98*, pp. 82–93.

66. Hurd, B. (2006). Water conservation and residential landscapes: Household preferences, household choices. *Journal of Agricultural and Resource Economics, 31*, pp. 173–192.

67. Vickers, A. (2006). Perspectives—New Directions in Lawn and Landscape Water Conservation. *Journal of the American Water Works Association, 98*, pp. 56–61.

68. Frumkin, H., Hess, J., Luber, G., Malilay, J., & McGeehin, M. (2008). Climate change: The public health response. *American Journal of Public Health, 98*, pp. 435–445.

69. Shuman, E. K. (2010). Global climate change and infectious diseases. *New England Journal of Medicine, 362*, pp. 1061–1063.
Haines, A., Kovats, R. S., Campbell-Lendrum, D., & Corvalan, C. (2006). Climate change and human health: Impacts, vulnerability, and mitigation. *Lancet, 367*, pp. 2101–2109.

70. Luber, G., & Prudent, N. (2009). Climate change and human health. *Transactions of the American Clinical and Climatological Association, 120*, pp. 113–117.

71. Zahran, S., Kim, E., Chen, X., & Lubell, M. (2007). Ecological development and global climate change: A cross-national study of Kyoto Protocol ratification. *Society & Natural Resources, 20*, pp. 37–55.

72. Selin, H., & VanDeveer, S. (2007). Political science and prediction: What's next for U.S. climate change policy? *Review of Policy Research, 24*, pp. 1–27.

73. Stavins, R. (2008). Addressing climate change with a comprehensive U.S. cap-and-trade system. *Oxford Review of Economic Policy, 24*, pp. 298–321.

74. Grimm, N. B., Faeth, S. H., Golubiewski, N. E., et al. (2008). Global change and the ecology of cities. *Science, 319*, pp. 756–760.

75. Byrne, J., Hughes, K., Rickerson, W., & Kurdgelashvili, L. (2007). American policy conflict in the greenhouse: Divergent trends in federal, regional, state, and local green energy and climate change policy. *Energy Policy, 35*, pp. 4555–4573.

76. Patz, J., Campbell-Lendrum, D., Gibbs, H., & Woodruff, R. (2008). Health impact assessment of global climate change: Expanding on comparative risk assessment approaches for policy making. *Annual Reviews of Public Health, 29*, pp. 27–39.

77. Füssel, H. (2007). Adaptation planning for climate change: Concepts, assessment approaches, and key lessons. *Sustainability Science, 2*, pp. 265–275.

78. Costello, A., Abbas, M., Allen, A., et al. (2009). Managing the health effects of climate change: Lancet and University College London Institute for Global Health Commission. *Lancet, 373*, pp. 1693–1733.

79. Gill, S., Handley, J., Ennos, A., & Pauleit, S. (2007). Adapting cities for climate change: The role of the green infrastructure. *Built Environment, 33*, pp. 115–133.

80. Gardner, G., & Stern, P. (2008). The short list: The most effective actions U.S. households can take to curb climate change. *Environment: Science and Policy for Sustainable Development, 50*, pp. 12–25.

81. Whitmarsh, L. (2009). Behavioural responses to climate change: Asymmetry of intentions and impacts. *Journal of Environmental Psychology, 24*, pp. 267–377.

Page references followed by *fig* indicate an illustrated figure; followed by *t* indicate a table.

A

Abandoned properties, 107–108
Accessibility: mobility versus, 69; as transportation policy driver, 69–70; unequal access to amenities, 201–202, 256
Active Living Research (ALR), 291–292
ADHD (attention deficit hyperactivity disorder), 83, 222
Adolescent substance abuse, 238*fig*
Advertising-behavior relationship, 241
Affordability (housing), 96–97, 109–110, 112
African Americans: defining race of, 196; dislocation and gentrification impacting, 44, 110–111, 220–222; food insecurity in households that include children, 175*fig*; housing segregation of, 31–32, 44, 111–112, 199–200; Jim Crow legislation against, 32; living near commercial hazardous waste facilities, 248*fig*; urban renewal elimination of neighborhoods of, 37;

vulnerabilities of, 195. *See also* Racial/ethnicity differences; Racism
Age-adjusted obesity rates, 52*fig*
Aging in place, 206
Agriculture: community-supported, 185–186; farm-residential interface, 186; Hartford Food System (HFS), 186; urban gardening, 187–188
Air pollutants: anti-idling campaigns to reduce, 142; asbestos, 145–146; carbon monoxide, 146–147; criteria, 139–140; environmental tobacco smoke, 149; Hazardous Air Pollutants (HAPS), 147–148; lead, 146; particulates (PM), 141*t*–143; radon, 143–144; school indoor air and, 148–149; VOCs (volatile organic compounds), 144–145
Air pollution: health conditions associated with, 149–153; regulatory framework on, 139–141; trends of, 138–139. *See also* Pollution
Air pollution-associated health issues: asthma, 150–151;

cardiovascular disease, 150; sick building syndrome, 144, 151–153
Air quality: air pollution relationship to, 139; anti-idling campaigns to improve, 142; indoor, 101; school indoor, 148–149
Alienation, anomie form of, 210–211
Alinsky, Saul, 236
Allostatic load, 219–220
Ambler, Euclid v., 31
American Apartheid (Denton and Massey), 32
American Community Survey, 73
American Household Survey, 92
American Public Health Association, 37
American Society of Civil Engineers, 130
Americans with Disability Act (1990), 207
Anomie, 210–211
Anti-idling campaigns, 142
Aquifers: description of, 166; overuse and contamination of, 166
Architecture, built environment association with, 10
Army Corp of Engineers, 131
Asbestos, 145–146

Asian/Pacific Islanders, 248*fig*
Assessment tools: The Community Toolbox, 282; cost-benefit analysis, 279–280; environmental impact assessment (EIA), 270–272; geographic information systems (GIS), 277–278; government data sources, 282–284; Health Impact Assessment (HIA), 272–275; International Physical Activity Questionnaire (IPAQ), 280; Neighborhood Walkability Assessment Survey (NEWS), 276–277; special equipment worn by study subjects, 281–282; System for Observing Play and Recreation in Communities (SOPARC), 281
Asthma, 150–151, 197
Automobiles: driving safety issue of, 74–75; EPA fuel efficiency standards for, 318; greenhouse gas emissions of, 317–318; hybrid and electric, 317; rates of household ownership of, 73–74; road rage and, 215. *See also* Driving;Transportation

B

Bauer, Catherine, 35
Behavioral Risk Factor Surveillance System (BRFSS), 55, 282, 283
Beverage and Soda taxes, 296
Bicycling: infrastructure and safety issues of, 81–82; lower traffic speed to encourage, 57; Portland (Oregon) policies encouraging, 84

Bike lanes: increasing safety using, 81–82; Portland (Oregon), 84
Bike-sharing programs, 82
Biological determinism, 228–229
Biophilia theory: on defensible space, 218–219; on density and health, 215–217; description of, 212–214; on high-rises and connections to the street, 217–218; on urban vs. rural living, 214–215
BMI (body mass index), 55, 295
Boston: Boston Schoolyard Institute (BSI), 295; Emerald Necklace of, 27
Boston Schoolyard Institute (BSI), 295
Bottled water, 160
Bowling Alone (Putnam), 233
Broadacre City, 32
Broken windows theory, 240
Brownfields: description of, 126–127; restoration of, 127
Brundtland Commission, 303
Bryant, Bunyan, 112
Built environment: air pollution relationship to, 139; Americans with Disability Act (1990) impact on, 207; cross-disciplinary nature of study of, 9–11; debate over health impacts of, 47; disaster response of restricting vs. building protective barriers, 127–129; disciplines associated with, 10–11; the elderly and, 205–206; environmental health questions about, 6–7; environmental tobacco smoke problem in, 149; how we evaluate, 7–8; influences

on the, 13–14; legal basis for health interventions related to, 297–298; particulate matter (PM) pollution impacted by features of, 143; placing analysis into broader context, 11–13; public perceptions and assumptions regarding, 8–9; race and, 198–199; reducing impervious surfaces, 130; understanding connections between health and, 3–4; vulnerability and, 195. *See also* Environment; Metropolitan structure
Built environment history: age of reform, 25–28; changing rates of life expectancy at birth, 25*fig*; current era (1980–2010), 38–39; era of industrialization and urbanization (1825–1930), 19–24; health effects in 19th century cities, 22–24; impact of immigration, 21; increased use of codes and zoning, 28–31; Industrial Revolution, 20–21; pre-Industrial Revolution era, 18–19; public housing and the New Deal, 35–38; twentieth-century architectural movements (1930–1980), 32–35; urbanization, 21–22
Burgess, Ernest, 210
Bus Riders Union (Los Angeles), 256, 265

C

Calhoun, John, 216
California Water Project, 157–158
Carbon dioxide emissions: efforts to limit, 317–318; not

covered by Clean Air Act, 138

Carbon monoxide, 146–147

Cardiovascular disease: air pollution impact on, 150; Latino immigrants to the U.S., 212*fig*

Cell phone use, 75

Centers for Disease Control and Prevention (CDC): BRFSS survey on obesity risk, 55; foodborne illnesses estimates by, 173; physical activity guidelines by, 80, 82

Central Park (New York), 27

Chadwick, Sir Edwin, 26, 28, 30

Children: access to open space and ADHD, 83, 222; encouraged to walk to school, 83–84; environmental health and vulnerabilities of, 203–205; food insecurity in households that include, 175*fig*; percentage with elevated blood lead levels, 101*t*; school-based health interventions aimed at, 293–296; walking benefits those with ADHD, 83. *See also* Schools; Vulnerable Populations

Chlorinated hydrocarbons (CFC), 105

Cholera: epidemics of 1832, 1846, 1854, 22–23; proven contagion of, 24

Cholorination by-products, 164

CIAM (Congrès International d'Architecture Moderne), 51

Cities: beginnings of urban planning (1825–1930) in, 25–31; creating healthy metropolitan structure, 58–63; environmental justice issues for, 249–265; era of industrialization and

urbanization (1825–1930), 19–24; features of a healthy community, 55–58; food deserts in, 179–182; Frank Lloyd Wright's Broadacre City, 32; health effects in 19th century, 22–24; health impacts of metropolitan structures of, 54–55; health in pre-Industrial Revolution, 18–19; higher density, 56; impact of immigration on, 21; impact of urbanization on, 21–22; inserting health into general plans of, 298; Le Corbusier's Ville Radieuse proposal, 34, 217; legal basis for built environment regulation by, 297–298; protecting from rising sea levels, 319; racial housing segregation (1825–1930) in, 31–32; shrinking city movement, 107–108; Spanish Law of the Indies on grid design of, 19; urban renewal of U.S., 36–38. *See also* Community; Neighborhoods; Urban communities; Urban renewal

City general plans, 298

The City in History (Mumford), 18

Clean Air Act, 138, 140, 271, 272

Clean Drinking Water Act, 156

Clean Water Act, 156, 271

Climate change. *See* Global climate change

Codes: earthquake, 122; enforcement of housing, 103–105; form-based, 53–54; housing regulation and, 103; inserting health into city general plans through, 298; introduction of housing, 28–31; planned

unit development (PUD), 50; smoke detectors, 102; urban sprawl solution through reform of, 60–61. *See also* Government regulations; Urban planning; Zoning

Collective efficacy, 230

Combined sewer overflows, 163

Commercial district rebuilding, 62–63

Communication infrastructure systems, 119–120

Community: broken windows theory on, 240; ecology research context of, 9; environmental justice issues for, 249–265; equity concept and gated, 13; features of healthy, 55–58; hazardous waste facilities acceptance by poorer, 263–264; health interventions, 292–293; health and sociological context of, 9; legal basis for built environment regulation by, 297–298; local sustainability movement in, 307–308; protecting from rising sea levels, 319. *See also* Cities; Neighborhoods

Community Development Corporations (CDCs), 98

Community legal advocacy, 105–106

The Community Toolbox, 282

Community-based participatory research, 239

Community-level health interventions, 292–293

Community-supported agriculture, 185–186

Commuting: description and data on, 71–72; health effects of, 72; suburban development impact on, 46–47; U.S. workers and

Commuting: (*continued*)
chosen mode of, 68*fig. See also* Driving; Traffic; Transportation
Compact metropolitan area, 56
Complete streets, 85
Composting toilets, 169
Concentrated poverty areas, 202, 227
Congestion charges, 69, 86
Congress for New Urbanism (CNU), 51
Connected street networks, 57
Connecticut Food Policy Council, 186
Consumer Product Safety Commission, 133
Contagion theory, 24
Contaminant-free housing, 105
Contamination: aquifers overuse and, 166; drinking water and sewage waste, 120–121, 158–159; foodborne illnesses due to, 172–174; lead/lead poisoning, 99–101*t*, 146, 164–165; pharmaceuticals in drinking water, 165–166. *See also* Pollution
Conventional development: description of, 44–45; new urbanism developed as alternative to, 50–51; problems with suburban and urban form of, 45–48
Cost-benefit analysis, 279–280
Crime: broken windows theory on, 240; defensible space to combat, 218–219; streetlights to lower, 58
Criteria air pollutants, 139–140
Cryptosporidium outbreak (Milwaukee, 1993), 159, 161
Cul-de-sacs street patterns, 72–73
Culture of poverty, 241–242
Cumulative risk, 194

D

Davis, Robert, 51
The Death and Life of Great American Cities (Jacobs), 38, 49
Decision making tools: environmental impact assessment (EIA), 270–272; Health Impact Assessment (HIA), 272–275. *See also* Information tools
Defensible space, 218–219
Demand management, 69
Dendritic street patterns, 72–73
Density: benefits of higher, 56; health and, 215–217; providing bonuses for healthier, 62
Desalination, 162
Design with Nature (McHarg), 309
Detroit's urban agriculture proposal, 182
Diabetes: Latino immigrants to the U.S., 212*fig*; stress as factor in development of, 220
Discrimination: description of, 196–197; housing segregation as, 31–32, 44, 111–112
Disease causation: contagion theory of, 24; miasma theory of, 24, 26
Diseases: asthma, 150–151, 197; cardiovascular disease, 150, 212*fig*; cholera, 22–23, 24; diabetes, 212*fig*, 220; flooding and waterborne, 121. *See also* Obesity
Displacement problem, 110–111
Disproportionate burden: accessing health effects of multiple exposures, 257–258; description of, 256–257; environmental enforcement issue of, 261–262; hazardous waste versus community growth issue of, 260–261; proximity versus unequal exposure, 258–260; race versus income, 258; West End Revitalization Association (WEBA) fight against, 262
Drinking water: bottled, 160; characteristics by suppliers, 157*t*; chlorination by-products, 164; composting toilets to conserve consumption of, 169; contamination by sewage waste, 120–121, 158–159; desalination, 162; impact on health by, 159–160; infrastructure for ensuring clean, 157*t*–159; lead found in, 164–165; nonpoint pollution of, 168–169; overuse and contamination of aquifers, 166; pharmaceuticals in, 165–166; reducing leaks, 168; reducing residential water use, 167*fig*–168; regulatory framework for, 156–157; sludge by-product of sewage treatment, 163–164; wastewater treatment, 162–163; water quality monitoring of, 160–161; water recycling, 161–162. *See also* Water quality
Driving: cell phone use while, 75; cost of, 75–76; increasing safety of, 74–75; road rage and, 215. *See also* Automobiles; Commuting; Traffic
Duany, Andres, 51, 52

Dudley Street Neighborhood Initiative (DSNI) [Boston], 237
Durkheim, Emile, 210

E

E. coli, 173
Earthquakes: disaster planning for, 122–123; Loma Prieta earthquake (1989), 115–116, 122; risk and damage from, 121–122
Ecological footprints: description of, 304–305; of rural versus urban residents, 307; selected national carbon, 305*fig*–306
Ecologically built environment, 11
Economics: built environment association with, 11; housing segregation related to poverty and, 111–112, 197; income inequality, 201–202, 256, 258; as influence on built environment, 14. *See also* Poverty
Elderly population: aging in place, 206; the built environment and vulnerabilities of, 205–206; extreme temperature events and, 123–124; housing needs of, 206
Electric and hybrid cars, 317
Emerald Necklace (Boston), 27
Emergency food assistance, 176
Eminent domain, 61
Environment: concerns over bottled water impact on the, 160; food production and farming impacts on the, 182–188; global climate change, 316–319; many meanings of, 4; physical,

4–5; social, 5; traditional meaning of, 6. *See also* Built environment
Environmental amenities access, 201–202, 256
Environmental design: green building design approach to, 313–316; green roofs, 310–311; greenbelts and land preservation, 56–58, 60, 132–133, 201–202, 223, 309–310; sustainability and the role of, 308–316; urban greening and, 312–313; xeriscaping, 168, 316
Environmental determinism, 228–229
Environmental health: children and, 203–204; process of creating, 204–205
Environmental health study questions: does risk occur outside body?, 6; is exposure or health risk voluntary, 6–7; is health risk caused by biological agent?, 7
Environmental impact assessment (EIA): characteristics of, 271*t*; overview of, 270–272
Environmental justice: definition of, 248; disproportionate burden issue of, 256–263; limitations of actions, 262–264; transportation justice component of, 80
Environmental justice movement: description of, 248–249; Executive Order (1994) impact on the, 253, 255–256; history of the, 249–252; lessons learned from the, 265; Principles of the Environmental Justice Network (1992), 252–253, 254–255; unequal access to

amenities issue of the, 201–202, 256. *See also* Hazardous waste facilities; Pollution
Environmental tobacco smoke, 149
Epidemiology: built environment association with, 10; transportation-related injuries, 71
Equity: built environment in context of, 12–13; sustainability and, 303–304; transportation justice issue of, 80; unequal access to amenities issue of, 201–202, 256
Euclid v. Ambler, 31
Evacuation plans, 118
Evidence-based urban design, 225
Executive Order (1994), 253, 255–256
Extreme temperature events, 123–124

F

Farm-residential interface, 186
Farmers markets, 185
Farming. *See* Food production/farming
Fast-food restaurant bans, 181–182
Federal Emergency Management Agency (FEMA), 120, 125, 128
Federal funding: financing infrastructure, 130–132; of housing, 95–98, 112; of mass transit, 79. *See also* Government regulations
Federal Housing Administration, 36
FHA (Federal Housing Administration), 94–95

Fires/fire injuries: household, 101–102; wildfire disasters and, 124–125

First National People of Color Environmental Leadership Summit (1991), 252–253, 254–255

Flooding: contamination from sewage problem of, 120–121; FEMA maps to estimate potential, 120; mold buildup following, 121; moving an entire town to prevent, 128; river restoration, 129–130; San Francisco Bay delta potential for, 119

Food deserts: description of, 179–180; strategies to address, 180–182

Food insecurity: percentage of households with children suffering, 175*fig*; as worldwide problem, 174–175

Food insecurity strategies: Detroit's urban agriculture proposal, 182; farm to school programs, 178; food pantries and emergency food assistance, 176; nutritional subsidy programs, 175–176; school gardens, 179; school vending machines as both problem and, 178–179; subsidized and free students lunches, 177–178

"Food miles" concept, 185

Food pantry programs, 176

Food production/farming: community-supported agriculture, 185–186; environmental effects of, 182–188; farm-residential interface, 186; farmers markets, 185; Hartford Food System (HFS), 186;

large-scale livestock operations, 183–184; locavore movement, 184–185; organic foods, 184; urban gardening, 187–188

Foodborne illnesses: challenges of preventing, 173–174; contamination causing, 172–173

Form-based codes, 53–54

Framingham Heart Study, 231

Fullilove, Mindy, 111

G

Garden Cities movement, 29

Gentrification, 44, 110–111, 220–222

Geographic information systems (GIS), 277–278

Global climate change: how health is impacted by, 316–317; hybrid and electric cars to slow down, 317; individual efforts to reduce, 319; limiting greenhouse gas emissions to slow down, 317–318; planning for, 318–319

Government data sources, 282–284

Government regulations: air quality, 139–141; environmental justice and enforcement of, 261–262; housing, 93–113; legal basis for built environment, 297–298; water quality, 156–157; water quality monitoring, 160–161; zoning, 30–31, 47–54, 60–61, 86–87. *See also* Codes; Federal funding; U.S. legislation

Graffiti, 240

Graywater (water distribution system), 161

Great Depression (1929), 36, 96

Green building design: LEED (Leadership in Energy and Environmental Design) promoting, 314–316; sustainability through, 313–314

Green roofs, 310–311

Greenbelts: healing gardens, 223; parks, 56–57, 132–133, 201–202; street trees, 57–58; sustainability promoted through, 309–310; urban greening, 312–313; as urban sprawl solution, 60. *See also* Land use

Greenhouse gas emissions, 317–318

Greenvich Village (New York City), 49

Griscom, John, 26, 30

Groups: collective efficacy of, 230; improving social capital by changing expectations of, 236–237; multilevel modeling of, 235; social support of, 230–231. *See also* Social capital

H

Hall, Edward, 216

Harlem (New York City), 251

Hartford Food System (HFS), 186

Hazardous Air Pollutants (HAPS), 147–148

Hazardous waste facilities: characteristics of neighborhoods near, 248*fig*; community growth around previously established, 260–261; environmental justice movement concerns with, 249–252; poorer community acceptance of, 263–264; proximity versus unequal exposure to, 258–260. *See also* Environmental justice movement; Pollution

Healing gardens, 223

Health: built environment in context of, 12; built environment influenced by beliefs of, 14; community in context of, 9; environmental, 203–205; in 19th century cities, 22–23; in pre-industrial era cities, 18–19; relationship of stress and, 219–220; role of active transport in, 80; understanding connections between built environment and, 3–4. *See also* Mental health

Health behaviors: advertising impact on, 241; how friends impact obesity and, 231; social norms influencing, 239–240

Health beliefs model, 289

Health disparities: housing segregation related to, 199–200; interventions to reduce racial, 199; poverty and, 200–203; racial, 197–198; of racism and discrimination, 196–197; U.S. infant mortality (2006), 198*fig*

Health effects: air pollution and related, 149–153; assessing multiple exposures and, 257–258; automobiles and, 73–77; changing metropolitan structure to improve, 58–63; of commuting, 72; debate over rural suburban, or urban,

47; global climate change, 316–317; healthy immigrant effect, 211–212; highways and, 77–78; mass transit and, 78–80; metropolitan structure's negative, 54–58; rural health advantage, 47; social capital, 235; suburban and urban development, 45–48. *See also* Public health interventions

Health facilities design, 224–225

Healthy community, 55–58

Healthy housing, 102–103

Healthy immigrant effect, 211–212

Heat waves, 123–124

The Hidden Dimension (Hall), 216

Higher densities, 56

Highways: health effects related to, 77–78; impact on urban communities, 76–77. *See also* Streets

Hill, Octavia, 26

Hispanics: air pollution impact and, 138; defining ethnicity of, 196; environmental justice movement leadership among, 250–251; food insecurity in households that include children, 175*fig*; key health indicators of immigrants to the U.S., 212*fig*; living near commercial hazardous waste facilities, 248*fig*; vulnerabilities of, 195. *See also* Racial/ethnicity differences

A History of Public Health (Rosen), 19

History. *See* Built environment history

HIV/AIDS education groups, 236

Homelessness problem, 109–110

HOPE VI program, 97, 219, 242

Household injuries, 102

Housing: attributes of healthy, 102–103; beginnings of urban planning (1825–1930) for, 25–31; decline of racial housing segregation (mid-1970s), 44; density of, 56, 62, 215–217; economic segregation of, 111–112; introduction of codes and zoning of, 28–31; Jim Crow legislation perpetuating segregated, 32; movement to fund public, 35–36; oriented toward streets, 58; racial segregation (1825–1930), 31–32, 111; regulatory framework of U.S., 93–113. *See also* Public housing

Housing affordability, 96–97, 109–110, 112

Housing problems: abandoned properties, 107–108; affordability, 96–97, 109–110, 112; displacement and gentrification, 44, 110–111, 220–222; fires/fire injuries and deaths, 101–102; gentrification, 44, 110–111, 220–222; history of, 92–93; homelessness, 109–110; household injuries, 102; housing for special needs populations, 108; indoor air quality, 101; lead, 99–101; mental health and housing, 112–113; mold, 99; occupied housing units and reported, 93*t*; pests, 106–107

Housing regulatory framework: abandoned properties, 107–108; code enforcement,

Housing regulatory framework: (*continued*) 103–105; codes and housing regulation, 103; Community Development Corporations (CDCs), 98; community legal advocacy, 105–106; current housing programs, 96–99; FHA (Federal Housing Administration), 94–95; HOPE VI program, 97; integrated pest management, 106–107; LHA (Local Housing Authority), 95, 97; public and publicly assisted housing, 95–96; Section 8 program, 97–98

Housing segregation: decline (mid-1970s) of, 44; economic-based, 111–112, 197; health disparities related to, 199–200; racism of (1825–1930), 31–32, 111

How the Other Half Lives (Riis), 26

Howard, Ebenezer, 29

Human capital, 228

Hurricanes: Hurricane Andrew (1992), 115, 126; Hurricane Katrina (2005), 115, 117–118, 125–126; inadequate communication during, 119–120; inadequate evacuation plans, 118; inadequate protective infrastructure, 118–119; storm surge of, 117

Hybrid and electric cars, 317

Hypertension, 212*fig*

I

Immigrants: anomie alienation experienced by, 210–211; healthy immigrant effect of, 211–212

Immigration: conceptual frameworks for understanding experience of, 211–212; impact on cities by, 21

Income inequality: access to environmental amenities and, 201–202, 256; environmental justice on race versus, 258. *See also* Poverty

Individual-level health interventions, 296–297

Indoor air quality: of schools, 148–149; sources of problems with, 101

Infant mortality: in 19th century cities, 23–24; in the U.S. by race (2006), 198*fig*

Information tools: The Community Toolbox, 282; cost-benefit analysis, 279–280; geographic information systems (GIS), 277–278; government data sources, 282–284; International Physical Activity Questionnaire (IPAQ), 280; Neighborhood Walkability Assessment Survey (NEWS), 276–277; special equipment worn by study subjects, 281–282; System for Observing Play and Recreation in Communities (SOPARC), 281. *See also* Decision making tools

Infrastructure: decaying, 130; earthquake disasters and failures of, 122–123; extreme temperature events and, 123–124; financing, 130–132; floods and issues of, 119, 120–121; highways,

76–78; hurricanes and inadequate communication, 119–120; hurricanes and inadequate protective, 118–119; long-term maintenance of, 132; parks and playgrounds, 56–57, 132–133; planning for global climate change by changing, 318–319; reducing impervious surfaces, 130; water quality and, 157*t*–159. *See also* Streets

Injuries: epidemiology of transportation-related, 71; fires/fire, 101–102; household, 102; wildfires, 124–125

Integrated Pest Management (IPM), 106–107

International Building Code, 103

International Code Council, 103

International Physical Activity Questionnaire (IPAQ), 280

International Style (or Modernism), 33–35

ISTEA (Intermodal Surface Transportation Efficiency Act), 78–79

J

Jacobs, Jane, 34, 38, 49

Jim Crow legislation, 32

Justice. *See* Environmental justice

K

Katz, Peter, 52

Kerner Commission report (1968), 199–200

Kyoto Protocol, 318

L

Lacavore movement, 184–185
Land use: air pollution relationship to, 139; eminent domain and, 61; intersection of transportation policies and, 70–71; urban gardening, 187–188. *See also* Greenbelts; Zoning
Landscape architecture, built environment association with, 11
Landslides, 125
Large-scale livestock operations, 183–184
Latinos. *See* Hispanics
Law, built environment association with, 11
Le Corbusier, 33, 34, 217
Lead: air pollution from gasoline containing, 146; drinking water and, 164–165; lead poisoning from paint with, 99–101*t*
LEED (Leadership in Energy and Environmental Design) promoting, 314–316
LEED-Neighborhood certification, 315
Legal issues. *See* Government regulations; U.S. legislation
Life expectancy at birth rates, 25*fig*
Liquefaction, 122
Liquor advertisements, 241
Livestock operations, 183–184
Local Housing Authority (LHA), 95, 97
Local mass transit funding, 80
Local sustainability movements, 307–308
Locavore movement, 184–185
Loma Prieta earthquake (1989), 115–116, 122
Los Angeles Bus Riders Union, 80

Los Angeles County Metropolitan Transportation Authority, 80
Louis, Oscar, 241
Low-income housing: Community Development Corporations (CDCs) promoting, 98; Local Housing Authority (LHA), 95, 97; Section 8 program for, 97–98. *See also* Public housing

M

McHarg, Ian, 46, 308–309
McKeown, Thomas, 23
Maintenance: importance of long-term infrastructure, 132; of water and sewer systems, 158–159
Marcuse, Peter, 303
Mass transit: federal funding of, 79; ISTEA (Intermodal Surface Transportation Efficiency Act) on, 78–79; Portland (Oregon), 84; role of active transport in health, 80; state and local financing of, 80
Massachusetts Bay Transportation Authority (MBTA), 265
Massachusetts Department of Public Health (Mass DPH), 290–291
Massachusetts Water Resources Authority (MWRA), 131
Mead, Margaret, 241
Medicine, built environment association with, 10
Mental health: biophilia theory on, 212–219; housing and, 112–113; nature deficit disorder, 213–214; rootshock and gentrification

effects on, 44, 110–111, 220–222; stressors and allostatic load roles in, 219–225; theory of anomie and, 210–211. *See also* Health
Methane, 317
Metropolitan structure: features of a healthy community, 55–58; finding solutions to, 58–63; negative health impacts of, 54–55. *See also* Built environment
Miasma theory, 24, 26
Mississippi River bridge collapse (2007), 130
Mississippi River Gulf Outlet (MRGO), 117–118
Model tenement movement, 26–27
Modernism (or International Style): origins and development of, 33–35, 217; public house designed using principles of, 36
Mold: flooding and buildup of, 121; housing problem of, 99
Mortality rates: of infants in 19th century cities, 23–24; racial disparities in, 197–198; U.S. infant mortality by race (2006), 198*fig*
Moses, Robert, 49
Mothers of East Los Angeles, 250
Moving to Opportunity Program (MTO), 227, 243–244
Moynihan, Daniel Patrick, 242
Mudslides, 125
Multilevel modeling, 235
Mumford, Lewis, 9, 11, 49
Municipal infrastructure funding, 130–132

N

National carbon footprints, 305*fig*–306
National Center for Health Statistics, 282
National Center for Healthy Housing (NCHH), 104
National Fire Protection Association, 103
National Health Interview Survey, 282
National Health and Nutrition Examination Survey (NHANES), 149, 282, 283
National Institute of Environmental Health Sciences (NIEHS), 253
National Latino and Asian American Survey, 282–283
Native Americans: environmentalism efforts in tribal lands of, 249; fighting for environmental justice of, 248. *See also* Racial/ethnicity differences
Natural disaster response: Brownfields restoration, 126–127; decaying infrastructure, 130; Federal Emergency Management Agency (FEMA) role in, 120, 125; federal and state responsibilities for, 125–126; financing infrastructure, 130–132; maintenance, 132; parks and playgrounds role in, 132–133; reducing impervious surfaces, 130; restricting buildings vs. building protective barriers, 127–129; river restoration, 129–130
Natural disasters: earthquakes, 115–116, 121–123;

extreme temperature events, 123–124; floods, 120–121, 128; hurricanes, 115, 117, 120, 125–126, 127–128; mudslides and landslides, 125; San Francisco Bay delta potential as, 119; wildfires, 124–125
Nature deficit disorder, 213–214
"Negro removal," 37
Neighborhood Walkability Assessment Survey (NEWS), 276–277
Neighborhoods: broken windows theory on, 240; commercial hazardous waste facilities and characteristics of, 248*fig*; disorder, social capital, adolescent alcohol/drug use in, 238*fig*; Dudley Street Neighborhood Initiative (DSNI) [Boston], 237; environmental justice issues for, 249–265; food deserts, 179–182; gentrification of, 44, 110–111, 220–222; hazardous waste facilities acceptance by poorer, 263–264; hazardous waste facilities unequal exposure vs. proximity of, 258–260; outdoor liquor and tobacco advertising in, 241; parks in, 56–57, 132–133, 201–202; playgrounds, 56–57, 132–133, 201–202; social capital for empowering, 238*fig*–239. *See also* Cities; Community
New Deal, 35–38
New Orleans: Hurricane Katrina (2005) destruction to, 115, 117–118, 125–126; protecting from rising sea levels, 319

New urbanism: developed as alternative to conventional development, 50–51; origins of, 38; public health and, 51–53
New York City: Central Park of, 27; first zoning ordinance adopted by, 30; Jane Jacobs' influence on urban planning in, 34, 38, 49; protecting from rising sea levels, 319; Triborough Bridge Authority of, 49; urban gardening issue in, 187; urban greening efforts by, 312; West Harlem Environmental Action (WEACT) in, 251
The New Yorker magazine, 11
Newman, Oscar, 218
Noise exposure, 222–223
Nursing-built environment relationship, 10
Nutritional subsidy programs, 175–176

O

Oakland Hills fire (1991), 124
Obesity: BMI (body mass index) measurement of, 55, 295; influence of friends on, 231; Latino immigrants to the U.S., 212*fig*; metropolitan structure impact on rates of, 54–58; school-based health interventions addressing childhood, 293–294; solutions through metropolitan structure changes, 58–63; urban sprawl relationship to, 55; U.S. age-adjusted rates of, 52*fig*. *See also* Diseases
Office of Management and Budget (OMB), 196

Ogallala aquifer (Great Plains), 166
Oglethorpe, Charles, 19
Olmstead, Frederick Law, 26, 27
On-street parking, 57
One-way streets, 87
Open space access, 222
Organic foods, 184
Ozonation, 159

P

Park, Robert, 210
Parking (on-street), 57
Parks: health benefits of, 132–133; neighborhood, 56–57; poverty and lack of access to, 201–202
Particulate matter (PM) pollution, 141t–143
Pedestrian zones, 86–87
Pedestrian-friendly street crossings, 57
Pedestrians: building amenities for, 63; epidemiology of transportation-related injuries of, 71; lower traffic speed to encourage, 57; sidewalks to encourage, 57; signal changes to better accommodate, 87–88. *See also* Walking
Penn, William, 19
People with disabilities: housing for, 108; transportation issues of, 73; vulnerabilities of, 207; walking safety policies for, 83
Perry, Clarence, 29, 44
Pests: ensuring pest-free housing, 104; IPM (Integrated Pest Management) enforcing codes on, 106–107
Pharmaceuticals in drinking water, 165–166

Physical activity: CDC guidelines for, 80, 82; interventions to increase school-related, 294–295; transit-oriented development to encourage, 62
Physical environment, 4–5
Planned unit development (PUD), 50
Plater-Zybeck, Elizabeth, 51
Playgrounds: health benefits of, 132–133; physical activity promoted by, 56–57; poverty and lack of access to, 201–202; safety issues of, 133
Pollution: carbon dioxide emissions, 138, 317–318; CFC (chlorinated hydrocarbons), 105; contaminant-free housing, 105; greenhouse gas emissions, 317–318; lead/lead poisoning, 99–101t; methane, 317; mold, 99, 121; noise exposure, 222–223; nonpoint pollution sources of water, 168–169; PAHs (polycyclic aromatic hydrocarbons), 105; restoration of Brownfields, 126–127; wastewater treatment of, 162–163; water contaminated by sewage waste, 120–121, 158–159. *See also* Air pollution; Contamination; Hazardous waste facilities
Polycyclic aromatic hydrocarbons (PAHs), 105
Poverty: access to environmental amenities and, 201–202, 256; built environment, income

inequality, and, 201; commercial hazardous waste facilities near poor neighborhoods, 248fig; Concentrated poverty areas, 202, 227; culture of, 241–242; dispersing communities of poor people to decrease, 242–243; spatial mismatch and, 202–203; vulnerabilities related to, 200–201. *See also* Economics; Income inequality
Pre-industrial era: health in cities of the, 18–19; historical account of cities during, 18
Public health: built environment association with, 10; current disconnect between urban planning and, 287–288; new urbanism and, 51–53; policies on asbestos-contaminated products by, 145–146; urban planning ideas adopted by, 38–39
Public health interventions: Active Living Research (ALR), 291–292; changing social norms approach to, 289–290; community-level, 292–293; health beliefs model of, 289; individual-level, 296–297; inserted into city general plans, 298; legal basis for built environment regulation, 297–298; Massachusetts Department of Public Health (Mass DPH) approach to, 290–291; school-based, 293–296; soda and beverage taxes as, 296. *See also* Health effects

Public housing: defensible space concept applied to, 218–219; HOPE VI program of, 97, 219, 242; origins and history of, 35–36; regulatory framework of, 95–96. *See also* Housing; Low-income housing

Public transportation systems: health impacts of, 56; transit-oriented development of, 62

Putnam, Robert, 233

R

Race: built environment and, 198–199; definition of, 195; environmental justice on income versus, 258; as social construct, 195–196; U.S. Census' self-reported, 196

Racial health disparities: causes of, 197–198; housing segregation related to, 199–200; interventions to reduce, 199; segregation and, 199–200

Racial/ethnicity differences: air pollution impact and, 138; food insecurity in households that include children, 175*fig*; neighborhoods with commercial hazardous waste facilities, 248*fig*; outdoor liquor and tobacco advertising in neighborhoods, 241; transportation justice and, 80; vulnerabilities based on, 195. *See also* African Americans; Hispanics; Native Americans

Racism: of current economic segregated housing, 111–112; decline of racial housing segregation (mid-1970s), 44; description of, 196; Jim Crow legislation, 32; racial housing segregation (1825–1930), 31–32, 111. *See also* African Americans

Radon, 143–144

Regional Plan Association of New York, 11

Rezoning, 62

Right-hand turn lanes, 88

Riis, Jacob, 26, 30

River restoration, 129–130

Road rage, 215

Robert Wood Johnson Foundation's Active Living Research (ALR), 291–292

Rootshock, 111, 220–222

Roundabouts, 87

Rules for Radicals (Alinsky), 236

Rural health advantage, 47, 214–215

Rural residents: comparing environmental impact of urban versus, 307; rural health advantage of, 47, 214–215

S

Safety issues: creating pedestrian zones, 86–87; defensible space to promote, 218–219; driving, 74–75; housing codes to ensure, 104; improving intersection, 88; infrastructure and bike, 81–82; pedestrian-friendly street crossings, 57; playground, 133

Salmonella, 173

San Francisco Bay delta, 119

San Jose, graywater (water distribution system) used in, 161

Sanitary science: built environment association with, 10; wastewater treatment, 162–163; water recycling, 161–162

School gardens, 179

School-based health interventions: addressing childhood obesity through, 293–294; Boston Schoolyard Institute (BSI), 295; to improve physical state of schools, 295; to increase physical activity, 294–295; promoting walking to schools, 295–296; soda and beverage taxes, 296

Schools: earthquake codes for construction of, 122; encouraging children to walk to, 83–84; EPA's Tools for Schools program, 149; farm to school programs of, 178; indoor air quality in, 148–149; school gardens sponsored by, 179; subsidized and free student lunches in, 177–178; vending machines available in, 178–179. *See also* Children

Sea level rising, 319

Seaside (Florida Panhandle), 51, 53

Secondhand smoke exposures, 149

Section 8 housing program, 97–98

Segregation. *See* Housing segregation

Self-efficacy, 230

Septic systems, 169

Sewage waste: combined sewer overflows problem, 163; flooding which causes contamination from,